Early Childhood Intervention

Early Childhood Intervention: Shaping the Future for Children with Special Needs and Their Families

Volume 1: Contemporary Policy and Practices Landscape

Volume 2: Proven and Promising Practices

Volume 3: Emerging Trends in Research and Practice

Early Childhood Intervention

Shaping the Future for Children with Special Needs and Their Families

Volume 2

Proven and Promising Practices

Susan P. Maude
Editor

Christina Groark, set editor

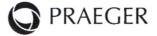 PRAEGER

AN IMPRINT OF ABC-CLIO, LLC
Santa Barbara, California • Denver, Colorado • Oxford, England

Northwest State Community College

Copyright 2011 by Christina Groark, Steven Eidelman, Louise A. Kaczmarek, and
Susan P. Maude

Library of Congress Cataloging-in-Publication Data

Early childhood intervention : shaping the future for children with special needs and their
families / Christina Groark, set editor.
   p. cm.
  Includes bibliographical references and index.
   ISBN 978–0–313–37793–8 (hard copy : alk. paper) — ISBN 978–0–313–37794–5 (ebook)
   1. Children with disabilities–Education (Preschool)—United States. 2. Children with
disabilities—Services for—United States. 3. Child development—United States. 4. Child
welfare—United States. I. Groark, Christina J.
LC4019.2.E25 2011
371.9–dc22   2011011997

ISBN: 978–0–313–37793–8
EISBN: 978–0–313–37794–5

15 14 13 12 11   1 2 3 4 5

This book is also available on the World Wide Web as an eBook.
Visit www.abc-clio.com for details.

Praeger
An Imprint of ABC-CLIO, LLC

ABC-CLIO, LLC
130 Cremona Drive, P.O. Box 1911
Santa Barbara, California 93116-1911

This book is printed on acid-free paper (∞)

Manufactured in the United States of America

For Paul, my son, and all children with special needs who deserve the best start in life that society in general, policy makers, professionals, and families can give them, and to those who advocate for them, thank you.

Contents

Preface and Acknowledgments

This series of three volumes is about special services known as *early intervention* or *early childhood special education* (EI/ECSE) provided to young children with special needs and their families. As the terms imply, these services provide support early in a child's life, even as early as birth, until the age of school entry. Specifically, early intervention as found in Part C of the IDEA 2004 Statute (P.L. 108-446) is defined as health, educational, and/or therapeutic services that are provided under public supervision and are designed to meet the developmental needs of an infant or toddler who has a developmental delay or a disability. At the discretion of each state, services can also be provided to children who are considered to be *at risk* of developing substantial delays if services are not provided. These services must be provided by qualified personnel and, to the maximum extent appropriate, must be provided in natural environments including the home and community settings in which children without disabilities participate. Early childhood special education (ECSE), as found in Part B, Section 619 of the IDEA, intends for smooth transition of a child from EI to ECSE. It stipulates that the local education agency will participate in the transition planning of a child from early intervention (Part C) to early childhood special education for a preschool-aged child the year she turns 3 years of age. The child may receive all the early intervention services listed on her service plan until her third birthday. Then she must be assessed as eligible for ECSE services

Why is this field important? First, it is scientifically known that early childhood is a time of significant brain development and substantial growth in every domain of all children's development. Second, it is widely accepted that at this time, all learning takes place in the context of relationships, and that families are central to these relationships. Therefore, for better child outcomes, short and long term, families must be involved at all levels. Third, professionals serving eligible children and families must be on the same page with the families, the children, and each other by coordinating their work and being focused on the skills that are important in the individual child's life. Fourth, this field is important because it demonstrates a connection between instruction and developmental outcomes that benefit children with or without disabilities. For example, the design of certain curricula, individualized educational programs, universal design for environments, tiered teaching methods, and other practices in these volumes are good strategies for all children, not only those with special needs.

But why attend to this particular population of children and families here and now? The prevalence of children with special needs worldwide as well as nationally is increasing. In 1991–1992, the prevalence of children with disabilities in the United States was estimated at 5.75 percent (http://www.cdc.gov/mmwr/PDF/wk/mm4433.pdf). In a more recent review (*Pediatrics* [2008], *121*, e1503–e1509) by Rosenberg, Zhang, and Robinson, the prevalence of developmental delays of children born in the United States in 2001 and eligible for Part C early intervention was indicated at 13 percent.

This growing prevalence also points to economic and public health concerns. Developmental delay, when attended to appropriately earlier in life, is shown to be lessened and thereby alleviate costs to the public. Typically, the estimated lifetime cost for those born in 2000 with a developmental disability is expected to total (based on 2003 dollars) $51.2 billion for people with intellectual disabilities, $11.5 billion for people with cerebral palsy, $2.1 billion for people who are deaf or have hearing loss, and $2.5 billion for people with vision impairment (http://www.cdc.gov/ncbddd/dd/ddsurv.htm). Early services work to significantly reduce these costs.

Also, as society, the economy, and all aspects of life are becoming more globally interdependent, it is our responsibility to help all children reach their potentials and contribute positively to our future. Our society needs a trained, talented, and diverse workforce. We cannot afford to lose the potential of such an important and large sector of children.

In addition to growing prevalence and the need for a diverse workforce, special needs affect all types of families. There is no culture, ethnic group, gender, geographic area, or socioeconomic status group that does not include children with special needs. Special needs and disabilities are inordinately diverse in terms of diagnosis, variability within a diagnosis, intensity, spectrum of characteristics, age of impact, multiplicity, and combinations of disabilities. Further, all children, typically developing or not, need some individualized attention, instruction, and care. They are not little adults. They learn by different styles and at different rates.

Because of this diversity and the importance of the development of this cohort of children, the editors worked diligently to be sure that the most current and best available research is combined with professional experiences, wisdom, and values; clinical expertise; and family-child perspectives. Although no rock was left unturned in the selection of topics and contributors, there was some difficulty in selecting topics. The advisors, editors, and publishers felt strongly that this series is to be of utility to a variety of professionals, parents, practitioners, policy makers, service trainers, students, academics, and scholars, including those not directly related to this field (e.g., a lawyer who is interested in policy, a parent who wants to know about the best supports for her child). Although we strongly intended to have the three volumes provide breadth to the readers, we still wanted them to be as comprehensive as possible. Once the topics were agreed upon, authors were easy to select because we invited the best in the field who could communicate the issues in an accurate, precise, and understandable way. Therefore, information was gathered from experience and scientific evidence by the best in the fields of early intervention and early childhood special education policy and law, medicine and health sciences, and education and child welfare, among others.

So the reader will find that the scope of this series is broad but still covers the critical components of early intervention and early childhood special education. It is organized into three volumes in such a way that readers can skim through each to find the areas of particular interest to them. The chapters within the three volumes are intended to answer key questions regarding how this field works. For instance, how do we identify children needing early intervention or early childhood special education and recognize them as early as possible? Where does this detection and subsequent service take place? Who works in early intervention, and what is their training? What is the families' role in all of this, and what are their rights? How does that role differ in early intervention compared to early childhood special education? Which programs, or what parts of programs, work best, and for whom? What does it cost to provide this service, and how effective is it? What are still some of the unknowns of this field (which is relatively young compared to other fields of study)?

Specifically, Volume 1, *Contemporary Policy and Practices Landscape*, begins with a historical perspective of this field. It then relates state policies and various attempts to implement them and international laws and sample country responses to the care, education, and development of children with disabilities. This volume also considers who provides these services; their training, background, and experiences; and evaluation of programs for quality and cost-effectiveness. Policies regarding children with special needs nationally and internationally tell us the rights of children and families. Sometimes they even tell us what should be provided and when. However, they do not tell us *how* to implement quality programs; thus, the need for Volume 2.

You will see, therefore, that the chapters in Volume 2, *Proven and Promising Practices in Early Intervention/Early Childhood Special Education*, cover the best available practices that are currently used and studied throughout the field of early intervention. These chapters include information on programs such as Early Head Start and Head Start and new, exciting model strategies and techniques in intervening with children with challenging behaviors, mental health diagnoses, sensory processing, and others. We were fortunate to find the best professionals in the fields of early intervention and early childhood special education, including individuals from occupational therapy, speech and language pathology, psychology, policy development, technology use with children, early literacy and math, teacher education, English-language learning, and specialists in visual and hearing impairments. Yet there is always room for new knowledge and improvement. That is what we hope we captured in Volume 3.

Volume 3, *Emerging Trends in Research and Practice*, creatively takes the reader into the realm of possibilities. It helps the reader think about needs of expanding or emerging populations such as culturally and linguistically diverse families and the need for schools to be prepared for learners with a wide range of needs and abilities. This volume also invites reflection on issues that are not totally resolved, like crossing systems in the delivery of services, how do we get over the financial and administrative silos in these public systems, and how do we get professionals and bureaucrats to work together to cross these systems? However, this volume also provides solutions to current issues that should be considered, advocated for, or debated, such as the Recognition and Response tiered model of instruction.

Finally, the chapters in Volume 3 point us in the direction of future research and trials of models and strategies. For instance, we need to make the best use of technology and research-based practices. Another example includes child progress monitoring and accountability. Monitoring and accountability have evolved over the years, and better practices actually may include simpler procedures. But are we capturing the complexities of teaching and learning? Do we really understand the needs of children with special needs and how to best engage their families and integrate a variety of professional recommendations for the most effective program? Finding these answers will demand a lot from professionals (e.g., to follow professional practices such as DEC-NAEYC), from researchers (e.g., to develop and test evidenced based practices), and from the public in general (e.g., to advocate).

All three volumes contain special features like matrices, graphs, and diagrams to stimulate readers not only in what is, but in what could be. They are different from other works in that they provide the state of the art in the field while considering the antecedents and the future prospective in the field. They are intended to be appealing to anyone interested in children, especially children with special needs, and to provide enough information to continue and grow that interest.

* * *

I would like to thank many people for their contributions to the creation, writing, editing, and production of this series. First, the volume editors, Steven Eidelman, Susan P. Maude, and Louise A. Kaczmarek, all of whom are first-rate professionals, child advocates, and early interventionists whom I relied upon heavily for chapter ideas, finding the best authors in the field, volume editing, writing chapters for the volumes, and fabulous contributions to the entire enterprise. There would be no series without them.

Second, my assistants, Mary Ellen Colella, Amy Gee, Mary Louise Kaminski, and Kaitlin Moore, who kept me organized, edited me and reedited me, and checked details when I could no longer see the trees through the forest.

In addition, thank you to our illustrious advisers. They came from so many different professions with the highest level of understanding of the nature of the children in these services and of what is needed by our readers. I appreciate their willingness to share their expertise openly and candidly.

And to my students, Amber Harris-Fillius, Claudia Ovalle-Ramirez, Robin Sweitzer, and Wen Chi Wang, thank you for their thorough reviews of the chapters. I learned a lot from them.

Finally, thank you to my family: Brian, Patti, Stephanie, and Paul, for teaching me about children and families and for their patience and encouragement throughout this work.

Chapter 1

Early Intervention—IDEA Part C: Service Delivery Approaches and Practices

Lynda Cook Pletcher and Naomi Younggren

THE CHILDREN AND FAMILIES

*A*J is the single dad of Damien, and they both live with AJ's mother. AJ's mother has expressed concern to AJ that Damien, now 14 months old, is not talking or walking. She feels that compared to other children, Damien is "behind." After seeing a brochure for the Happy Steps program, she gave information to AJ to schedule a free evaluation of Damien's development. AJ called Happy Steps and spoke with an intake coordinator, who gave him information about Happy Steps and how to schedule a screening of Damien's overall development. If the screening indicates there may be delays, Damien will be referred for a more in-depth evaluation. Based upon those results, Damien and his family may be eligible for services and supports either through early intervention or other community programs. AJ then made an appointment for a developmental screening of Damien at the family home.*

For the past two years, 2-1/2-year-old Jessica has received early intervention services to help her and her family adapt to her hearing loss. Jessica wears aids in both ears and now uses whole sentences in both verbal and signed communication. Although her services were first at home, she also receives services now at the same child care center she attends with her baby sister. A primary service provider (PSP) from the early intervention program, a speech language pathologist (SLP), visits with the family monthly. They (family and PSP) discuss Jessica's Individualized Family Service Plan (IFSP) outcomes and how things are going, as well as identifying new outcomes and activities. The PSP also makes consultative visits to the child care center three times a month to assist Jessica's service providers on her IFSP activities. There, he models activities for the staff, helps them design learning activities, and works directly with

Jessica as she engages in play with her peers. Altogether, they have begun to plan for her transition out of early intervention into preschool special education when Jessica turns 3 years old.

These are just two examples of the many types of families and children who receive early intervention services under the Individuals with Disabilities Education Act (IDEA) Part C Infants and Toddlers program. In 2006, the families of approximately 298,000 infants and toddlers were enrolled in Early Intervention programs across the United States (Goode, Lazara, & Danaher, 2008). This chapter will further discuss these key underpinnings to the section of IDEA that supports our very youngest children and their families.

CONCEPTUAL FRAMEWORK: PRINCIPLES AND POLICIES, PRACTICES, AND PROGRAM DESIGN

Figure 1.1 shows a conceptual framework of the Early Intervention system under Part C of IDEA and the organizational content for this

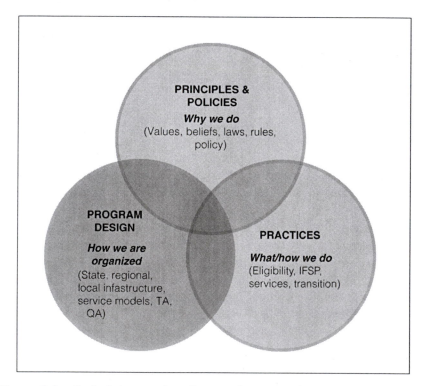

Figure 1.1   Early Intervention System Framework.

chapter. Collectively, the system is designed to achieve positive impacts, also known as desired results, for children like Damien and Jessica and their families.

The three concentric circles signify the system's necessary components. The top circle representing *Principles and Policies* is comprised of the values, beliefs, laws, and rules that define *why* a state Part C program delivers the services it provides. Values and beliefs should influence programs and practices. In turn, principles and policy should facilitate demonstration of essential values and beliefs.

The practices circle represents the *ways* in which service providers work with children and families. Practices are the day-to-day interactions between a service provider and a family, as well as broader practices used by the state for activities such as child-find, assessment, or other activities related to service delivery. Practices also demonstrate *what* a system does and what children and families actually receive as they participate in early intervention services. The values and beliefs of the early intervention system and the federal and state policies all directly influence practices that are operationalized within homes and communities.

The program design circle encompasses *how* a state or local program is organized to deliver services. There is wide variation from state to state and even within states as to their organization and administrative structures. However, the federal law does require specific systemic components that must be in place for a state to receive federal funding for early intervention, but allows for flexibility in how these programmatic functions are carried out.

External to these three core components are contextual features such as current research and evidence, funding reductions or increases, and new laws or regulations, which can have an impact on these intermingled early intervention system components. For example, new research and evidence can drive changes in practices, which simultaneously influence reflection and revision of values and beliefs and necessitate revision of the policies and procedures that are guided by those ideals. Concurrently, organizational structures might require realignment to complement the desired new practice approach. The momentum of such change also demands ongoing professional development to promote the knowledge, skills, dispositions, and confidence of service providers to implement such changes in service delivery approaches.

In this chapter, we examine the driving federal policy, major key principles, and resulting practices for approaching the delivery of services to infants, toddlers, and families enrolled in state early intervention programs. More than 40 years of research, demonstration projects, and direct service provision have contributed to variations in the way services are organized and delivered under the Individuals with Disabilities Education Improvement Act Part C (IDEA, 2004) and the Early Intervention Program for Infants and Toddlers with Disabilities and their Families. The intent of this chapter is not to promote one particular service delivery model or approach, but rather to supply the reader with pertinent information to understand service delivery approaches widely used today and to realize the influences of policy, practice, and research in their promotion.

PRINCIPLES: VALUES AND BELIEFS

Individual values and beliefs of service providers, administrators, and family members influence what they feel is a good or bad idea. People are shaped by their assumptions and expectations (Manning, Curtis, & McMillen, 1996). Often, events such as being exposed to new life experiences, gaining new knowledge, putting beliefs into practice, and engaging in self-reflection can influence individual discovery. Changing personal values and beliefs is not easy. This is important to recognize as the legislation, themes, approaches, and models explored in this chapter have evolved over the past three decades and are heavily value-laden and call for personal change. The changes in early intervention service delivery has been fueled by the articulation of values and beliefs through research, publications, training events, demonstration projects, position statements from advocacy groups, and families sharing personal stories. Changing practice is in part confounded by what an individual thinks about the ideas at a core level.

POLICIES: FEDERAL LEGISLATION

In 1968, almost 20 years prior to the federal legislation that created the Program for Infants and Toddlers with Disabilities, the Bureau of Education for the Handicapped (BEH), the precursor to the current Office of Special Education Programs (OSEP), provided competitive federal dollars to fund 20 centers across the country. These centers used the funds to explore and demonstrate best practice ideas and to develop models for working with young children with disabilities (Gallagher, Danaher, & Clifford, 2009). These efforts marked the beginning of what continues today as competitive federal grant opportunities for research, model demonstration projects, and technical assistance, all contributing toward the pool of sound research supporting evidence-based practices.

During this same time period, with an emphasis provided by President Johnson's War on Poverty, other federal bureaus and divisions promoted significant legislation affecting young children, including the Head Start and Economic Opportunity Act (1965) and the Early and Periodic Screening Diagnosis and Treatment Act (Title XIX of the Social Security Act, 1967). Federal funding in these areas added emphasis on the importance of helping young children to "get a good start" on their health and development, thereby providing prevention and treatment services for the most vulnerable populations. Federal funds were used to establish the network of University Disability Centers, once referred to as University Affiliated Programs (UAPs), and now called the University Centers for Excellence in Developmental Disabilities (UCEDD). The Division of Maternal Child Heath provided funding for hospital programs around the country for children with disabilities, thereby establishing the Children's Special Health Clinics (CSHC) network. Although these important programs focused on life span issues of the population with disabilities, they also provided valuable research, demonstration models, and services for very young children with disabilities.

In the following decades, federal dollars and interest in young children with disabilities, and families, continued to increase. This created a plethora of research, treatment options, and new ways of providing services outside institutional settings. These early programs and centers were instrumental in developing many of the underlying themes that became the foundational principles for the initial legislation and subsequent reauthorizations. This initial legislation (Part H of Public Law 99-457), passed in 1986, set in place the system of services for infants and toddlers with disabilities (birth to age 3) and their families. The 1997 Amendments renamed the legislation the Individuals with Disabilities Education Act (IDEA), and the Infants and Toddlers section was moved from Part H of the legislation to Part C of the bill. In 2004, IDEA was once again reauthorized and renamed the Individuals with Disabilities Education Improvement Act (IDEIA). The Infant and Toddlers section remained in Part C of the Act.

Unique Features of the Legislation

A number of features in the federal legislation support the direction taken by particular approaches to service delivery. It is important to understand these features of the law in order to have the broad view of what early intervention services are to be and provide before exploring specific concepts and practice models. The following section highlights a few of the unique features of IDEA Part C, early intervention services.

Variation in State and Local Design

From its inception, Part C was not intended to be a new and separate program. The intent of the law was to use federal dollars to fill gaps by creating coordinated, interagency systems building upon what was already in place within each state. Federal dollars are used to pay for the services that are not provided by another federal or state program such as Head Start; Title V; Early Periodic Screening, Diagnosis, and Treatment (EPSDT); Child Health Specialty Clinics (CHSCs); Supplemental Social Security Insurance (SSI); Medicaid; Women, Infants, and Children (WIC) Program; or special education services provided by the state education agency. Another variation found among the states applies to the lead agency requirement of the law. The governor from each state is required to name one state agency to be the single line of authority responsible for the implementation, maintenance, and oversight of the system. Lead agencies could be the Department of Education, Health, Developmental Disabilities, Human Services, or a combination of departments and bureaus. The lead agency and the partners involved in providing services vary from state to state.

Who Receives Services?

Children *and* families are the focus of Part C. The law specifies this dual focus by stating that "services means services that are designed to meet the developmental needs of each child eligible . . . *and the needs of the family* related to enhancing the child's development" (IDEA Regulations, 1999, 34 C.F.R. § 303.12 [a] [1]; emphasis added). Eligibility for the program is required, and each state defines its own eligibility criteria. At a minimum, states must serve children who demonstrate a state-defined measure of delay in one or more areas of development, or have a known condition that has a high probability of resulting in a later delay. The term early intervention, used to describe the policy

and services of Part C, reinforces and recognizes the critical importance of providing assistance as soon as possible.

Over time, the focus on helping families enhance their child's development has evolved. In the 1970s, parents often played a subordinate
role in early intervention as the professionals took charge (Peterander,
2000). In the 1980s, parents became recognized as co-therapists following the professionally prescribed regime of treatment. Partnership
became the focus in the 1990s and into the twenty-first century. Today,
a focus remains on building quality relationships with families and
recognizing that it is through this relationship that effective early intervention services are provided (Kelly & Barnard, 1999; McWilliam,
2010; Rush, Shelden, & Hanft, 2003; Turnbull & Turnbull, 2001).

The law specifies the active participation of families in all aspects of
service delivery. Parents are listed as a primary referral source and can
ask for an eligibility evaluation without having to have a professional
make the referral. The Federal regulations introduce the term *family-
directed* (20 U.S.C. 635 [a] [3]) as families are to be involved in the
evaluation and assessment of their child as well as identification of
their own needs and concerns. Families are listed as team members
and are active participants in determining services during the Individualized Family Service Plan (IFSP) meeting. Procedural safeguards
support parent rights to receive appropriate, individualized services
as the law stipulates. Therefore, families as well as the child are key
recipients of services.

What Services Are Included?

There are 16 specified early intervention services that each state system must make available to children and their families. Multidisciplinary teams, with active parent participation, determine how to
address the identified concerns and document the agreed-upon services on the IFSP. The general role of all service providers includes consulting with parents and other community partners, as well as
providing developmental services to the child. Table 1.1 provides a
listing of the services, based on the needs of the child and family as
outlined on their IFSP, specified in the law. Table 1.2 provides a list of
the professionals that may provide those services.

Every child and family receives service coordination beginning at
referral and continuing until the child exits early intervention. Service
coordination is an active, ongoing process that involves helping families gain access to early intervention and other needed community

Table 1.1   Early Intervention Services

I.	Family training, counseling and home visits
II.	Special instruction
III.	Speech-language pathology and audiology services, and sign language and cued language services
IV.	Occupational therapy
V.	Physical therapy
VI.	Psychological services
VII.	Service coordination
VIII.	Medical services for diagnostic or evaluation purpose only
IX.	Early identification, screening and assessment services
X.	Health services necessary to enable the child to benefit from other Early intervention services
XI.	Social work
XII.	Vision
XIII.	Assistive technology devices and AT services
XIV.	Transportation and related cost that are necessary to enable the child and child's family to receive another services listed above

Source: 20 U.S.C.S. 1432(E).

services. Service coordination activities include assisting the family to be part of the entire process from referral through evaluation, eligibility determination, IFSP development, service delivery, and transition.

Where Services Occur

All services the child receives are to be provided in the *natural environment*, described as the "home or community settings in which children

Table 1.2   Qualified Personnel in Early Intervention

I.	Special educators
II.	Speech language pathologists and audiologists
III.	Occupational therapists
IV.	Psychologist
V.	Social workers
VI.	Nurses
VII.	Registered dietitians
VIII.	Family therapist
IX.	Vision specialists including ophthalmologists and optometrists
X.	Orientation and mobility specialist
XI.	Pediatricians and other physicians

Source: 20 U.S.C.S. 1432(F).

of the same age without disabilities participate" (20 U.S.C. 632 [4] [G]). This term, supported by the concept of full inclusion, appeared in the original legislation in 1986. Services go to where each child and family is actively engaged within their own community. This may include the family's home, grandparents' home, child care center, preschool, park, or other community settings. This construct of natural environments extends beyond the location of service provision to the methodology of using natural family and community routines and activities as opportunities for children's learning (Dunst & Bruder, 1999; Dunst, Trivette, Humphries, Raab, & Roper, 2001; Hanft, Rush, & Shelden, 2004; McWilliam, 2000; Sandall, McLean, & Smith, 2000; Tisot & Thurman, 2002). All of these environments are thought to be rich in learning opportunities from which children with disabilities can benefit. The concept of natural environment as more than a location of service provision is explored later in this chapter.

How Services Are Provided

The services and supports needed by very young children and their families are delivered from state health, human services, and education programs. These could be public and/or privately funded agencies and from formal (e.g., programs, agencies, organizations) and informal (e.g., family members, friends, churches) sources of help. No single professional or program can be the sole source of meeting the needs of the child and family. Infants and toddlers at risk for or with disabilities need the combined expertise from a variety of professionals, disciplines, and types of agencies (Bruder & Bologna, 1993). The expectation in the law is that service providers within and across the specified agencies and programs work as a team with the family in meeting both the child's and the family's identified needs. Teams (made up of two or more disciplines and the family) evaluate the child, conduct the IFSP team meeting, develop the IFSP, provide direct and ongoing services, and meet at least every six months and annually to evaluate and rewrite the IFSP.

MAJOR FOUNDATIONAL CONCEPTS UNDERGIRDING EARLY INTERVENTION PRACTICES

As the field of early intervention has evolved over the past three decades, a number of key concepts have resulted from contributions in research, advances in practice, and modifications in policy. Although each are interrelated, they also have individual influences on current thinking guiding practice. The following section briefly addresses the major key concepts that represent a major shift in the design and direction of the service system over the last 20 years, based upon research and evidence and supported by the intent of the federal legislation.

FAMILY-CENTERED PRACTICES

The term *family-centered* generally implies the use of "a set of interconnected beliefs and attitudes that shape program philosophy and behavior of personnel as they organize and deliver services" (Pletcher & McBride, 2000, p. 1). This term appears in almost all help-giving fields with slightly differing definitions (Adams & Nelson, 1995; Allen, Brown, & Finlay, 1992; Cohen & Syme, 1985; Kretzmann & McKnight, 1993; Schorr, 1988). However, there are common descriptions, including terms such as strengths-based, consumer-driven, family support, empowerment, proactive service delivery, competency-focused, partnerships, collaborative relationships, and family-driven, that distinctly define family-centered practices in early intervention (Baird & Peterson, 1997; Dunst, 2002; McWilliam, 2010; Mahoney & Wheeden, 1997; McWilliam, Snyder, Harbin, Porter, & Munn, 2000; Pletcher & McBride, 2000).

Family-centered practices draw from social system theory, ecological perspective to human growth and development, positive proactive help-giving, and empowerment principles. Dunst, Trivette, and Deal (1988) developed an early intervention model in which service providers use specific help-giving practices that are tied to positive results. These practices include skills such as building trust and rapport with families, using active reflective listening, providing open and positive communication, displaying nonjudgmental attitudes about the family, providing assistance that is wanted or desired by the family, and helping the family learn or display capabilities and new competences. In addition to the use of specific skills of positive help-giving, family-centered early intervention practices provide assistance that are based upon family-identified needs and concerns, use specific family strengths and functioning styles, and employ both formal and informal support available to the family from their own community to mobilize resources to meet the unique needs of the child and family (Dunst, Johanson, Trivette, & Hamby, 1991; Pletcher, 1997).

Building upon the work of Dunst and his colleagues, other researchers and authors also describe family-centeredness as a set of principles or specific attitudes and beliefs. These descriptions include treating families with respect; tailoring supports and services to each family; being flexible, and responsive to family concerns, priorities and cultures; building upon strengths; including families as equal partners; providing information in clear, concise ways; and using the families' activities and interests to encourage child learning (Bruder, 2000; Bruder & Dunst, 2008; Jung & McWilliam, 2005; McWilliam et al., 2000).

RELATIONSHIP-BASED APPROACH

Working with families who are caring for infants and toddlers is all about relationships. Every domain of development is affected by the caring and nurturing relationships that happen in the early childhood years (Shonkoff & Phillips, 2000). These relationships first apply to immediate family members but then extend to others, including family members, friends, child care providers, and other significant people in the child's immediate community. The relationship-based approach is built upon the premise that all children learn and grow from supportive relationships with family and caregivers. In turn, families and caregivers grow and learn from supportive relations with service providers and other community members. This approach focuses on early learning theory and theories of social and emotional development in young children (Greenspan & Wieder, 1998; Kelly & Barnard, 1999; Mahoney, Boyce, Fewell, Spiker, & Wheeden, 1998).

There are similarities between relationship-based and family-centered practices as both approaches have common foundations. Many of the skills that service providers use with families to build positive relationships are similar to those described in family-centered practices. Service providers use strategies that support parents in their relationships with their child as the vehicle for intervention. Service providers support parents' competence and confidence to increase their child's learning and participation in daily life (Bruder & Dunst, 2000). In essence, to be family-centered requires relationship-based practices, and to have relationship-based practices, one must be family-centered.

NATURAL ENVIRONMENTS

The term *natural environment* was first introduced in the original 1986 federal legislation to refer to a location where early intervention services should be provided, the home or community setting, and to state that infants and toddlers should not be separated from their same-age peers without disabilities. Prior to the passage of initial legislation, federally funded research studies and model demonstration projects—often housed on university campuses—demonstrated the benefits of inclusion and reinforce the premise that young children with disabilities did not need to be removed from their home or community and placed in special purpose schools or private clinics to benefit from help, as was often the norm in 1986. The evidence obtained from these studies and projects guided and shaped policy in support of inclusion. It is not a choice or a philosophical belief for early intervention programs to provide services in natural environments; it has been a legal requirement since 1986. Only when the child's goals cannot be achieved satisfactorily in the home or community setting can another location be used. When this does occur, there must be written justification on the IFSP as to why this other setting is more appropriate for meeting the outcome or goal.

The construct of natural environments extends beyond the location of service provision to using natural family and community routines and activities as opportunities for children's learning. Traditional intervention services were child-centered and typically occurred within the context of lesson plans designed and implemented by educators and therapists (Mahoney & Filer, 1996; McBride & Peterson, 1997; Peterander, 2000; Weston & Ivins, 2001). The provision of early intervention services in natural environments involves working in partnership with families and caregivers to encourage naturally occurring activities that promote learning and to apply agreed-upon development-enhancing modifications that fit into existing family or child care everyday routines and typical activities. Conceptualized in this way, families, caregivers, and early intervention service providers work side by side to discover and to build upon children's interests that occur naturally throughout the day.

Moving services out of already established clinics or programs into a family's home or their community presents challenges for service providers and for parents. Professional organizations such as the American Speech-Language-Hearing Association (ASHA), American

Physical Therapy Association (APTA), American Occupational Therapy Association (AOTA), and Infant and Toddler Coordinator Association (ITCA) have developed clear statements and position papers endorsing the benefits of providing services in natural environments (ITCA, 2000, Pilkington, 2007; Vanderholf, 2004; Woods, 2008a, 2008b). However, early intervention service providers continue to describe challenges, such as time spent driving, visits to homes and neighborhoods they feel are not safe, availability of team members for consultation, transporting equipment, and feeling that the activities they provide in a family's home are not as effective as those they could provide in a clinic (Campbell, Sawyer, & Muhlenhapt, 2009). Administrators describe challenges in supervising staff, providing professional development, rewriting policy, and funding difficulties also attributed to the limitations of or barriers in providing services in natural environments (Campbell et al., 2009).

Parents generally express satisfaction with services provided in natural environments as it is often more convenient (Campbell et al., 2009). Doing so minimizes the need to take children to many appointments in a variety of places. Parents understood that natural environments provided many opportunities for learning but, most importantly, that the home and community afford the child and family with full inclusions, places to make friends, and opportunities to become active participants in community life (Campbell et al., 2009).

ACTIVITY-BASED APPROACH

In an activity-based approach, behavioral learning principles are used to encourage children to interact in meaningful daily activities that have the specific purpose of helping a child to gain, generalize, strengthen, and use skills to meet functional goals and objectives (Pretti-Frontczak & Bricker, 2004). The activities are child-directed with multiple learning opportunities embedded into the *real* daily activities in which the child is involved. The activity-based approach follows the child's lead rather than directing a child through adult-created and adult-presented activities designed to address specific instructional objectives or a sequence of curriculum goals in a preset order.

In an activity-based approach, the learning objectives are designed for each child based upon the individual child's strengths, needs, and interests. Research supports that children's learning and development occurs more rapidly when their interests engage them in social and nonsocial interactions. This provides them with opportunities to practice existing abilities, explore their environments, and learn new competencies through all opportunities that occur naturally throughout each child's day (Dunst, Hamby, Trivette, Raab, & Bruder, 2000; Hanft & Pilkington, 2000; McWilliam, 2010).

NATURAL LEARNING OPPORTUNITIES

Natural learning opportunities help families and service providers understand that services provided in natural environments are not just about the locations where the service provider goes, but what occurs in those places constitutes meaningful engagement and learning for the child (Bronfenbrenner, 1979). Dunst and Bruder (1999, 2002) have conducted extensive research on the effects of personal interactions and environmental settings on children's opportunities for learning. They have helped the early intervention field recognize that families' lives are filled with natural opportunities for a child's learning (Dunst et al., 2000). Using natural learning opportunities also reinforces learning in contexts where the competencies are necessary and desired (Bricker, Pretti-Frontczak, & McComas, 1998; Dunst, Bruder, et al., 2001; Woods, Kashinath, & Goldstein, 2004).

The use of natural learning opportunities shifts the focus from interventionists working directly with the child and implementing professionally prescribed activities, to interventionists partnering with parents and caregivers to identify and enhance opportunities occurring within the family's and caregivers' daily activities. By supporting families to embed the child's learning goals within the family routines and activities, the frequency of intervention extends beyond periodic sessions with the early intervention service providers (Mayhew, Scott, & McWilliam, 1999). Mayhew and colleagues specifically reinforce the concept that "all intervention occurs between visits" (p. 16). This focus reinforces family involvement and heightens families' confidence and competence, which, in turn, positively influences the entire family (Ketelaar, Vermeer, Helders, & Hart, 1998).

FUNCTIONAL OUTCOMES AND GOALS

Functional outcomes represent integrated skills across the developmental domains. Functional outcomes improve the child's ability to participate in activities that are relevant to the child and family, capitalize on natural motivations, and lead to practical improvements in child and family life. Identifying functional outcomes require understanding of the family's routine-based concern (e.g., mealtime is difficult and hectic because it is hard to feed the twins; bedtime is a challenge because he will not stay in his bed) or outcomes they want to accomplish. Listening to the family's descriptions of their routines and activities provides valuable information about what is most important to the family and helps to plan intervention that is functional, realistic, and relevant to the family (Bernheimer & Keogh, 1995; Dunst et al., 2000; McCormick & Noonan, 2002; Roper & Dunst, 2003; Schuck & Bucy, 1997).

For children involved in child care, it is also indispensable to take the time to learn about the caregiver routines and any routine-based concerns they may have. Involving caregivers in the development of the IFSP is vital for success in identifying and developing appropriate and "doable" strategies to accomplish key outcomes. Through their participation, caregivers can provide valuable input, thereby assisting with the buy-in needed to accomplish the agreed-upon strategies. Without their investment and involvement, it is difficult to ascertain if strategies will be implemented. Acknowledging and capitalizing on caregivers' expertise is a central construct needed to include them as valued team members.

To ensure development of a functional IFSP, outcomes must be grounded on family priorities and framed in the context of family life, not based upon the child's developmental deficits from standardized evaluation. IFSP outcomes that are written to address functional goals look different from traditional service-driven outcomes. The early intervention services listed on the IFSP are specific to the outcomes and provide information, resources, and support to the family and other caregivers.

TEAM-BASED SERVICE DELIVERY

Teamwork is a cornerstone component of early intervention because by design, it represents multiple professionals and agencies coming together to meet the diverse needs of eligible infants and toddlers and their families. The interrelated nature of early intervention requires that support personnel and agencies work together while embracing each family they meet as equal members of the team

(Sandall et al., 2000). To achieve this collaboration, multidisciplinary, interdisciplinary, and/or transdisciplinary teaming models are structures most frequently implemented when delivering early intervention services.

A multidisciplinary team is characterized as a group of professionals working independently of each other, yet sharing a common goal (Gargiulo & Kilgo, 2000; Woodruff & McGonigel, 1988). The professionals work as specialists focusing on domain-specific aspects of the child (e.g., the speech therapist designs and delivers services focused on the communication goals for the child, while the physical therapist separately attends to the child's gross motor goals). Service delivery is often professionally driven, with the professionals identifying the problems and designing the ameliorating intervention. Family input is primarily for sharing information specific to the child, rather than giving ideas, solving problems collaboratively, or discussing concerns. In this model, professionals are essentially the key decision makers, and intervention focuses on the child.

The difference between the multidisciplinary and interdisciplinary teaming models is most evident in the interaction among team members (Gargiulo & Kilgo, 2000; Woodruff & McGonigel, 1988). In the interdisciplinary team, the professionals conduct independent evaluations but come together to share results. Intervention strategies are collaboratively designed but separately implemented by domain-specific specialists (e.g., the physical therapist [PT] supports the child on his/her crawling; the speech and language pathologist [SLP] supports the child on his/her requesting food by pointing). Although the family is more readily involved as a team member, its input remains secondary to that of the professionals. This model sees families as involved, but it is limited in the application of family-centered practices.

The transdisciplinary model involves professionals sharing roles and seeing the child as a whole within the context of the family (Gargiulo & Kilgo, 2000; Mayhew et al., 1999; Woodruff & McGonigel, 1988). Within this type of teaming model, it is believed that sharing the expertise of all team members, including the family, provides a well-rounded approach without fragmenting services by professional specialty area or developmental domain (Dinnebeil, Hale, & Rule, 1999). The family on the transdisciplinary team is valued as an active member with a recognized and respected decision-making role.

Transdisciplinary team members accept and build upon each other's knowledge and skills. Often the term *role release* is used in describing the actions of team members, as any member of the team may be working with the child and family or with other caregivers. Members of a transdisciplinary team cross professional discipline boundaries to achieve service integration by consulting or coaching one another. They do not *abandon their* discipline, but blend specific skills with other team members to focus on achieving integrated outcomes.

One member on a transdisciplinary team works the most frequently with the family. In the approaches described later in this chapter, this person is referred to as the primary service provider (PSP). This individual works collaboratively with the other team members to integrate information to deliver efficient and comprehensive services to a child and family. The assignment of a primary service provider to a specific child and family should be based upon the IFSP outcomes. They must have access to all other team members on a regular basis to receive information, consultation, and coaching from their other team members related to child and family outcomes and intervention strategies. The use of a PSP on a transdisciplinary team is not a *watered-down* version of services but, rather, a method that emphasizes service delivery that is unified around functional family needs, uses specialists as effectively as possible, and allows for families to form a close and helpful relationship with one primary person (McWilliam, 2004).

The dual focus in early intervention of providing services to young children and assisting families requires service providers to understand and use adult learning principles as they work with family members and caregivers. Adult learning principles are also important for team members to use with one another and to use in the design of staff development activities. Principles of adult learning theory focus on practices such as involving adults in all aspects of learning, including planning, practicing, evaluating, and reflecting, which lead to mastery (Trivette, 2009).

For adults, all life experiences (including mistakes) provide opportunities for learning. Adult learning can be formal or informal, planned or unplanned, and can take place in an endless array of settings. Adults' desires to learn new skills or strategies for handling certain situations are often influenced by external occurrences, such as having a child with a disability or a need to learn new skills to participate on a transdisciplinary team. Adult learning is an interactive process, which not only encompasses the relationship between a *teacher* and *learner*, but also the environmental influences and the social situation at the particular time (Knowles, 1980). Many early intervention service providers have not received formal coursework or experiences in their personnel preparation programs about adult learning. Yet, it is essential to gain an understanding of how adults learn to engage families and other caregivers or team members in acquisition and use of new skills.

COMMUNITY OF PRACTICE—CONSENSUS THINKING: AGREED-UPON PRINCIPLES

A national community of practice (CoP) was formed in 2005 to study the various service delivery approaches and models advocated by lead researchers in early intervention and to develop a consensus set of evidence-based practices (Buysee & Wesley, 2006). The purpose of this work was to focus not on the differences in the models and approaches, but on the points of agreement, and to provide national guidance in the form of agreed-upon principles and practices. The workgroup developed a mission statement and articulated seven key principles as the necessary foundation to support the system of family-centered early intervention (see Table 1.3).

Table 1.3 includes the mission of early intervention services and key principles developed by this workgroup. Table 1.4 further clarifies one of the seven key principles noted in Table 1.3: the role of the primary service provider. This table identifies the key concepts behind the principle and provides a sample of indicators or what it might "look like/ doesn't look like" in practice.

MOST COMMONLY NAMED APPROACHES OR MODELS FOR DELIVERING EARLY INTERVENTION SERVICES

Terminology Confusion

The field of early intervention currently uses various words to describe how early intervention services are structured and delivered. A myriad of terminology is also used to discuss the changes state systems and programs are making or would like to make to advance their service delivery structure and practices. Just as Peterson (1987) noted about early childhood and early childhood special education programs can vary across the state, city, and/or the hallway from one another, so do the terms and practices used in early intervention vary across and often within states. This discrepancy adds to the confusion about what is being operationalized. Furthermore, sometimes a term such as "model"

Table 1.3   Mission of Early Intervention Services and Key Principles

Mission

Part C early intervention builds upon and provides supports and resources to assist family members and caregivers to enhance children's learning and development through everyday learning opportunities.

Key Principles

- Infants and toddlers learn best through everyday experiences and interactions with familiar people in familiar contexts.
- All families, with the necessary supports and resources, can enhance their children's learning and development.
- The primary role of a service provider in early intervention is to work with and support family members and caregivers in children's lives.
- The early intervention process, from initial contacts through transition, must be dynamic and individualized to reflect the child's and family members' preferences, learning styles and cultural beliefs.
- IFSP outcomes must be functional and based on children's and families' needs and family-identified priorities.
- The family's priorities, needs and interests are addressed most appropriately by a primary service provider who represents and receives team and community support.
- Interventions with young children and family members must be based on explicit principles, validated practices, best available research, and relevant laws and regulations.

Source: Workgroup on Principles and Practices in Natural Environments (2008b).

is used, and other times the word "approach," "concept," "philosophy," or "theme" is used to describe the particular ways a state system or program delivers their early intervention services.

State-Named Approaches

In 2009, the National Early Childhood Technical Assistance Center (NECTAC) gathered information from states describing their early intervention approaches or models in practice or in development (Pletcher, 2009). This information was gathered through a review of state Web sites, documents, and results from a survey sent to all state Part C coordinators asking them to name currently endorsed practice models or models toward which they were considering moving. Each state coordinator was given the opportunity to review and validate compiled state-specific information for accurate representation. States could name more than one approach if there was not a statewide endorsement of one particular approach. The aggregate of this

Table 1.4   Exemplar of One of the 7 Principles: Looks Like/Does Not Look Like

The primary role of the service provider in early intervention is to work with and support the family members and caregivers in a child's life.

Key Concepts
- EI service providers engage with the adults to enhance confidence and competence in their inherent role as the people who teach and foster the child's development
- Families are equal partners in the relationship with service providers
- Mutual trust, respect, honesty, and open communication characterize the family–service provider relationship

This principle DOES look like this
- Using professional behaviors that build trust and rapport and establish a working "partnership" with families
- Valuing and understanding the service provider's role as a collaborative coach working to support family members as they help their child; incorporating principles of adult learning styles
- Providing information, materials, and emotional support to enhance families' natural role as the people who foster their child's learning and development

Source: Workgroup on Principles and Practices in Natural Environments (February 2008c).

information, presented in Table 1.5, provides a comprehensive look at how states describe their service delivery approach. This table reports the approaches identified by states and frequency of occurrences. As indicated, the primary service provider approach is the most frequently cited as either an approach under investigation by a state or used at varying degrees as a practice within the state.

All states that mentioned endorsing a particular approach, commented that it was *not* standard or consistent practice across the state. Based upon these data, it appears that rather than adopting one particular model, states are adapting multiple concepts and various subcomponents of a range of approaches to make practices work within their state structures. States reporting similar words in their named approaches (e.g., primary service provider) may in fact have differing practice interpretations, perhaps depending upon which national leader has been assisting the state in policy and/or professional development efforts. In the next section, several of the nationally recognized approaches or models will be briefly explained.

Twenty-three states did not name a specific approach, yet their Web sites and statewide professional development materials included

Table 1.5   Service Delivery Approaches Identified by Part C Coordinators

State-Named Approaches	Frequency
Primary Service Provider	8
Primary Service Provider/Coaching Model	6
Transdisciplinary Team with a Primary Service Provider	6
Consultative Team Model	4
Multidisciplinary Team Model	2
RBI with a Primary Service Provider	2
Everyday routines and activities	2
Relationship-based approach	1
Direct Therapy–consultative model	1
Interdisciplinary Model with independent providers or vendor system	1
Early Intervention Teams (EIT) with a Primary Service Provider approach	1
Everyday Routines and Activities and Places (ERAP)/Transdisciplinary Team	1
No approach named	23

Source: Pletcher (2009).

reference to specific concepts or practices, such as family-centered, relationship-based, transdisciplinary teaming, routines-based interview (RBI), routines-based assessment, functional outcomes, eco-mapping, and use of the CoP principles described earlier in this chapter. Many of these terms appear as specific descriptors included in the nationally recognized approaches described below.

FIVE MOST COMMON RECOGNIZED OR USED APPROACHES OR MODELS

The five approaches or models and their components explored in this section are the ones most frequently mentioned in the previous NECTAC-sponsored survey of states (2009). Please note, these are not the only approaches of or models for working with children and families in early intervention, nor is it our intent to imply endorsement of any particular approach. All of these approaches have foundational links to the major principles discussed earlier in this chapter; therefore, similar concepts and words are evident. However, each approach has distinct practices, tools, or processes that define how it is put into practice in the context of early intervention. Recognizing that each of the approaches is built upon a strong line of research and many supporting and defining principles, it would be impossible to address all the nuances of these highly regarded approaches in the context of this chapter. We believe it is important to provide the reader with a brief overview of each model or approach as well as resource links for learning more about the specifics of each model or approach presented.

Approach #1: Primary Coach Approach to Teaming or PSP with Coaching

Hanft, Rush, and Shelden (2004) are credited with describing the primary coach approach to teaming, or the PSP with coaching approach, in their research and publication *Coaching Families and Colleagues in Early Intervention* (2004). Shelden and Rush (2009) define the primary coach approach as "the use of a geographical based team, where one member is selected as the primary coach (to the family), receives coaching support from other team members and provides direct support to the parents and other care providers using coaching and natural learning environments practices to strengthen parenting competence and confidence and promote child learning and development" (p. 2). This approach is further described as a family-centered, capacity-building method of intervention with young children who have disabilities or developmental delays. In addition, there is a significant emphasis on natural learning environment practices and functional outcomes. The two major definers of this approach, coaching and primary coach, are described in the next section.

Coaching

The methodology of "coaching" is focal to this approach. Hanft et al. (2004) reinforce the value of a coaching approach and define it as "an interactive process of observation, reflection, and action in which a coach promotes, directly and/or indirectly, a learner's ability to support a child's participation in family and community contexts" (p. 4). The early interventionist works side by side with the family or other caregivers, to focus on building the confidence and competence of the parent/caregiver to ultimately identify, refine, and reflect on development-enhancing strategies so that they can be used throughout the family's daily activities. Emphasis on respecting parents and caregivers as adult learners and applying principles of adult learning are cornerstone to this model, which reinforces a support-based approach that empowers families and caregivers. It is important to note that any team member or service provider can use coaching strategies in their work, not only with families and other caregivers, but also with colleagues.

Primary Coach

There is one team member who works most closely with all the family members and other caregivers, called the primary coach. This person can be a team member of any discipline. In partnership with the family, the primary coach works collaboratively with other members of the team to coordinate consultation and joint visits and to receive coaching support as needed from other team members. This ensures that each family has the right mix of direct and/or indirect access to all team members. Intervention is recognized as a dynamic practice requiring active involvement of the coaching and collaborating team members to facilitate creative solutions by pooling the knowledge and expertise of all partnership members (Hanft et al., 2004; Turnbull & Turnbull, 2001). The reader is also directed to http://www.coachinginearly childhood.org/index.php to learn more about the specifics of this model.

Approach #2: Family-Centered Intervention in NATural Environments (FACINATE)

The Family-Centered Intervention in NATural Environments (FACI-NATE) model, developed by McWilliam (2010), is grounded by philosophy and research and designed for practical application. Although FACINATE was not specifically named as a state approach, several components associated with the model were named (e.g., RBI, eco-mapping, routine-based intervention). This model contains the following five components and associated practices.

1. *Understanding the Family Ecology*: The eco-map is the practice used to implement this component. An eco-map is a visual illustration of who is in the family's life and the degree of support (or stress) they provide. It is used to identify all the support networks available to the family.

2. *Functional Intervention Planning*: The Routines Based Interview (RBI) is a detailed interview focusing on the family and their unique mix of routines and activities that can be used to promote functional growth and development of the child. Its three purposes are to develop a list of functional outcomes, to assess child and family functioning, and to establish a positive relationship with families (McWilliam, Casey, & Sims, 2009). When the RBI is implemented as designed, it results in a list of concrete goals and outcomes for the child that can be used to write the IFSP outcomes.

3. *Integrated Services*: Within the FACINATE model, the primary service provider (PSP) is the assigned professional who provides ongoing support to the family with backing and assistance from a team of other professionals, in the form of consultation and joint visits. The PSP, who can be a generalist or a specialist, ultimately addresses the IFSP outcomes with the family.

4. *Support-Based Home Visits*: During ongoing visits with the family, the PSP uses the Vanderbilt Home Visiting Script (VHVS) (McWilliam, 2010) to provide emotional, material, or informational support to the family. The VHVS offers a template for service providers to use in conjunction with the IFSP functional outcomes and activities.

5. *Collaborative Child Care Consultation*: This component of the model refers to the support between the early intervention service providers and the child care staff in the program where the child is enrolled. The goal of consultation is to model incidental teaching methods and embedding interventions within daily routines in the early care and education setting, thus increasing child engagement and learning (McWilliam & Casey, 2008).

The reader is also directed to http://www.siskin.org/www/docs/112.180 to learn more about this model.

Approach #3: Therapists as Collaborative Team Members for Infant/Toddler Community Services (TaCTICS), Family Guided Approaches to Early Intervention (FACETS), and Family Guided Routines Based Intervention (FGRBI)

These three models were developed by Dr. Juliann Woods and build upon family-centered practices through natural routines and by collaborative teaming. The first two models, *TaCTICS* (Therapists *as* Collaborative *Team* members for *Infant/Toddler Community Services*) and *FACETS* (Family-guided Approaches to Collaborative Early-intervention Training and Services) reinforce the values that families are the center point of intervention, and children learn functional skills through daily routine activities and interactions. These models support team collaboration, including cross-agency integration. They acknowledge the importance of understanding sociocultural diversity as service providers work with families. Professional development resources and topical modules provide practical tools for service providers and can be found online at http://tactics.fsu.edu and http://www.facets.lsi.ku.edu.

The third model developed by Woods, *FGRBI* (Family Guided Routines Based Intervention) draws upon the resources included in TaCTICS and FACETS and adds five distinct processes with resources for each process (Bricker & Cripe, 1992; Cripe & Venn, 1997). This model integrates embedded intervention with the day-to-day challenges of implementing interventions that meet the spirit of natural environment legislation. The basic premises of the five processes are as follows:

1. *Introduction of Natural Environments and Welcoming the Family*: Within this process, the interventionist welcomes the family, introduces the early intervention steps, and describes and defines how daily routines can be used to promote children's learning.
2. *Routines Based Assessment in Natural Environments*: The assessment process includes gathering information about families' daily routines and children's activities. In doing so, the interventionists gain a concrete understanding of the family's concerns, priorities, and resources.
3. *Linking Assessment to Intervention*: Using the information gathered through the routines based assessment, the team develops a plan that addresses the priorities that are most meaningful

and pertinent to the child and family. The outcomes are contextually relevant to the family's routines and activities, and learning opportunities correspond to the family's current events and interactions.

4. *Involving Caregivers in Teaching and Learning*: This process reinforces the importance of meeting parents and caregivers where they are, respecting their individual learning styles, and creating opportunities to actively engage them in the teaching and learning that is a natural part of early intervention.

5. *Monitoring Progress*: Continuous monitoring ensures that intervention is effectively meeting the dynamic needs of the child and family. Without progress monitoring, the team runs the risk of intervention slippage away from family needs and priorities.

Information and staff development resources for this model can be found at http://fgrbi.fsu.edu.

Approach #4: Everyday Routines and Activities

Dunst and Bruder (1999, 2002) organized their ideas from social system and activity-learning theory for conceptualizing a way of using everyday family and community opportunities, experiences, and events to help young children with disabilities develop everyday knowledge and skills. Figure 1.2 conceptualizes this model and extends beyond the narrow focus of *locations* represented at the top of the triangle, to *activity settings*, at the midsection, and then to the wealth of *learning opportunities*, at the broad base of the triangle. Within this framework, the focus of intervention moves from delivering service provider-directed and child-centered intervention to promoting children's functional participation in development-enhancing activity settings.

Locations are defined as the physical places and social contexts in which the child and family find themselves each day. Each location provides for multiple activity settings for learning. Activity settings are defined as happening whenever a child is in a particular situation where people, materials, or objects in those settings either encourage or discourage a child from "doing something" (Dunst & Bruder, 1999). Activity settings can be identified in everyday family routines such as mealtimes, bedtimes, or through special routines such as going to the beach or weekly swimming lessons. Activity settings offer many more opportunities for learning and for enjoyable mastery of a new skill through meaningful practice (Dunst, Bruder, Trivette, Raab, &

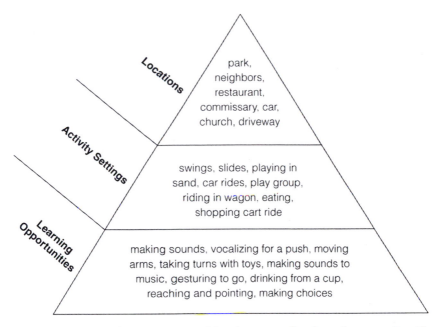

Figure 1.2   Learning opportunities in everyday locations and activities (http://www.ssa.gov/OP_Home/ssact/title19/1900.htm); family and community as a source of learning (http://www.everydaylearning .info/lov1-2php).

McLean, 2001). The learning opportunities that happen in activity settings can be planned or happen spontaneously. Figure 1.2 provides exemplars of a plethora of learning opportunities that can emerge in activity settings.

Research conducted by Dunst and Bruder found that although all families have activity settings and routines, they are not all the same. Family routines, activities, and the places where they spend time are unique to each family. Children experience different kinds of learning opportunities depending on where they live, the cultural and rituals of their families, and the unique activities that different families participate in and enjoy (Dunst, Trivette, et al., 2001). Therefore, the triangle framework representing everyday routines, activities, and learning opportunities will be unique for each family and will be different over time as changes occur in the child's life and their family's life.

Early intervention service providers can use this concept as a tool as they work with families to identify the places families go, the activity settings within these locations, and the potential learning opportunities afforded to their child. Everyday family and community settings are the real-life natural environments for each family. The Everyday Children's Learning Opportunities Institute provides a broad range of information on young children's everyday learning opportunities and natural learning environments. More information about the institute and additional resources can be found at http://www.everyday learning.info/index.php.

Approach #5: Community of Practice (CoP): The Agreed-upon Practices

While each of the above-mentioned approaches share similarities, they each advocate different tools and processes to implement the particular model or approach. The Community of Practice (CoP), previously explained in this chapter, brought the nationally recognized researchers who developed the models presented with other key stakeholders to focus on the commonalities of delivering services. The third document produced by this group, "The Agreed-upon Practices," is built upon the work outlined in their first two companion documents (see Tables 1.3 and 1.4) and should be utilized in conjunction with them to be fully understood. This third document reflects an extensive list of model neutral implementation practices. Model neutral means that the practices do not align with or endorse any one particular model or approach; rather, they reflect the consensus opinion of the nationally recognized workgroup members. Although not an exhaustive list of everything that should happen while a family is in early intervention, and not intended as a sequential checklist, the practices suggest a flow of best practice–endorsed activities, beginning with the first contacts between the family and the service provider through the family's transition out of Part C services. All together, the document suggests 37 practices and 166 activities to support the provision of quality early intervention services in natural environments.

Table 1.6 provides an example of 4 of the 10 suggested practices included in section three of the document entitled "Ongoing intervention with families and other caregivers." Even within this partial example, it is possible to see many of the foundational principles defined earlier in the chapter as well as a blending of implementation practices from various models and approaches just described.

Table 1.6   Example from Agreed-Upon Practices

Section 3: Providing Ongoing Intervention

1. Build on or establish trust and rapport.

- Before each visit, reflect on your own beliefs and values and how they might influence your suggestions and strategies with this particular family or caregiver.
- Use communication styles and social behaviors that are warm and welcoming and respectful of family culture and circumstances.
- Conduct yourself as a guest in the family's home or caregiver's setting.
- Respectfully provide complete and unbiased information in response to requests or questions.
- Be credible and follow through on plans you made with the family.
- If you don't know the answer to a question, tell the family you do not know but will find out for them. Tell them when you will get back to them with the information.

2. During the first visit, review the IFSP and plan together how the time can be spent.

- Describe the practical aspects of a visit and what the family or caregiver can expect. For example: the length of the typical visit, that other people are always welcome at the family's invitation, the variety of places in which visits can occur, the program's cancellation policy, etc.
- Describe examples of visits in various home and community settings where the family participates. You might want to offer to share clips from commercial or videos produced by your program.
- Invite the family to reflect on their experience with the IFSP process to date and share any concerns or questions.
- Review the IFSP document and assessment information.
- Consider each agreed-upon outcome—is it what the family is still interested in? Prioritize again, if necessary, where to begin; change wording if needed; provide any explanations to help family understand purpose, etc.
- Discuss how outcomes, activities, and strategies can be a starting place for each home visit.
- Clarify who will work on each outcome—family, friends, other caregivers, service providers.
- Talk about community activities and events that can be used to support practice and mastery for the specific outcomes.
- If not previously done, ask the family to sign the IFSP, consent forms, and any other necessary documentation.
- Provide information about family-to-family support and parent groups that are available.

3. For ongoing visits, use the IFSP as a guide to plan how to spend the time together.

- Begin each visit by asking open-ended questions to identify any significant family events or activities and how well the planned routines and activities have been going.

(Continued)

Table 1.6   (Continued)

- Ask if there are any new issues and concerns the family wants to talk about. Explore if these concerns need to be addressed as new outcomes; if so, plan an IFSP review.
- Decide which outcomes and activities to focus on during the visit.

4. Participate with the family or other caregivers and the child in the activity and/or routine as the context for promoting new skills and behaviors.

- Offer a variety of options to families for receiving new information or refining their routines and activities, such as face-to-face demonstrations, video, conversations, written information, audios, CDs, diaries, etc.
- Gather any needed toys and materials and begin the selected activity or routine.
- Listen, observe, model, teach, coach, and/or join the ongoing interactions of the family and child.
- Encourage the family to observe and assess the child's skills, behaviors, and interests (a continual part of ongoing functional assessment). For example, ask the family if behaviors are typical, if they've seen new behaviors (suggesting emerging skills), or how much the child seems to enjoy the activity.
- Use a variety of consulting or coaching strategies throughout the activity, including: observing, listening, attending, acknowledging, expanding, responding, probing, summarizing, etc.
- Reflect with the family on what went well, what they want to continue doing, and what they would like to do differently at the next visit.

Source: Workgroup on Principles and Practices in Natural Environments (February 2008a).

CONSIDERATIONS OR CHALLENGES FOR IMPLEMENTING A PARTICULAR STATEWIDE MODEL OR APPROACH

Exploring and implementing these approaches is all about change. Although there is an abundance of literature about change, it is not our intent in these final paragraphs to review system change theory. Rather, this concluding section shares a few thoughts about implementing and sustaining statewide change of new practices. "Change" can be thought of as a verb encompassing all the actions necessary for developing and adopting new ideas associated with an alternative practice and for establishing reorganization necessary to support the changes (Smale, 1998). Implementation of change is all about people; what they believe and value, what they understand and can do in practice, and how they feel supported to manage the required changes. Changing a service delivery approach and putting in place all the infrastructures needed to support the change and sustain implementation is no quick or simple task (Fixsen, Naoom, Blasé, Friedman, & Wallace, 2005; Smale, 1998).

"Implementation" is the terminology and science of putting a new idea, model, or practice into actual use at a program level. Fixsen et al. (2005) define implementation as "a specific set of activities designed to put into practice an activity or program of known dimensions" (p. 5). They define six stages of implementation, which include: exploration and adoption, program installation, initial implementation, full operation, innovation, and sustainability. Each stage has specific activities or processes. If a state is endorsing a particular approach and desiring all early intervention programs to use this endorsed approach when delivering services, the state would need to carefully address each of these six stages.

Taking a model that has been put into practice in one program or location and replicating it broadly throughout a geographical area or state is referred to as *going to scale* or *scaling-up*. This too often requires changes in program design, new policy or even laws, and new funding mechanisms to support the changes (Harris, 2010; Weiss & HFRP, 1988). As states move to adopt or adapt a new service delivery approach, it will require a working knowledge of both implementation and scaling-up procedures if their efforts are to improve their service delivery system and result in positive sustainable change.

Whether it is one particular agency or an entire state that is perusing service delivery change, it is essential to keep the Early Intervention System Framework (see Figure 1.1) clearly in mind as the three interconnected circles, Principles, Practices, and Program Design, must be examined, addressed, and aligned to develop and/or maintain an effective and coherent system. Any change in one component will impact the other components. Programs or states will need to clearly articulate the purpose and supporting principles of their early intervention system to service providers, families, referral sources, and other community partnership agencies. Statements such as those proposed by the consensus work of the CoP may prove helpful as programs or states embark upon service delivery change.

As noted above, this work will require multifaceted actions. From a principles and policies perspective, there will likely be a need to realign or even rewrite state rules and regulations that support the direction of their work. At a practices level, there will be a need for many concrete examples of practice and procedural guidance on what the approach will *look like* or *not look like* as it is put into practice. This will require ongoing professional development and support on the tools suggested by the approach being adopted and/or on the use of best practices described in the CoP Agreed-upon Practices documents. Early intervention service providers will not only need ongoing opportunities to gain and refine their knowledge and skills for their day-to-day work with children and families; they will also need ongoing support, mentoring, reflective supervision, and encouragement to put these practices into action competently and confidently within the context of early intervention processes from referral through transition.

Finally, at a systems design level, both local and state early intervention programs will need adjustments to support the changes in principles and practices. Team delivery, consultation time, new funding structures to support the changes in service delivery, new public awareness materials, supervision, and ongoing professional development are just a few of the program design system components that will need attention. Collectively, early intervention system principles, practice, and program design must be grounded on research-based evidence and function harmoniously if children like Damian and Jessica and the millions of other current and future families participating in early intervention are to truly benefit from early intervention services.

We believe the complexity and ultimate value of service delivery system change can be summed up by a final comment made by a State Part C Coordinator at the 2009 National Early Childhood Conference in the session on "Service Delivery Models" when she challenged others by stating, *"This is no easy task to implement change in practice consistently across the state. This will take years. You must plan carefully and make that plan known to others throughout the state. It is hard but very exciting work. To know that we will have service providers using practices that have years of research and evidence supporting them, based on values and beliefs we feel are fundamental, and that all families will receive services and supports consistently across our state will be worth it in the end. Yes!!"* (Part C Coordinator).

REFERENCES

Adams, P., & Nelson, K. (Eds.) (1995). *Reinventing human services; community-and family-centered practice*. New York: Aldine de Gruyer.
Allen, M., Brown R., & Finlay, B. (1992). *Helping children by strengthening families: A look at family support programs*. Washington, DC: Children's Defense Fund.

Baird, S., & Peterson, J. (1997). Seeking a comfortable fit between family-centered philosophy and infant-parent interaction in early intervention: Time for a paradigm shift? *Topics in Early Childhood Special Education, 17*(2), 139–164.

Bernheimer, L. P., & Keogh, B. K. (1995). Weaving interventions into the fabric of everyday life: An approach to family assessment. *Topics in Early Childhood Special Education, 15*(4), 415–433.

Bricker, D., & Cripe, J. W. (1992). An activity-based approach to early intervention. Baltimore: Paul H. Brookes.

Bricker, D., Pretti-Frontczak, K., & McComas, N. (1998). *An activity-based approach to early intervention* (2nd ed.). Baltimore: Paul H. Brookes.

Bronfenbrenner, U. (1979). *The ecology of human development: Experiments by nature and design.* Cambridge, MA: Harvard University Press.

Bruder, M. B. (2000). Family-centered early intervention: Clarifying our values for the new millennium. *Topics in Early Childhood Special Education, 20*(2), 105–115.

Bruder, M. B., & Bologna, T. M. (1993). Collaboration and service coordination for effective early intervention. In W. Brown, S. K. Thurman, & L. Pearl (Eds.), *Family-centered early intervention with infants and toddler: Innovative cross disciplinary approaches* (pp. 103–127). Baltimore: Paul H. Brookes.

Bruder, M. B., & Dunst, C. J. (2008). Factors related to the scope of early intervention service coordinator practices. *Infants & Young Children, 21*, 176–185.

Buysee, V., & Wesley, P. W. (2006). *Evidence-based practice in the early childhood field.* Washington, DC: Zero to Three.

Campbell, P. H., Sawyer, B., & Muhlenhaupt, M. (2009). The meaning of natural environments for parents and professionals. *Infants and Young Children, 22*(4), 264–278.

Cohen, S., & Syme. S. L. (Eds.) (1985). *Social support and health.* New York: Academic Press.

Cripe, J. W., & Venn, M. L. (1997). Family-guided routines for early intervention services. *Young Exceptional Children, 1*(1), 18–26.

Dinnebeil, L. A., Hale, L., & Rule, S. (1999). Early intervention program practices that support collaboration. *Topics in Early Childhood Special Education, 19*(4), 225–235.

Dunst, C. J. (2002). Family-centered practices: Birth through high school. *Journal of Special Education, 36*(3), 139–147.

Dunst, C. J., & Bruder, M. B. (1999). Family and community activity settings, natural learning environments, and children's learning opportunities. *Children's Learning Opportunities Report, 1*(2).

Dunst, C. J., & Bruder, M. B. (2002). Valued outcomes of service coordination, early intervention, and natural environments.Exceptional Children, 68, 361–375.

Dunst, C. J., Bruder, M. B., Trivette, C. M., Raab, M., & McLean, M. (2001). Natural learning opportunities for infants, toddlers, and preschoolers. *Young Exceptional Children, 4*(3), 18–25.

Dunst, C. J., Hamby, D., Trivette, C. M., Raab, M., & Bruder, M. B. (2000). Everyday family and community life and children's naturally occurring learning opportunities. *Journal of Early Intervention, 23*(3), 151–164.

Dunst, C. J., Johanson, J., Trivette, C. M., & Hamby, D. (1991). Family-oriented early intervention policies and practices: Family-centered or not. *Exceptional Children, 58.*

Dunst, C. J., Trivette, C. M., & Deal, A. (1988). *Enabling and empowering families: Principles and guidelines for practice*. Baltimore: Paul H. Brookes.

Dunst, C. J., Trivette, C. M., Humphries, T., Raab, M., & Roper, N. (2001). Contrasting approaches to natural learning environment interventions. *Infants and Young Children, 14*(2), 48–63.

Fixsen, D., Naoom, S. F., Blasé, D. A., Friedman, R. M., & Wallace, F. (2005). *Implementation research: A synthesis of the literature*. University of South Florida, Louis de la Parte Florida Mental Health Institute, The National Implementation Research Network (FMHI Publication #231).

Florida State University, Department of Communication Disorders. (n.d.). *Family Guided Routines Based Intervention (FGRBI)*. Retrieved from http://fgrbi .fsu.edu

Gallagher, J. J., Danaher, J. C., & Clifford, R. M. (2009).The evolution of the national early childhood technical assistance center. *Topics in Early Childhood Special Education, 29*(1), 7–23.

Gargiulo, R. M., & Kilgo, J. L. (2000). *Young children with special needs: An introduction to early childhood special education*. Albany, NY: Delmar.

Goode, S., Lazara, A. & Danaher, J. (Eds.). (2008). *Part C updates* (10th ed.). Chapel Hill: University of North Carolina, FPG Child Development Institute, National Early Childhood Technical Assistance Center.

Greenspan, S. I., & Wieder, S. (1998). *The child with special needs: Encouraging intellectual and emotional growth*. Reading, MA: Perseus Books.

Hanft, B. E., & Pilkington, K. O. (2000). Therapy in natural environments: The means or end goal for early intervention. *Infants and Young Children, 12*(4), 1–13.

Hanft, B. E., Rush, D. D., & Shelden, M. L. (2004). *Coaching families and colleagues in early childhood*. Baltimore: Paul H. Brookes.

Harris, E. (2010, Spring). Six steps to successfully scale impact in the nonprofit sector. *The Evaluation Exchange, Harvard Family Research Project XV*(1).

Individuals with Disabilities Act of 1986, 20 U.S.C. § 1400 *et seq* (Part H). Retrieved from http://codes.lp.findlaw.com/uscode/20/33/I/1400

Individuals with Disabilities Act Regulations, 1999, 34 C.F.R. § 303.400–460. Retrieved from http://www.nectac.org/idea/303regs.asp

Individuals with Disabilities Education Act of 2004, Pub. L. No 99-457, 20 U.S.C. § 1436. Retrieved from http://codes.lp.findlaw.com/uscode/20/33/III/1436

Individuals with Disabilities Education Improvement Act of 2004, 20 U.S.C. § 1400 *et seq*. Retrieved from http://www.wrightslaw.com/idea/idea.2004.all.pdf.

Individuals with Disabilities Education Improvement Act of 2004, Pub. L. No. 101 -476, 20 U.S.C. §§ 1400 *et seq.*

ITCA. (2000). *Position paper on the provision of early intervention services in accordance with federal requirements on natural environments*. IDEA Infant Toddler Coordinators' Association Board of Directors, April 3, 2000.

Jung, L. A., & McWilliam, R. A. (2005). Reliability and validity of scores on the IFSP rating scale. *Journal of Early Intervention, 27*(2), 125–136.

Kelly, J. F. & Barnard, K. E. (1999). Parent education within a relationship-focused model. *Topics in Early Childhood Special Education, 19*(3), 151–157.

Ketelaar, M., Vermeer, A., Helders, P. J. M., & Hart, H. (1998). Parental participation in intervention programs for children with cerebral palsy: A review of research. *Topics in Early Childhood Special Education, 18*(2), 108–117.

Knowles, M. (1980). *The modern practice of adult education: From pedagogy to andragony.* Chicago: Associated Press/Follett.

Kretzmann, J. P., & McKnight, J. L. (1993). *Building communities from the inside out: A path towards finding and mobilizing a community's assets.* Chicago: ACTA Publications.

Mahoney, G., Boyce, G., Fewell, R. R., Spiker, D., & Wheeden, C. A. (1998). The relationship of parent-child interaction to the effectiveness of early intervention services for at-risk children and children with disabilities. *Topics in Early Childhood Special Education, 18*(1), 5–17.

Mahoney, G., & Filer, J. (1996). How responsive is early intervention to the priorities and needs of families? *Topics in Early Childhood Special Education, 16*(4), 437–457.

Mahoney, G., & Wheeden, A. (1997). Parent-child interaction—the foundation for family-centered early intervention practice: A response to Baird and Peterson. *Topics in Early Childhood Special Education, 17*(2), 165–184.

Manning, G., Curtis, K., & McMillen, S. (1996). *Building community: The human side of work.* Cincinnati, OH: Thomas Executive Press.

Mayhew, L., Scott, S., & McWilliam, R. A. (1999). *Project INTEGRATE: A training and resource guide for speech and language pathologists.* Chapel Hill: Frank Porter Graham Child Development Center, University of North Carolina.

McBride, S. L., & Peterson, C. (1997). Home-based early intervention with families of children with disabilities: Who is doing what? *Topics in Early Childhood Special Education, 17*(2), 209–233.

McCormick, L., & Noonan, M. J. (2002). Ecological assessment and planning. In M. M. Ostrosky & E. Horn (Eds.), *Young Exceptional Children Monograph Series No. 4 Assessment: Gathering meaningful information* (pp. 47–60). Longmont, CO: Sopris West.

McWilliam, R. A. (2000). It's only natural . . . to have early intervention in the environments where it's needed. In S. Sandall & M. M. Ostrosky (Eds.), *Young Exceptional Children Monograph Series No. 2: Natural environments and inclusion* (pp. 17–26). Denver, CO: Division for Early Childhood of the Council for Exceptional Children.

McWilliam, R. A. (2004). Enhancing services in natural environments. Retrieved from http://www.nectac.org/~ppts/calls/2004/partcsettings/mcwilliam.ppt

McWilliam, R. A. (2010). Support-based home visiting. In R. A. McWilliam (Ed.), *Working with families of young children with special needs* (pp. 203–236). New York: Guilford Press.

McWilliam, R. A. & Casey, A. M. (2008). *Engagement of every child in the preschool classroom.* Baltimore: Paul H. Brookes.

McWilliam, R. A., Casey A. M., & Sims, J. (2009). The routines-based interview as method for gathering information and assessing needs. *Infants and Young Children, 22*(3), 224–233.

McWilliam, R. A., Snyder, P., Harbin, G. L., Porter, P., & Munn, D. (2000). Professionals' and families' perceptions of family-centered practices in infant-toddler services. *Early Education and Development, 11*(4), 519–538.

Peterander, F. (2000). The best quality cooperation between parents and experts in early intervention. *Infants and Young Children, 12*(3), 32–45.

Peterson, N. L. (1987). *Early intervention for handicapped and at-risk children; An introduction to early childhood special education.* Denver, CO: Love.

Pilkington, K. (2007). American Occupational Therapy Association (AOTA). *Side by side: Transdisciplinary early intervention in natural environments.* Retrieved from http://www.aota.org/Pubs/OTP/1997-2007/Features/2006/f-040306 .aspx?css=print

Pletcher, L. C. (1997). *Family centered practices: A training guide.* Chapel Hill, NC: ARCH National Resource Center.

Pletcher, L. C. (2009). *Survey of state approaches to service delivery and materials developed.* National Early Childhood TA Center. Retrieved from http://www .tacommunities.org/getfile/view/id/1005/cid/5009/p/folder_5186 http:// www.tacommunities.org/document/list/p/%252Ffolder_5186

Pletcher, L. C., & McBride, S. (2000). *Family-center services: Guiding principles and practices for delivery of family centered services.* Retrieved from http://nectac.org/ topics/families/famctrprin.asp

Pretti-Frontczak, K., & Bricker, D. D. (2004). An activity-based approach to early intervention (3rd ed.). Baltimore: Paul H. Brookes.

Roper, N., & Dunst, C. J. (2003). Communication intervention in natural learning environments guidelines for practice. *Infants and Young Children, 16*(3), 215–226.

Rush, D. D., Shelden, M. L., & Hanft, B. E. (2003). Coaching families and colleagues: A process for collaboration in natural settings. *Infants and Young Children, 16*(1), 33–47.

Sandall, S., McLean M. E., & Smith, B. J. (2000). *DEC recommended practices for early intervention/early childhood special education.* Longmont, CO: Sopris West.

Schorr, E. B. (1988). *Within our reach: Breaking the cycle of the disadvantaged.* New York: Doubleday.

Schuck, L. A., & Bucy, J. E. (1997). Family rituals: Implications for early intervention. *Topics in Early Childhood Special Education, 17*(4), 477–493.

Shelden, M. L., & Rush, D. D. (2009). Checklist for implementing a primary-coach approach to teaming. FIPP CASE tools, 5(1) Center for the Advanced Study of Excellence in Early Childhood and Family Support Practices, Family Infant and Preschool Program, J. Iverson Riddle Developmental Center, Morganton, NC. Retrieved from http://www.fippcase.org/casetools/casetool_vol5 _no1.pdf

Shonkoff, J., & Phillips, D. (2000). *From neurons to neighborhoods: The science of early childhood development.* Washington, DC: National Academy Press.

Smale, G. (1998). *Managing change through innovation.* London: The Stationery Office.

Social Security Act. (1965). Title XIX, § 1900. Retrieved from http://www.ssa.gov/ OP_Home/ssact/title19/1900.htm

TaCTICS: Therapists as Collective Team members for Infants/Toddler Community Services, Project TaCTICS. (n.d.). Retrieved from http://tactics.fsu.edu

Tisot, C. M., & Thurman, S. K. (2002). Using behavior settings theory to define natural settings: A family-centered approach. *Infants and Young Children, 14*(3), 65–71.

Trivette C. M. (2009). Participatory adult learning profession development strategies. Conference presentation at the 9th Annual Early Childhood Inclusion Institute, Chapel Hill, NC.

Turnbull, A., & Turnbull, R. (2001). *Families, professionals, and exceptionality collaborating for empowerment* (4th ed.). Columbus, OH: Merrill Prentice Hall.

University of Kansas Life Span Institute. (n.d.). Family-guided approaches to collaborative early-intervention training and services (FACETS). Retrieved from http://www.facets.lsi.ku.edu

Vanderholf, M. (2004). American Physical Therapy Association (APTA). *Maximizing your role in early intervention*. Retrieved from http://www.apta.org/AM/Template.cfm?Section=search&template=CM/HTMLDisplay.cfm&ContentID=8534

Weiss, H. B. and Harvard Family Research Project (HRFP). (1988). *Going to scale: Issues in the development and proliferation of community-based family support and education programs*. Cambridge, MA: Author.

Weston, D., & Ivins, B. (2001). From testing to talking: Linking assessment and intervention through relationships with parents. *Zero to Three, 21*, 47–50.

Woodruff, G. & McGonigel, M. J. (1988). Early intervention team approaches: The transdisciplinary model. In J. Jordan, J. Gallagher, P. Hutinger, & M. Karnes (Eds.), *Early childhood special education: Birth to three* (pp. 163–182). Reston, VA: Council for Exceptional Children.

Woods, J. (2008a). American Speech-Language-Hearing Association (ASHA). *Providing early intervention services in natural environments*. Retrieved from http://www.asha.org/Publications/leader/2008/080325/f080325b.htm

Woods, J. (2008b). American Speech-Language-Hearing Association (ASHA). *Roles and responsibilities of speech language pathologist in early intervention*. Retrieved from http://www.asha.org/docs/html/GL2008-00293.html

Woods, J., Kashinath, S., & Goldstein, H. (2004). Effects of embedding caregiver-implemented teaching strategies in daily routines on children's communication outcomes. *Journal of Early Intervention, 26*(3), 175–193.

Workgroup on Principles and Practices in Natural Environments (February 2008a), *Agreed upon practices for providing services in natural environments*. OSEP TA Community of Practice—Part C Settings. Retrieved from http://www.nectac.org/topics/families/families.asp

Workgroup on Principles and Practices in Natural Environments (February 2008b), *Mission and key principles for providing early intervention services in natural environments*. OSEP TA Community of Practice—Part C Settings. Retrieved from http://www.nectac.org/topics/families/families.asp

Workgroup on Principles and Practices in Natural Environments (February, 2008c), *Seven key principles: Looks like/doesn't look like*. OSEP TA Community of Practice–Part C Settings. Retrieved from http://www.nectac.org/topics/families/families.asp

Early Childhood Special Education Methods and Practices for Preschool-Aged Children and Their Families

Lynette K. Chandler, Robin Miller Young,
and Nasiah Cirincione Ulezi

HISTORICAL PERSPECTIVE OF EARLY CHILDHOOD SPECIAL EDUCATION

ECSE has roots in several fields, including special education for school-aged students with exceptionalities, behavior analysis, and early childhood education. It has been influenced by a variety of theories and philosophies regarding child development and learning and by initiatives to support the learning and development of young children.

Special Education and Behavior Analysis

Special education and behavior analysis research has documented the significant influence of the environment in promoting learning and development. Variables within the environment set the occasion for behavior to occur, and the consequences that follow behavior influence how well behavior is learned. Behavioral theorists emphasize the importance of positive consequences (positive reinforcement) in promoting skill acquisition, maintaining learned skills, and generalization of learned skills to different situations. Skills and behaviors that are followed by positive reinforcement are strengthened and will be more likely to occur again in similar environmental situations.

Behaviorists and special educators believe that adults and peers are critical components of the child's environment and that adults directly influence learning in two ways. First, they purposefully arrange environmental variables to draw out and then reinforce new and appropriate skills and behaviors (Chandler & Dahlquist, 2009). Second, adults directly teach and reinforce skills using research-based teaching strategies and adapting materials and activities to meet the needs of each child. Many of the research-based practices currently used in ECSE have been adapted from those employed with older individuals with disabilities and will be discussed later in this chapter. Examples of these are task analysis (Carter & Kemp, 1996), shaping (Peterson, 2004), tiered models of instruction (Stewart, Martella, Marchand-Martella, & Benner, 2005), positive behavior support (Carr et al., 1999), and universal design for learning (CAST, 2008).

Early Childhood Education

Early childhood education and the constructivist theory of learning have contributed much to the current practices in ECSE. Central to the theory is the belief that learning is an active, constructive process that occurs through self-initiated actions within activities and interactions with peers and adults. Children construct an understanding of and knowledge about their worlds through experiences and reflections about those experiences (Darragh, 2010; Grennon Brooks, n.d.). Several theorists have contributed to the theory. Piaget (1937/1954) believed that children are self-motivated to discover and construct knowledge from their own actions on and experiences within their world. Learning occurs through processes of assimilation and accommodation of new information that alters mental schemes or existing knowledge. As children interact with their environments, they assimilate new concepts into an existing scheme. When they acquire information that does not fit within the current scheme, they accommodate the new information, leading to new or expanded schemes. Piaget also described stages of cognitive development during early childhood, positing that each stage provides a foundation for subsequent learning. The role of the teacher or other practitioners within Piaget's approach is to develop effective physical environments to support assimilation and accommodation at each stage of learning.

John Dewey (2004) underscored the importance of using children's interests in effective teaching. He advocated for the use of child-centered curricula that built on children's interests and incorporated "hands-on" experiences rather than predetermined, inflexible, teacher-directed instruction. Dewey felt that it was important to teach children "how to learn" and problem-solving skills versus simply teaching academic content. The role of the practitioner is to observe, guide, and encourage as needed.

Maria Montessori believed that intelligence was influenced by children's interactions with their environments, and that sensory-based learning was especially critical for young children (Edwards, 2002). Montessori focused on the individualized nature of learning, recognizing that all children were capable of learning, but they needed to learn at their own pace. This could be accomplished by allowing children to repeat activities until concepts and skills were mastered. She described a strong relationship among children's innate drive to interact with their environment, adults' facilitation of learning, and the environment. The role of the practitioner is to observe individual children and prepare activities and materials for each child based on those observations (Hull, Goldhaber, & Capone, 2002; Malaguzzi, 1996).

Vygotsky explored sociocultural theory, which pointed to the importance of social interactions and interpersonal relationships in learning and development. He stressed the importance of adults and peers and reciprocal relationships in the child's environment. Vygotsky's focus on social relationships as well as information from attachment theory, which asserts that the quality of early relationships influences lifelong social competence, helped early childhood educators recognize positive social-emotional development as a significant outcome of early childhood. Another contribution from Vygotsky is the concept of the Zone of Proximal Development (ZPD): the distance between what a child can do independently and what a child can do with support or the next skill to be learned. The teacher's role is to guide and support learning through scaffolding (e.g., prompting, assistance, feedback) to help the child move from one level or skill to another. Vygotsky also believed that children with disabilities were capable of learning, and that they would learn best by participating in environments that were designed to facilitate learning for typically developing children (Gargiulo & Kilgo, 2005).

Compensatory Programs Initiatives

Toward the end of the twentieth century, the federal government provided funding for several programs for young children who were at risk for academic failure and their families. These compensatory programs were designed to minimize the effects of poverty and other risk factors on development and to promote success in school. Three

well-known research initiatives are the Perry Preschool Project
(High Scope, 2005), the Chicago Child-Parent Center (CPC) Program
(Reynolds, 2008), and the Abecedarian Project (Campbell, Ramey,
Pungello, Sparling, & Miller Johnson, 2002). Each of these initiatives
provided center-based preschool programs for children living in poverty and evaluated the effects of their preschool experiences through
high school and into adulthood. These programs documented positive
short- and long-term effects. Children who participated in these programs had higher IQ scores and academic achievement, had fewer
grade retentions, and received fewer special education services than
children who did not receive preschool services. Evaluation of students in the Perry Preschool project at ages 27 and 40 revealed that
these children had lower rates of teen pregnancy, fewer arrests, and
use of social services, and they were more likely to graduate from high
school, attend college, own a home, and have higher incomes and
more positive work histories than children who did not participate in
the program (Darragh, 2010). Moreover, the programs were cost-
effective in terms of the amount of money invested in preschool and
the outcomes obtained (Parks, 2000). For example, a recent study of
prekindergarten (pre-K) programs in New Mexico estimated that
$5.00 in benefits was generated for every dollar invested in pre-K
programs (Hustedt, Barnett, Jung, & Goetze, 2009). Current research
regarding preschool programs continues to document both short-
and long-term benefits of high-quality preschool programs (Partnership for America's Economic Success, 2010).

In the 1960s, Head Start programs were designed to address multiple influences that can negatively impact child development. These
comprehensive programs focused on nutrition, health, and safety;
development across domains (e.g., physical, cognitive, social-
emotional, communication, and adaptive) and academic areas (e.g.,
early literacy and math); parent involvement and support; economic
issues; and other areas of family need (Peterson, 1987). Services were
provided by multiple disciplines, including teachers, therapists, psychologists, and social services personnel. In 1972, federal law required
Head Start programs to reserve 10 percent of their slots for children
with disabilities. Head Start programs now have disability service
plans that include strategies for identifying and meeting the needs of
children with disabilities.

The compensatory programs demonstrated that early intervention
can have a positive and enduring impact on child development and
learning (Borman, n.d.). They also underscored the importance of

involving parents as partners in their child's program and collaborative team-based service delivery, two values that guide ECSE today.

CURRENT INFLUENCES ON EARLY CHILDHOOD SPECIAL EDUCATION

ECSE incorporates philosophies, values, and practices from each of the fields and theories described above to create a distinct discipline that addresses the needs of young children who have or are at risk for developmental disabilities from birth to 8 years of age and their families. ECSE also is influenced by (1) federal and state laws and regulations; (2) federal, state, and local initiatives; (3) national organizations and their recommended practices, frameworks for learning, and position statements; and (4) research on effective practices.

FEDERAL AND STATE LAWS AND REGULATIONS AND INITIATIVES

Individuals with Disabilities Education Act

The primary federal legislation related to ECSE is the Individuals with Disabilities Education Act (IDEA). The IDEA law and clarifying regulations identify state requirements and responsibilities for providing a free and appropriate education (FAPE) to children and youth with disabilities, and delineate the rights of children with disabilities and their families. This chapter is limited to our discussion to those aspects of IDEA that influence early childhood special education practices at the preschool level (also see Council for Exceptional Children [CEC], 2006; IDEA, 2004).

IDEA establishes procedures and criteria for determining eligibility to receive special education and related services. States are mandated by IDEA to provide special education and related services to eligible children from ages 3 through 21. Special education services are defined as specially designed instructional services to meet the needs of the child and to allow access to the general education curriculum (e.g., adaptations and modifications of materials, teaching strategies, and goals and alternative assessment methods). Related services are additional supports that allow a child to benefit from special education services (e.g., speech, occupational, or physical therapy, assistive technology, transportation, and counseling).

Special education and related services can be delivered to preschool-aged children in a variety of early childhood settings, including community child care, Head Start programs, and preschool programs provided by local school districts or cooperatives (Dinnebeil, McInerney, & Hale, 2006). IDEA requires that special education and related services be delivered in the Least Restrictive Environment (LRE). LRE is defined as providing services to children with disabilities in settings that are as close as possible to the general education environment, that include peers who are typically developing, and that meet the needs of the individual child (Grisham-Brown, Hemmeter, & Pretti-Frontczak, 2005). The LRE decision is made by a team that includes school-based professionals and the child's parents or guardians. This team first reviews information obtained from assessment about the child's strengths and needs and then determines the annual developmental, educational, and early academic and behavioral goals to be addressed and the special education and related services that will be provided. Only then does the team determine which type of setting would best meet the needs of the child.

Although IDEA does not require that all children receive services in inclusive settings or programs (i.e., settings that blend children with disabilities and children who are typically developing into heterogeneous groups), the team must first consider if an inclusive setting would be appropriate for the child (i.e., is the child likely to make adequate progress on annual goals in an inclusive setting?) (CONNECT, 2009). If the team agrees that the child is not likely to make adequate progress in an inclusive placement, even with special education and related services and supports, then the team may consider a continuum of placement options such as dual placement in an inclusive classroom and a segregated classroom or resource room or full-time placement in a segregated classroom (Etscheidt, 2006). When an alternative placement option is identified as the LRE, the team must justify the placement decision and identify opportunities for the child to interact with peers who are typically developing.

IDEA requires teams to identify parent concerns related to their child and to consider those concerns when making decisions about the child's program. Teams must document parent participation in making decisions and describe procedures for informing parents about their child's progress. The team documents decisions about the frequency and type of special education and related services and the LRE on an Individualized Education Plan (IEP). The IEP also (1) identifies annual developmental, educational, and behavioral goals for the child; (2) documents the link between child goals and the general education curriculum and state standards; and (3) specifies how the team will evaluate child progress.

Finally, the use of person-first language as a recommended practice is reflected in the title of this law. Person-first language is based on the philosophy that individuals with disabilities are not defined by their disabilities. Disability is just one of many characteristics of an individual, and children with disabilities are more like their same-age peers than they are different. Person-first language dictates that when we refer to a child who has a disability, we refer to the child first instead of labeling the child by his or her disability (Snow, 2009). So, for example, a teacher would say that she has a child with autism in her class versus an autistic child. Person-first language has been embraced by early childhood special education and professional organizations such as the Division for Early Childhood as a recommended practice that focuses on the whole child and his or her abilities.

State Initiatives for Universal Preschool

Demonstrations of the effectiveness of early intervention provided by compensatory programs and current research demonstrating the effectiveness of high-quality preschool programs has led to *Preschool for All* or *Universal Preschool* initiatives across the country. Many states have developed or are developing state-sponsored programs for preschool-aged children. In 2008, more than 80 percent of 4-year-olds in the United States were enrolled in some type of preschool program. Almost 40 percent of those children attended public programs such as Head Start or school-based programs. Thirty-eight states currently provide state-funded preschool programs for almost 1.4 million 4-year-old children with and without disabilities (Barnett, Epstein, Friedman, Stevenson Boyd, & Hustedt, 2008). The growth of state-funded programs has provided new opportunities for serving children with disabilities in settings with peers who are typically developing or are at risk. For example, in 2007, almost half of the preschoolers with disabilities spent more than 80 percent of their day and received special education services in inclusive early childhood programs (IDEAdata, 2007).

The development of early learning standards also can be traced to the universal preschool or Pre-K movement and other federal initiatives. For example, Head Start developed the Child Outcomes Framework, which identifies skills, abilities, knowledge, and behaviors that young children should acquire before they enter kindergarten programs

(Head Start Bureau, 2003). The federally funded Good Start, Grow Smart initiative sought to improve program quality through the development of state standards for early learning and support for professional development (Grisham-Brown, Pretti-Frontczak, Hawkins, & Winchell, 2009). The No Child Left Behind law requires states to establish standards for early literacy and math for 4-year-old children.

Standards are statements of the knowledge and skills that children should achieve across developmental domains (physical, cognitive, communication, social-emotional, and adaptive) or academic content areas (e.g., early literacy, math, science) at various ages or grades (Brovoda, Leong, Payner, & Seminov, 2000). Standards guide (1) the identification of general education goals for all children, (2) the selection or development of early childhood curricula and teaching strategies to meet those goals, and (3) the development of assessment procedures to determine progress in meeting goals (McCormick, Grisham-Brown, & Hallam, 2007). Thirty-five of the 38 states with pre-K programs have developed early learning standards (Barnett et al., 2008).

NATIONAL ORGANIZATIONS

Two organizations have greatly influenced the philosophies and practices within early childhood special education. The National Association for the Education of Young Children (NAEYC) is the largest national organization focusing on early childhood education. It is "dedicated to improving the well-being of all young children, with particular focus on the quality of educational and developmental services for all children from birth through age 8" (NAEYC, 2010). NAEYC membership is available to individuals who "desire to serve and act on behalf of the needs and rights of all young children" (NAEYC, 2010). The Division for Early Childhood (DEC) of the Council for Exceptional Children is an international organization whose members include individuals who work with or on behalf of young children with disabilities and other special needs, birth through age 8, and their families. The mission statement indicates that "DEC promotes policies and evidence-based practices that support families and enhance the optimal development of young children who have or are at-risk for developmental delays and disabilities" (DEC, 2010).

Both NAEYC and DEC believe that early childhood education should be available to all children; children who are typically developing, children with special needs and/or who are at risk, and children with cultural and linguistic diversity. These two organizations frequently collaborate in advocacy and legislative efforts. They have developed several joint position statements and other publications, and often endorse publications and position statements developed by each organization.

Developmentally Appropriate Practice

NAEYC and DEC have developed two important documents that work together to guide the philosophy, values, and practices in ECSE. The first is Developmentally Appropriate Practice (DAP), written by NAEYC (Copple & Bredekamp, 2009). DAP provides a framework of principles and practices that promote learning and development for young children and that guide the development of early childhood programs and services. The goals of DAP are to teach in ways that "meet children where they are as individuals and as a group; and help each child reach challenging and achievable goals that contribute to his or her ongoing development and learning" (Copple & Bredekamp, 2006, p. 3). To meet these goals, DAP must be age appropriate, individually appropriate, and appropriate to children's social and cultural contexts.

Age appropriate refers to developing goals, providing experiences, and selecting teaching strategies based on knowledge of the scope and sequence of child development and likely interests of children across different ages. DAP preschool programs provide materials and activities that are of interest to 3- and 4-year-olds and that address skills that are typically attained during the preschool years. For example, children begin to develop early literacy skills such as rhyming, writing their name, and retelling a story during the preschool years. Therefore, it would not be developmentally appropriate to expect preschoolers to write an essay about a book they read. It would be developmentally appropriate, however, to ask children to talk about a field trip taken by the class or to provide materials that children can use to draw a picture about the field trip and write or scribble their name on their picture.

Individually appropriate practices are responsive to the unique needs of individual children with and without disabilities, regardless of their chronological age. There can be great variability across children in their interests and abilities, learning style, rate of learning, and amount of support needed to learn. Goals for learning and materials, activities, and experiences should address the range of interests and abilities of children in a program, and teaching strategies must provide the level and type of support needed to foster learning for individual children (Horn, Lieber, Sandall, Schwartz, & Wolery, 2002; Copple & Bredekamp, 2009). For example, while many of the 4-year-olds in a classroom enjoy playing together and sharing materials, a few children are not developmentally ready to share with their peers. Rather than forcing these children to share, the teacher provides each child with his or her own set of materials. She also plans activities that promote cooperation or turn-taking so that the children experience the joy of playing with peers. For instance, she introduces a board game, helps small groups of children make props for the class play, and praises children when they play together. Strategies and activities such as these will support children as they move from parallel (side by side) to cooperative play and sharing with peers (Chandler & Maude, 2009).

Culturally appropriate practices are responsive to the social and cultural contexts of the children in a program. Teachers learn about social, linguistic, and cultural contexts from children's families and by observing each child during daily activities and routines. They consider children's linguistic and cultural backgrounds and experiences as they develop activities and routines, select materials, and provide instructional and emotional supports (Copple & Bredekamp, 2006). For example, a teacher posts common words in Spanish in each center so that adults can use those words when interacting with a child who speaks Spanish.

DEC Recommended Practices

The Division for Early Childhood supports the use of DAP and believes that high-quality, developmentally appropriate environments and experiences are necessary for all children and should be the foundation of all early childhood programs. However, for some children, high-quality DAP environments and experiences may not be sufficient to meet their unique needs (Clawson & Luze, 2008; Horn et al., 2002). For these children, individualized strategies and varying levels and types of supports may be needed. DEC builds on the work of NAEYC and the DAP framework by providing a set of Recommended Practices for working with children with disabilities and children at risk (Sandall, Hemmeter, Smith, & McLean, 2005). The DEC Recommended Practices (DEC RPs) provide practitioners with guidelines and effective practices that can be used to meet the unique needs of children with disabilities and to support their families. DEC RPs are divided into five direct-service areas—Assessment, Child-Focused Practices, Family-Based Practices, Interdisciplinary Models, and Technology Applications—and two areas of indirect service—Policies, Procedures, and Systems Change and Personnel Preparation.

The DEC RPs are derived from research evidence regarding the effectiveness of specific practices, the experience or wisdom of practitioners and families regarding the effectiveness of strategies for which there is not yet sufficient research support, and core values regarding children and families. Some of these core values are (1) all children have the right to participate actively and meaningfully within their families and communities; (2) children have the right to participate in high-quality programs that provide individualized experiences to promote the development of each child; and (3) services and supports should be family-centered, recognizing the importance of the family in the child's life and the importance of family-professional relationships to achieving optional outcomes for children and their families. Examples of the DEC RPs will be presented later in this chapter.

There is general consensus between early childhood and early childhood special educators that DAP and DEC RPs are applicable to meeting the needs of all children within early childhood settings (Buysse & Hollingsworth, 2009; Odom & Wolery, 2003). Thus, the DAP guidelines and DEC RPs work together to support the needs of all young children, including those with developmental disabilities, children who are gifted, children at risk, and children who present social, cultural, and linguistic diversity. Both of these guidelines and practices, and a shared philosophy that values the right of all children to participate in experiences that maximize their learning and development, must be part of any program that serves preschool-aged children. This focus on meeting the needs of all children within their families and communities is congruent with the movement to provide supports and services in inclusive settings.

INCLUSION

In the past, children with disabilities were largely taught in segregated settings that served only children with disabilities. There were few opportunities for children with disabilities to participate in settings and activities with peers who are typically developing (Odom, 2000). In situations in which children did attend the same programs as their peers, they routinely were taken out of the classroom for varying amounts of time to receive special education services, or they were isolated from peers for large parts of the day to work on individual goals. Over time, practitioners, families, and researchers began to explore alternatives to segregated classrooms, calling for all children to have opportunities to participate in inclusive settings. Support for inclusion has increased in recent years, and today many children with disabilities participate in settings and activities together with peers who are typically developing, and they receive special education services in those inclusive settings (DEC/NAEYC, 2009). Although increasing numbers of children with disabilities have access to inclusive programs, full access to inclusive programs has not yet occurred (National Professional Development Center on Inclusion [NPDCI], 2007).

Inclusion is a core value that is supported by DEC and NAEYC. Both organizations believe that children with disabilities and special needs should have access to classrooms and programs that they would attend if they did not have a disability. Both organizations believe that all children should have access to the general education curricula, be included in meaningful experiences with same-age peers, and receive individualized supports to help them reach their full potential. Inclusion also is supported by IDEA legislation, which requires teams to consider inclusive settings when determining the LRE and to provide opportunities for children with disabilities to interact with peers who are typically developing if an inclusion setting is not selected. The effectiveness of inclusion has been confirmed by research documenting positive outcomes for children with and without disabilities, families, and practitioners who participate in high-quality inclusive programs (Guralnick, 2001; NPDCI, 2007; Odom, 2002; Odom, Schwartz, & ECRII Investigators, 2002).

DEC and NAEYC recently developed a joint position statement regarding early childhood inclusion (2009). The definition of inclusion from this position statement is presented in Box 2.1. The definition focuses on three features of inclusion: access, participation, and supports. *Access* refers to assuring that children and families have access to a range of learning environments and settings within their community; that they have opportunities to participate in daily activities, routines, and experiences; and that they have access to the general education curriculum. *Participation* refers to using individualized supports to help each child actively and meaningfully participate in the settings and activities to which they have access. The greatest benefits

---

Box 2.1   Definition of Inclusion

Early childhood inclusion embodies the values, policies, and practices that support the right of every infant and young child and his or her family, regardless of ability, to participate in a broad range of activities and contexts as full members of family, communities, and society. The desired results of inclusive experiences for children with and without disabilities and their families include a sense of belonging and membership, positive social relationships and friendships, and development and learning to reach their full potential. The defining features of inclusion that can be used to identify high-quality early childhood programs and services are access, participation, and supports (DEC/NAEYC, 2009, p. 2).

---

from inclusion occur when practitioners plan for and support participation; they promote a sense of belonging and membership, help children engage in positive interactions and develop friendships with peers, and foster the development of each child through individualized adaptations, accommodations, and supports (Chandler & Maude, 2009; Horn et al., 2002). Fiscal and administrative *supports* provide the foundation for inclusive programs that promote a shared vision and philosophy for inclusion and that provide resources and guidance to practitioners and families as they design, implement, and evaluate inclusive services.

Each of these features contributes to high-quality inclusive experiences for all children and families, as indicated in Figure 2.1, and they can be used for developing and identifying high-quality inclusive programs. Inclusive preschool programs may occur in a variety of settings (e.g., public school, community child care, and Head Start) and there can be considerable differences across programs based on resources, values, community standards, and personnel. There is no single model for developing an inclusion program or for delivering services within inclusive settings. The challenge for staff is to develop and maintain high-quality, developmentally appropriate programs that are individually appropriate and promote access and participation for all children. Fortunately, there are evidence-based strategies and practices within each of the defining features of inclusion to guide our efforts to develop high-quality inclusive programs.

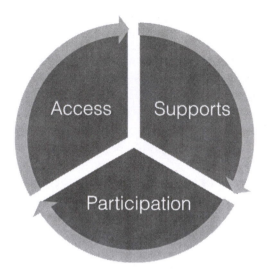

Figure 2.1   Defining features of high-quality inclusive programs.

Access

Children with disabilities and those who are at risk for developing disabilities or experiencing problems in school are more alike than they are different from their same-age peers. They generally are interested in and learn from the same types of experiences, activities, and materials as preschoolers who are typically developing and have the same or similar learning needs and goals (Strain, Bovey, Wilson, & Roybal, 2009). Therefore, one of the first steps in developing high-quality programs is to provide all children with access to the learning environment, including the physical setting; general education curricula, materials, activities, and routines; teacher-guided instruction and experiences; and interactions with peers and adults. One of the most effective strategies for providing access to all children is universal design.

Universal Design

Universal design is a proactive practice employed in the field of architecture that considers the needs of diverse individuals in the conceptualization, design, and construction of products and environments so that they are accessible to those who might use them. For example, buildings are designed to include wide hallways, ramps, and elevators to accommodate wheelchairs and building elevators, and rooms often include Braille next to printed words and numbers so that individuals with vision impairments or who are blind can identify their floors and rooms. These same considerations are used to design preschool environments so that they are accessible to all children, including those with vision impairments, who are deaf/hard of hearing, have motor disabilities, or a combination of these. A universally designed setting provides all children with access to materials and all indoor and outdoor areas (Center for Community Inclusion & Disability Studies, 2007; Orkwis, 2003).

The practice of universal design also can be applied to educational activities and adult-guided instruction to address the diverse needs of children who may attend the program (Kame'enui & Simmons, 1999). The Universal Design for Learning (UDL) is a proactive approach that promotes access to and participation in the general education curriculum by considering the diverse abilities and needs of all children when developing centers, selecting materials, planning activities and routines, establishing expectations and learning goals for children, and identifying teaching and assessment strategies (CEC, 2005). The UDL approach is the opposite of a "one-size-fits-all" approach to education. Rather, it is based on differentiation; consideration of the differences between children and adjusting the curriculum, goals, and teaching strategies to meet the unique needs of each child. Differentiation allows teachers to respond to the learning needs of increasingly diverse classrooms of children.

In a UDL program, the teacher's job is to provide multiple and diverse paths to learning by (1) providing a variety of carefully selected materials, activities, and experiences; (2) developing and supporting alternative ways of using materials and participating in activities and routines; and (3) using a variety of instructional strategies that are responsive to the range of abilities, interests, and needs of children in their classrooms (Orkwis, 2003). As stated in the DEC/NAEYC joint position statement on inclusion (2009), UDL procedures help provide every child with access to learning environments, the general education curriculum, daily activities, routines, and experiences that provide opportunities for child-guided and teacher-guided learning.

Participation

While providing children with access to inclusive settings and experiences is an essential first step in developing high-quality inclusive programs, access alone does not guarantee that children will benefit from inclusive settings and experiences. Many children will need specialized and individualized instructional strategies and supports to help them actively and meaningfully participate in the settings and experiences to which they have access (Buysse & Hollingsworth, 2009; Wolery, 2005). This requires educators to be intentional in planning and providing instructional strategies and supports for all children, especially those with unique needs and abilities. Intentional teaching and other evidence-based strategies work together to promote participation for all children. These strategies are described in the sections that follow.

Intentional Teaching

Intentional teaching is based on the understanding that both children and teachers actively contribute to children's learning (Copple & Bredekamp, 2006). Intentional teachers use their knowledge about the scope and sequence of skill acquisition during the preschool years to identify goals for learning, and they select classroom activities and teaching strategies that will enable children to achieve those goals (Notari-Syverson & Sadler, 2008). This is the essence of intentional teaching. Intentional teachers first identify what to teach. Then they plan when, where, and how they will teach and support learning. Finally, they design a system for monitoring children's progress in meeting goals and using progress-monitoring outcomes to make decisions during subsequent planning (Grisham-Brown et al., 2005).

This is not to say that all experiences need to be planned and guided by adults. Intentional teachers recognize that children learn much from child-initiated exploration and engagement with materials and peers (Epstein, 2007; Wolery, 2005). For example, children learn many social, play, and communication skills such as taking turns, holding conversations, problem solving and persistence, and pretend play through engagement in child-initiated activities and interactions with peers during those activities. However, children also learn much from teacher-initiated and guided activities in which teachers use specific instructional strategies and supports to promote engagement and learning. For example, children learn many early literacy skills such as naming letters of the alphabet, identifying the sounds letters make, and how to write their name through adult-guided instruction and support in developmentally appropriate activities. An intentional teacher determines which type of skills are best learned through teacher-initiated and guided instruction and which type of skills are best learned through child-initiated exploration with strategic adult support. Intentional teachers use a blend of child-initiated and teacher-initiated and guided activities, and they vary these based on the content or skills being addressed as well as the unique needs of individual children (Copple & Bredekamp, 2009; Epstein, 2007). An important part of intentional planning and teaching is developing children's sense of belonging and positive social relationships with peers and adults (Ostrosky, McCollum, & SeonYeong, 2007). These, too, require active planning. Simply placing children with and without special needs in the same setting does not guarantee that they will interact with each other, be successful in their interactions, or acquire a sense of belonging. Adults must demonstrate positive attitudes regarding all children in the program; arrange opportunities for children to interact with each other; and provide guidance and support to make those interactions positive, effective, and mutually rewarding (Guralnick, 2001). Many children may benefit from teacher-guided instruction to facilitate learning positive social-emotional skills that are necessary for developing and maintaining reciprocal, satisfying relationships with peers and adults (Fox, Carta, Strain, Dunlap, & Hemmeter, 2010).

Embedded Instruction

This strategy builds on intentional teaching by strategically embedding instruction and opportunities for children to acquire and practice functional and meaningful skills within daily activities and routines throughout the day (NPDCI, 2007; Odom & Wolery, 2003). Embedded instruction reflects the belief (and evidence from research) that children learn some skills best when they are taught and practiced during authentic activities or contexts in which the skills are useful and should naturally occur and that provide natural reinforcement or logical consequences for learning (Pretti-Frontczak & Bricker, 2004; Wolery, 2005). Natural reinforcement or logical consequences are those events that logically follow a behavior and affect the future occurrences of a behavior. Consequences that are desired will increase future occurrences, and consequences that are punishing will decrease future occurrences of behavior. For instance, the natural consequence for Ann when she asks a peer to share is receipt of the desired item. On the other hand, the natural punishing consequence for Ann when she takes a friend's toy without asking might be that the child hits her.

Embedding instruction provides children with multiple opportunities to practice skills during a variety of activities and routines, including circle time, centers activities, caretaking routines, snack or mealtime, outdoor play, and teacher-planned activities (Chandler et al., 2008; Grisham-Brown et al., 2009). For example, children can practice counting during dramatic play when they count the number of play dollars needed to buy a pizza, during a group activity in which they count how many cups of flour are needed to make brownies, and when they count the number of circles on the dice and the number of spaces their pawn gets to move in a board game. In another example, children in the Bunny classroom practice early writing (or scribbling) when they sign in and out of the classroom at the beginning and end of the day, put their name on art work, and write a grocery list while playing in the housekeeping center. Opportunities to practice skills in a variety of activities and over time will strengthen skill acquisition and mastery, and promote generalization of the skill to new activities and routines.

Teachers often plan embedded activities by examining the daily schedule to determine which activities and routines could provide authentic opportunities to apply knowledge and practice important skills and behaviors. They then plan specific strategies and instructional procedures to assure that children have opportunities to practice skills during selected activities and routines (Pretti-Frontczak & Bricker, 2004; Sandall, Giacomini, Smith, & Hemmeter, 2006). This can be done for a class of children as well as for individual children. For example, Jodi has an IEP goal to talk to her peers. Her teacher, Mr. Burke, decides that this skill could be practiced during arrival, snack, and science-center time. Mr. Burke helps Jodi say hello to peers and adults when she arrives in the morning. As snack helper, Jodi asks each friend if they want crackers or cereal and then gives each peer the requested item. Finally, Mr. Burke limits the number of magnifying glasses in the science center and then models sharing by asking another child to share with him, and he praises peers when they ask each other to share the magnifying glass. If Jodi does not imitate these models, Mr. Burke reminds her to ask a friend to share.

Embedding also facilitates the teacher's ability to address multiple goals for one child as well as different goals for several children during activities. For instance, when the teaching assistant (TA) is in the block center, she helps Jacob work on his goal of color identification by asking for a red block or a blue block. She poses strategic questions to Enrique to help him describe what he is building. The TA prompts Wendy to interact with peers by suggesting she ask Enrique for a block, and she prompts Wendy to share when peers ask for materials that she is using. The TA also models oral language by describing what she and they are building, and she expands on the children's words (e.g., Jacob says "blue" when asked what color block he wants, and the TA says "here is a big blue block").

A final defining feature of embedded or activity-based practices is the provision of specialized services within the classroom setting. Rather than removing a child from the classroom to address IEP goals or working individually with a child in a segregated area of the classroom, early childhood special educators, therapists, and other specialists now are more likely to address IEP goals within the classroom during meaningful and functional activities (Childress, 2004). For example, the speech and language pathologist sits at Rory's table during snack and provides multiple opportunities for Rory to practice pronouncing "s"-blends correctly (e.g., sn-ack, sp-oon, and sc-oop). She also joins Rory in the book center and helps Rory and other children in the center pronounce and describe new vocabulary words.

Evidence-Based Instructional Strategies and Supports

Educators promote participation in the general education curriculum and daily activities and routines, acquisition of individualized (e.g., IEP) and general goals, and the development of positive social relationships and a sense of belonging by using evidence-based, specialized instructional strategies and supports (Odom et al., 2002). These are selected and individualized for each child based on the child's characteristics and learning style, current skills, and unique needs and abilities. Several of these are described in Box 2.2 (Chandler & Dahlquist, 2009; Chandler & Maude, 2009; Milbourne & Campbell, 2007; NPDCI, 2007; Odom & Wolery, 2003; Wolery, 2005).

Response to Intervention

A relatively new practice for promoting participation and supporting learning and development is Response to Intervention (RtI) (Barnett, VanDerHeyden, & Witt, 2007; VanDerHeyden & Snyder, 2006). RtI is a proactive, preventative, collaborative, multitiered assessment and instructional approach for identifying and meeting the needs of all children (Coleman, Buysse, & Neitzel, 2006). RtI programs are designed to "catch" children as early as possible who are at risk or have delays in developmental domains, early academic skills, and

Box 2.2 Evidence-Based Instructional Strategies to Promote Learning and Development	
Instructional Strategy	**Definitions and Examples**
Accommodations and Modifications	Adjustments to and modification of the environment, activities and routines and tasks, materials, instructional strategies, and expectations and goals that maximize access and participation for each child. *Environment*: Ms. Carter rearranges furniture in the housekeeping area so that Serafina can move about the area with her wheelchair. *Activities, routines, and tasks*: Alec has a hard time paying attention and sitting through circle. So Ms. Nancy makes circle more active by adding movement opportunities and giving Alec frequent turns to participate. She also assures that he is one of the first children to move to activity centers to reduce waiting at the end of circle. *Materials*: Ms. Gingerich puts pictures of the steps to be followed in conducting the science experiment to the science center and she adds rubber grips to pencils so that children can better grasp the pencils as they record experiment results. *Instructional strategies*: Ms. Julia uses preteaching to help Les understand new vocabulary in a book that she will read to the whole class. She reads the book with Les the day before and sends the book home for Les's parents to read with her. *Expectations and goals*: Most children are expected to request objects using 3-5 word sentences (e.g., I want more red paint). The goal for Jared, whose primary language is Spanish, is to request in English by naming the object (e.g., paint).
Partial Participation	Adapting the degree to which a child participates in an activity or how a child participates in an activity. This strategy is *(Continued)*

based on the belief that children should not be excluded from an activity if they are not able to participate in the same way as other children. Rather, all children should be allowed to participate to some degree in all activities. For instance, Colleen, who has health problems, is not able to dance with her peers during the "stop and freeze when the music stops" activity. Rather than excluding Colleen from this activity, her teacher puts her in charge of starting and stopping the music.

Scaffolding

Providing the amount and type of assistance a child needs to acquire and practice a new skill or perform a task at a higher level. Scaffolding entails identifying what a child knows and is able to do, identifying the next skill the child should learn, and then providing support to help the child achieve the new skill or perform the skill at a higher level. Teachers provide the least amount and most helpful type of scaffolding that the child needs. As the child is able to do the skill independently, the teacher reduces the amount and type of scaffolding provided. Scaffolding includes *open-ended questions* to help a child make connections between events and problem-solve ("What is going to happen in this story? "How are we going to fix this?"); *expansions* of a child's utterances by adding new information; *feedback* that helps a child perform the skill correctly ("remember to ask your friend to play"); and *positive reinforcement* that provides a desired consequence following appropriate behavior and identifies appropriate skills or behavior ("That's great; you asked Al for help, and he helped you").

Prompts and Prompt Fading

Cues that provide assistance or information to support learning. Prompts can be provided before or during an activity. They

(Continued)

may be *verbal* ("ask your friend to open the door"), *visual* (the teacher points to the item she requests, Luke follows the sequence card that shows a picture of each step in hand washing), *modeled* (the teacher claps two times as she says Sasha's name and tells children that "Sasha" has two parts (Sasha), *physical* (the teacher uses hand-over-hand assistance to help Mariah hold the fishing pole). Prompts also can be *combined* as they are in social stories that are developed to address specific problems a child might be experiencing. They use pictures (visual) and words (vocal, written) to describe a challenging social situation and what a child can try to do in that situation (Gray, 2000). For example, Mr. Bolen developed a social story with Shawn that describes how Shawn feels when a peer has his favorite toy, suggests that he can try asking his friend for a turn, and then shows Shawn and his friend taking turns with the toy. The story also indicates that if his friend says no, Shawn can try waiting or find a different toy to use. Teachers provide only as much prompting as is necessary to help the child be successful. They then withdraw or fade prompts as the child is able to perform the skill independently. Mr. Bolen and Shawn initially read his social story daily. When Shawn was consistently asking friends for a turn and waiting for a turn, Mr. Bolen faded the frequency of reading the story to every other day, then weekly, and so forth until it was no longer needed.

Naturalistic Prompting Strategies

This includes a variety of strategies in which adults use specialized prompting strategies to help children acquire and practice communication skills in the natural environment. *Incidental teaching* involves arranging the environment so that a child is

(Continued)

likely to initiate, and then requesting an expanded or more sophisticated response. For example, the juice is visible during snack but out of reach of the child. Luke says "juice." The teacher says, "You want orange juice?" If Luke elaborates by saying "orange juice," the teacher gives him the juice. If he does not elaborate, the teacher prompts and then reinforces elaboration (e.g., "tell me orange juice"). The *Mand-Model strategy* often is used with children who do not initiate. The teacher asks the child a question or tells the child what to do and then waits for a response. If the child responds, the teacher provides reinforcement. If the child does not respond, the teacher models the skill and reinforces if the child responds to the model. For instance, the teacher sees Garret looking at the slide. She tells him to ask for help climbing the slide. If Garret asks for help, she helps him. If he does not ask for help, the teacher models, "I want help please." She helps Garret if he imitates her model. *Time delay* strategies begin with adults providing prompts until a child is able to perform a skill. After this, the adult waits for a specific amount of time before providing a prompt. For instance, the teacher prompts Hannah to request a ride on the swing. Once Hannah is able to do this, the teacher waits a few seconds before prompting Hannah to request a ride. As Hannah's requesting skills improve, the amount of time the teacher waits before prompting increases. Eventually, Hannah does not need a prompt to request rides on the swing.

Peer Mediation or Support

Peers provide support to help children participate in activities and routines. Peers may model skills or behavior and provide scaffolding and reinforcement. In some cases, peers are taught specific strategies

(Continued)

to support their friends. For instance, Alexis uses a wheelchair, has poor grasping abilities, holds her head upright for short periods of time, and uses pictures to communicate. Alexis's teacher taught several peers specific strategies for interacting with Alexis, including responding to her requests when she points to pictures, laying materials flat on her tray so she can see them, and helping her with fine motor tasks such as turning the pages of a book.

Assistive Technology and Specialized Equipment

This includes a variety of materials and equipment that increase, maintain, or improve the capabilities of a child with disabilities. Assistive technology (AT) can include simple, low-cost materials such as adaptive grips that make it easier for children to grasp objects such as crayons and spoons, and the Picture Exchange Communication System (PECS), in which children use pictures to communicate with other individuals. AT also can include high-cost equipment such as touch screens that allow access to computer programs without operating a mouse or keyboard.

Shaping

Reinforcing small steps or successive approximations of a skill or behavior. Teachers identify a child's current skill and abilities and then build on these to achieve a final goal. For example, Sheela is able to participate in circle for about three minutes before she becomes disruptive and is removed from circle. The teacher identifies staying in circle for four minutes as her first goal. She allows Sheela to leave circle after four minutes, before she is disruptive. When Sheela is able to participate in circle for four minutes, the teacher gradually increases her expectations to 5, 7, 10 minutes, and so forth until finally, Sheela participates throughout the entire circle.

(Continued)

Task Analysis	Dividing a task into small steps, teaching one step at a time, and providing assistance with the remaining steps that are not currently being taught. For example, Ms. Valor develops a task analysis of hand washing (e.g., turn on the water, wet hands, put soap on hands, rub hands, rinse hands in water, turn off water, grab towel, and dry hands). She first teaches Grady to turn on the water and then helps Grady complete the remaining steps in the task. When Grady is able to turn on the water independently, Ms. Valor next teaches Grady the next step in the task analysis. As Grady is able to perform each step, Ms. Valor adds a new step to the sequence. By the end, Grady is performing each step in the task.

social-emotional skills, and to intervene early by providing additional instructional supports and strategies to meet children's needs (Buysse & Hollingsworth, 2009).

Many programs using RtI employ two or more tiers of instruction in which the intensity of supports and services and the frequency of progress monitoring increases with each ensuing tier (Young, Shields, & Chandler, 2009). RtI begins with Tier 1, which addresses early childhood standards or outcomes for all children. Tier 1 includes practices that are fundamental to high-quality early childhood programs, such as accessible environments, evidence-based and developmentally appropriate curriculum, embedded experiences, intentional planning and teaching, scaffolding, and child goals linked to early learning standards and progress monitoring outcomes (Chandler et al., 2008). Tier 1 also includes universal screening and progress monitoring to identify individual children who are not making adequate progress and might benefit from more intensive and frequent instruction and support provided through subsequent tiers. Tiers 2 and 3 might include additional small-group instruction; additional practice on goals embedded within activities and routines; more teacher-initiated and guided instruction; modification of curriculum, materials, teaching methods, and goals; increased collaboration with and use of specialists; frequent progress monitoring; and collaborative problem-solving (VanDerHeyden & Snyder, 2006).

The RtI framework links goal identification, universal screening and progress monitoring assessment outcomes, and instruction through a collaborative problem-solving approach conducted by a team of practitioners and family members. Teams (1) examine child outcome data to determine progress; (2) analyze concerns for individual and small groups of children, develop individualized goals, and plan the type and intensity of instructional strategies and supports to be used in Tiers 2 and 3; (3) implement instructional strategies within tiers; and (4) examine child outcome data to determine child progress and next steps within the RtI program (Center for Response to Intervention in Early Childhood [CRTIEC], 2009).

Many preschool programs have implemented RtI models to address early language and literacy, early math skills, and social-emotional literacy. Currently, there is no single RtI model that has been adopted across programs in the United States. Many programs are developing RtI models (Buysse, Winton, & Zimmerman, 2007), some are adopting existing models such as Recognition and Response, and others are adapting models that have been implemented in elementary school programs (e.g., Illinois ASPIRE, 2010). It is up to individual programs to develop, adapt, or adopt an RtI model that best meets the needs of children, families, and staff and that makes best use of existing resources. Future guidance may come from the joint position statement on RtI that is being developed by DEC, NAEYC, and Head Start. An example of an RtI process for two children is included in Box 2.3.

Community-based and public school preschool programs should use the practices and strategies previously discussed to promote access to and meaningful participation in preschool settings for all children, including those with disabilities and who are at risk for developmental delays. However, the ability of staff to provide access and promote participation is largely dependent on the resources and support they receive from their administration and programs.

Support

Effective inclusion programs are built on a strong foundation of administrative infrastructure and program supports (DEC/NAEYC, 2009). Lieber and her colleagues (2002) identified several system-level supports that are critical to effective inclusion programs. These include (1) shared philosophy and vision regarding inclusion,

Box 2.3   The RtI Process at Happy Days Preschool

The Happy Days preschool has developed an RtI model to meet the needs of all children. For Tier 1, they provide a high-quality program using an evidence-based general education curriculum and activities designed to promote early language and literacy and early math skills and social-emotional development. After three months of participating in the Tier 1 curriculum, Reggie and Eric both were identified as not making adequate progress in early math skills because they scored below the 25% on the universal screening assessment. They were selected to receive Tier 2 instruction in addition to continuing to participate in Tier 1. The problem-solving team analyzed each child's strengths and needs and developed a Tier 2 plan that consisted of daily adult-guided small-group games that targeted early math skills and additional targeted opportunities to practice math skills were embedded throughout daily activities and routines. The boys' families also provided practice on early math skills during family activities and routines. The team collected weekly progress monitoring data during the math games and administered a general early math progress monitoring assessment every six weeks. They used information from weekly progress monitoring to make changes to Tier 2 interventions. For example, they added additional prompting strategies for Reggie during the math game and increased the number of embedded practice opportunities he received each day. At the end of the second six-week progress monitoring period, Eric had made great progress and the team decided that he no longer needed Tier 2 instruction. Reggie's progress was not as great as the team had hoped. As a result, they decided that Reggie would receive Tier 3 interventions. The team developed a Tier 3 plan that included teacher-guided instruction provided individually to Reggie on a daily basis. The team also modified goals for Reggie so that he was expected to learn a smaller number of early math skills. The team collected daily progress monitoring data and planned to administer the general progress monitoring assessment at the end of four weeks. At that point, the team would make decisions about next steps for Reggie. He might continue to receive Tier 3 intervention, return to Tier 2 instruction, return to Tier-1-only instruction, or be referred to determine eligibility for special education services.

(2) shared instructional approaches and strategies for teaching and supporting all children, (3) administrative support, (4) collaboration among team members, and (5) positive relationships with families.

Program Philosophy

A program-wide philosophy that celebrates inclusion is the core of a sound inclusive program. Shared philosophies, beliefs, and values regarding inclusion foster a sense of "ownership" across staff (DeStefano, Maude, Crews, & Mabry, 1992; Peterson, 1987). Program staff believe that all children and families belong and are welcomed members of the school and classroom, and that educating all children well is everyone's responsibility (DEC/NAEYC, 2009). A strong inclusion philosophy emphasizes that children with disabilities and who are at risk do not have to meet prerequisite developmental and educational skills and behavior before they are accepted into an inclusive program (Odom et al., 2002). Rather, programs and staff must be ready to teach all children based on the concept of social equity (Schwartz, Sandall, Odom, Horn, & Beckman, 2002). A program philosophy that supports inclusion also promotes similar beliefs regarding how children learn and the teacher's role in supporting learning for children with and without disabilities (Lieber et al., 2002). Staff hold similar beliefs about DAP and strategies to promote access and participation for all children as well as specialized knowledge to meet the needs of diverse children. A program philosophy also sets the stage for parent/family and staff relationships and family options for participation.

Administrative Support

Administrative support is the key to effective inclusion programs. Administrators provide leadership in establishing a program-wide philosophy and ensuring that the philosophy is reflected in all parts of the program, including the mission statement and action plan to support inclusion (Lieber et al., 2002; Odom et al., 2002). Administrators also are important to fostering positive attitudes and dispositions regarding diversity and inclusion. Administrator attitudes influence staff attitudes and acceptance of children with ability, linguistic, and cultural diversity. In turn, staff attitudes and acceptance influence the reactions of children and families.

Administrators are responsible for ensuring that staff are prepared to meet the needs of all children by providing or arranging for ongoing professional development followed with in-class coaching, mentoring, and/or consultation (Chandler & Maude, 2009; Odom, 2009). Administrators make sure that teams have sufficient time to engage in planning, collaboration, and evaluation (Horn & Jones, 2005). They also allocate fiscal and other resources and staffing patterns and assign children to classrooms based on the concept of natural proportions (Schwartz et al., 2002). Natural proportions suggest that the proportion of children with disabilities in the preschool classroom should match the proportion of individuals with disabilities in the general population. Finally, administrators develop and institutionalize evaluation systems to identify (1) the impact of the program on general child outcomes, (2) the impact of the program on individual children, (3) how well the curriculum and instructional strategies are implemented (fidelity), and (4) staff and family satisfaction (Hollingsworth, Able Boone, & Crais, 2009).

Collaboration

Many children with disabilities and children who are at risk for developmental delays are likely to receive services from a variety of staff including early childhood and early childhood special educators, bilingual educators, teaching assistants, and related services personnel. In some inclusive programs, classrooms may be co-taught by an early childhood educator and an early childhood special educator, with support provided by a number of teaching assistants. When this occurs, both teachers generally are responsible for working with all children, and both collaborate in planning the general education curriculum and individualized strategies for children.

More often than not, however, inclusive classrooms are staffed by an early childhood teacher and teaching assistants, and the special education teacher and related services personnel work as itinerant staff who provide services for a number of children across different programs, schools, and classrooms (Dinnebeil et al., 2006). During visits to a preschool setting, itinerant staff may work directly with one child or a small or large group of children, as well as provide consultation to early childhood classroom staff. When itinerant staff work directly with children, they typically do so for brief periods of time (e.g., Samantha receives speech therapy for 20 minutes, two times per week). If that were the only time that IEP or other individualized goals were addressed, it is unlikely that the dosage (40 minutes per week) would be sufficient to result in expected levels or rates of progress. One way to address this is for all team members to collaborate in developing plans for early childhood staff to employ specialized teaching strategies and to embed practice on IEP and other goals throughout daily activities and routines between itinerant visits (Childress, 2004; Dinnebeil et al., 2006; Lieber et al., 2002; McWilliam, 2005). This is consistent with the practice of embedding multiple opportunities to practice skills during meaningful and functional activities and routines throughout the day.

Collaboration in preschool programs should be reciprocal. Each member of the team, including family members, contributes to the development of child goals, instructional strategies, and evaluation of progress in meeting goals. Collaboration helps team members focus on the "whole child" and the use of skills within functional activities in the classroom setting rather than focusing only on their narrow area of expertise (e.g., motor skills, communication skills). Team members may share information, jointly plan lessons and adaptations for individual children, teach each other specific strategies, provide coaching and mentoring, and examine progress monitoring and assessment outcomes, engage in problem solving, and make decisions about goals and strategies (Chandler & Maude, 2009).

Collaboration is not always easy to do. The ability to function as an effective member on various teams is an essential skill for early childhood staff members. Team members must develop trusting relationships so they (1) are willing to share information with others about their area of expertise and teach others to implement specific strategies, (2) are flexible in adopting new roles and using new strategies, and (3) are able to give and receive feedback from one another. Collaboration also takes time, and as mentioned above, administrators must assure that teams have time to engage in team building and collaborative planning.

Collaboration with Families

The importance of collaborating with families and the development of positive relationships with families is supported by federal law (IDEA) and DEC and NAEYC. DEC promotes the use of a family-centered approach that recognizes that families are the constant in a child's life and that families and homes are the primary nurturing contexts for learning and development (Trivette & Dunst, 2005). Program staff should interact with families in ways that are respectful and responsive to cultural and linguistic diversity, socioeconomic and education backgrounds, and family beliefs, values, and priorities for their child and family.

Families and service providers should develop partnerships in which they work together to determine and achieve child and family goals. Families are important members of their child's team. They can provide valuable information about their child's strengths and needs, the family's priorities, and strategies that have been effective at home and in the community (Chandler & Dahlquist, 2009). In light of this, IDEA requires teams to consider parent concerns for their child when determining IEP goals, and it supports the parent's right to participate in making decisions about their child's program (Stowe & Turnbull, 2001). Families also have many opportunities to extend practice on goals from the preschool setting to home and community settings. This is supported by both IDEA and the DEC RPs. IDEA stipulates that families can request training to assist them in addressing their child's IEP goals, and the DEC RPs indicate that program staff should provide families with resources and supports that enable them to promote their child's development (Trivette & Dunst, 2005). The practice of embedding applies to teaching and providing practice on skills within home and community settings as well as classroom settings. Families and other team members can examine the activities and routines in which the family participates and embed practice on goals within those natural learning opportunities.

Family experiences with inclusion are more positive when (1) they are included as important members of the team and participate in making decisions about their child's program, (2) they receive information that is understandable (i.e., without jargon) and that helps them make informed decisions, (3) they feel that their child receives services that meet his or her needs, (4) they have options for participation versus expectations imposed by program staff, and (5) there is honest and ongoing communication between families and other team members (Beckman, Hanson, & Horn, 2002; Erwin, Soodak, Winton, & Turnbull, 2001).

Inclusion at the preschool level is successful to the extent that teachers and other practitioners, caregivers, and families are supported and have access to appropriate resources (Dinnebeil et al., 2006). When these supports are in effect, they lead to effective inclusive preschool programs. When they are not in effect, they may serve as barriers to providing access and promoting meaningful participation within inclusive programs (Chandler & Maude, 2009).

SUMMARY

Although inclusion is not available or provided for every preschooler with disabilities in the United States, the option to participate in inclusive programs to the extent that it is beneficial for the child and family is supported by federal and state laws and the DEC and NAEYC professional organizations. Research has documented that children with disabilities can and do benefit from participation in inclusive settings, as do children who are typically developing and children at risk (NPDCI, 2007; Odom, 2002). The outcomes for children with disabilities in early academic and developmental areas generally are equal to or exceed those obtained in self-contained settings, and some children make greater gains in communication, play, and social-emotional skills and appropriate behavior (Guralnick, 2001; Hollingsworth et al., 2009; Odom et al., 2002). As stated earlier, positive outcomes for children who participate in inclusive programs are not guaranteed. Optimal outcomes are most often associated with high-quality programs that provide systems-level supports to develop and sustain inclusion efforts and in which service providers actively plan for inclusion and employ the types of strategies and recommended and evidence-based practices that promote access and participation for children and families.

REFERENCES

Barnett, D. W., Epstein, D. J., Friedman, A. H., Stevenson Boyd, J., & Hustedt, J. T. (2008). *The state of preschool 2008: State preschool yearbook*. New Brunswick, NJ: Rutgers University, National Institute for Early Education.

Barnett, D. W., VanDerHeyden, A. M., & Witt, J. W. (2007). Achieving science-based practice through response to intervention: What it might look like in preschools. *Journal of Educational and Psychological Consultation, 17*, 31–54.

Beckman, P. J., Hanson, M. J., & Horn, E. (2002). Family perceptions of inclusion. In S. L. Odom (Ed.), *Widening the circle: Including children with disabilities in preschool programs* (pp. 98–108). New York: Teachers College Press.

Borman, G. D. (n.d.). *Compensatory education–United States*. Retrieved from http://education.stateuniversity.com/pages/1877/Compensatory-Education.html

Brovoda, E., Leong, D., Payner, D., & Seminov, D. (2000). *A framework for early literacy instruction: Aligning standards to developmental accomplishments and student behaviors* (Rev. ed.). Retrieved from http://www.mcrel.org/PDF/Literacy/4006CM_EL_Framework.pdf

Buysse, V., & Hollingsworth, H. L. (2009). Program quality and early childhood inclusion: Recommendations for professional development. *Topics in Early Childhood Special Education, 29*, 119–128.

Buysse, V., Winton, P., & Zimmerman, T. (Eds.). (2007). RtI goes to Pre-K: An early intervening system called recognition and response. *Early Developments, 11*, 6–10.

Campbell, F. A., Ramey, C. T., Pungello, E., Sparling, J., & Miller-Johnson, S. (2002). Early childhood education: Young adult outcomes from the Abecedarian Project. *Applied Developmental Science, 6*(1), 45–57.

Carr, E. G., Horner, R. H., Turnbull, A. P., Marquis, J. G., Magito-Mclaughlin, D., McAfee, M. L., et al. (1999). *Positive behavior support for people with developmental disabilities.* Washington, DC: American Association on Mental Retardation Monograph Series.

Carter, M., & Kemp, C. R. (1996). Strategies for task analysis in special education. *Educational Psychology*, 1469-5820, *16*(2), 155–170.

CAST. (2008). *Universal design for learning guidelines version 1.0.* Wakefield, MA. Retrieved from http://www.udlcenter.org/sites/udlcenter.org/files/UDL_Guidelines_v2%200-Organizer_0.pdf

Center for Community Inclusion & Disability Studies. (2007). *Growing ideas: Increase access: Universal design in early care and education.* Retrieved from http://www.ccids.umaine.edu/ec/growingideas/univdeslg.pdf

Center for Response to Intervention in Early Childhood. (2009). Tiered prevention model. Retrieved from http://www.crtiec.org/tiered_prevention_model

Chandler, L. K., & Dahlquist, C. M. (2009). *Functional assessment: Strategies to prevent and remediate challenging behavior in school settings* (3rd ed.). Columbus, OH: Merrill.

Chandler, L. K., & Maude, S. (2009). Teaching about inclusive settings and natural learning environments. In P. J. Winton, J. A. McCollum, & C. Catlett (Eds.), *Practical approaches to early childhood professional development: Evidence, strategies, and resources* (pp. 207–226). Washington, DC: Zero to Three.

Chandler, L., Miller Young, R., Nylander, D., Shields, L., Ash, J., Bauman, B., et al. (2008). Promoting early literacy skills within daily activities and routines in preschool classrooms. *Young Exceptional Children, 11*, 2–16.

Childress, D. (2004). Special instruction and natural environments: Best practices in early intervention. *Infants and Young Children, 17*(2), 162–170.

Clawson, C., & Luze, G. (2008). Individual experiences of children with and without disabilities in early childhood settings. *Topics in Early Childhood Special Education, 28*, 132–147.

Coleman, M. R., Buysse, V., & Neitzel, J. (2006). *Recognition and response: An early intervening system for young children at-risk for learning disabilities.* Chapel Hill: University of North Carolina, FPG Child Development Institute.

CONNECT: The Center to Mobilize Early Childhood Knowledge. (2009). *Policy advisory: The law on inclusive education.* Chapel Hill: University of North Carolina, FPG Child Development Institute.

Copple, C., & Bredekamp, S. (2006). *Basics of DAP: An introduction for teachers of children 3 to 6.* Washington, DC: National Association for the Education of Young Children.

Copple, C., & Bredekamp, S. (Eds.). (2009). *Developmentally appropriate practice in early childhood programs serving children from birth through age 8.* (3rd ed.). Washington, DC: National Association for the Education of Young Children.

Council for Exceptional Children. (2005). *Universal design for learning: A guide for teachers and education professionals.* Upper Saddle River, NJ: Merrill/Prentice Hall.

Council for Exceptional Children. (2006). *CEC's comparison of IDEA 2004 regulations to 1996 regulations*. Arlington, VA: CEC. Retrieved from http://www.dec -sped.org

Darragh, J. (2010). *Introduction to early childhood education: Equity and inclusion*. Upper Saddle River, NJ: Pearson Education.

DEC/NAEYC. (2009). *Early childhood inclusion: A joint position statement of the Division for Early Childhood (DEC) and the National Association for the Education of Young Children (NAEYC)*. Chapel Hill: University of North Carolina, FPG Child Development Institute.

DeStefano, L., Maude, S. P., Crews, S. H., & Mabry, L. (1992). Using qualitative evaluation methods to identify exemplary practices in early childhood education. *Early Education and Development, 3*(2), 173–187.

Dewey, J. (2004). *Democracy and education*. New York: Macmillan. (Original work published 1916).

Dinnebeil, L., McInerney, W., & Hale, L. (2006). Understanding the roles and responsibilities of itinerant early childhood special education teachers through Delphi research. *Topics in Early Childhood Special Education, 26*, 153–166.

Division for Early Childhood (DEC). (2010). *DEC Mission Statement*. Retrieved from http://www.dec-sped.org

Edwards, C. (2002). Three approaches from Europe: Waldorf, Montessori, and Reggio Emilia. *Early Childhood Research and Practice, 4*(1). Retrieved from http:// ecrp.uiuc.edu/v4n1/edwards.html

Epstein, A. S. (2007). *The intentional teacher: Choosing the best strategies for young children's learning*. Washington, DC: National Association for the Education of Young Children.

Erwin, E. J., Soodak, L. C., Winton, P. J., & Turnbull, A. (2001). "I wish it wouldn't all depend on me": Research on families and early childhood inclusion. In M. J. Guralnick (Ed.), *Early childhood inclusion: Focus on change*. (pp. 127–158). Baltimore: Paul H. Brookes.

Etscheidt, S. (2006). Least restrictive and natural environments for young children with disabilities: A legal analysis of issues. *Topics in Early Childhood Special Education, 24*, 167–178.

Fox, L., Carta, J., Strain, P. S., Dunlap, G., & Hemmeter, M. L. (2010). Response to Intervention and the Pyramid model. *Infants and Young Children, 23*(1), 3–13.

Gargiulo, R., & Kilgo, J. (2005). *Young children with special needs* (2nd ed.). Clifton Park, NY: Thompson/Delmar.

Gray, C. (2000). *The new social story book*. Arlington, TX: Future Horizons.

Grennon Brooks, J. (n.d.). Constructivism as a paradigm for teaching and learning. Retrieved from http://www.thirteen.org/edonline/concept2class/ constructivism/index.html

Grisham-Brown, J., Hemmeter, M. L., & Pretti-Frontczak, K. (2005). *Blended practices for teaching young children in inclusive settings*. Baltimore: Paul H. Brookes.

Grisham-Brown, J., Pretti-Frontczak, K., Hawkins, S. R., & Winchell, B. N. (2009). Addressing early learning standards for all children within blended preschool classrooms. *Topics in Early Childhood Special Education, 29*, 131–142.

Guralnick, M. J. (Ed.). (2001). A framework for change in early childhood inclusion. In M. J. Guralnick (Ed.), *Early childhood inclusion: Focus on change*. (pp. 3–35). Baltimore: Paul H. Brookes.

Head Start Bureau. (2003). *The Head Start path to positive child outcomes.* Retrieved from http://www.hsnrc.org/CDI/pdfs/hsoutcomespath28 ppREV.pdf

High Scope. (2005). *High Scope preschool study.* Retrieved from http://www.highscope.org/Content.asp?ContentId=219

Hollingsworth, H. L., Able Boone, H., & Crais, E. R. (2009). Individualized inclusion plans at work in early childhood classrooms. *Young Exceptional Children, 13,* 19–35.

Horn, E., & Jones, H. (2005). Collaboration and teaming in early intervention and early childhood special education. In E. Horn & H. Jones (Eds.), *Young Exceptional Children Monograph Series No. 6: Interdisciplinary teams* (pp. 11–20). Missoula, MT: Division for Early Childhood.

Horn, E., Lieber, J., Sandall, S. R., Schwartz, I. S., & Wolery, R. A. (2002). Classroom models of individualized instruction. In S. L. Odom (Ed.), *Widening the circle: Including children with disabilities in preschool programs* (pp. 46–60). New York: Teachers College Press.

Hull, K., Goldhaber, J., & Capone, A. (2002). *Opening doors: An introduction to inclusive early childhood education.* Boston: Houghton Mifflin.

Hustedt, J. T., Barnett, W. S., Jung, K., and Goetze, L. D. (2009). New Mexico Pre-K evaluation: Results from the initial four years of a new state preschool initiative. Retrieved from http://nieer.org/pdf/new-mexico-initial-4-years.pdf

IDEA: Individuals with Disabilities Education Improvement Act of 2004, Pub. L. No. 101-476, 20 U.S.C. §§ 1400 *et seq.*

IDEAdata. (2007). *Table 2-1:* Children ages 3 through 5 served under IDEA, Part B, by disability category, educational environment and state: Fall 2007. Retrieved from https://www.ideadata.org/arc_toc9.asp#Grants

Illinois ASPIRE (Alliance for School-based Problem-solving and Intervention Resources in Education). (2010). Retrieved from http://www.illinoisaspire.org

Kame'enui, E. J., & Simmons, D. C. (1999). *Toward successful inclusion of students with disabilities: The architecture of instruction: An overview of curricular adaptations.* Reston, VA: Council for Exceptional Children.

Lieber, J., Wolery, R. A., Horn, E., Tschantz, J., Beckman, P. J., & Hanson, M. J. (2002). Collaborative relationships among adults in inclusive preschool programs. In S. L. Odom (Ed.), *Widening the circle: Including children with disabilities in preschool programs* (pp. 81–97). New York: Teachers College Press.

Malaguzzi, L. (1996). *The hundred languages of children: Narrative of the possible.* Reggio Emilia, Italy: Reggio Children.

McCormick, K. M., Grisham-Brown, J., & Hallam, R. (2007). Embedding state standards and individualized instruction in young children's investigations. In E. Horn, C. Peterson, & L. Fox (Eds.), *Linking curriculum to child and family outcomes* (pp. 29–45). Missoula, MT: Division for Early Childhood.

McWilliam, R. (2005). Recommended practices: Interdisciplinary models. In S. Sandall, M. E. McLean, & B. J. Smith (Eds.), *DEC recommended practices in early intervention/early childhood special education* (pp. 127–146). Longmont, CO: Sopris West.

Milbourne, S. A., & Campbell, P. H. (2007). *CARA's Kit: Creating adaptations for routines and activities.* Philadelphia: Child and Family Studies Research Programs, Thomas Jefferson University.

NAEYC. (2009). *Developmentally appropriate practice in early childhood programs serving children from birth through age 8.* Retrieved from http://www.naeyc.org/files/naeyc/file/positions/position%20statement%20Web.pdf

NAEYC. (2010). About NAEYC. Retrieved from http://www.naeyc.org/content/about-naeyc

National Professional Development Center on Inclusion (NPDCI). (2007). *Research synthesis points on early childhood inclusion.* Chapel Hill: University of North Carolina, FPG Child Development Institute.

Notari-Syverson, A., & Sadler, F. (2008). Math is for everyone: Strategies for supporting early mathematical competencies in young children *Young Exceptional Children, 11,* 2–16.

Odom, S. L. (2000). Preschool inclusion: What we know and where we go from here. *Topics in Early Childhood Special Education, 20,* 20–27.

Odom, S. L. (2009). The tie that binds: Evidence-based practice, implementation, science, and outcomes for children. *Topics in Early Childhood Special Education, 29,* 53–61.

Odom, S. L. (Ed.). (2002). *Widening the circle: Including children with disabilities in preschool programs.* New York: Teachers College Press.

Odom, S. L., Schwartz, I. S., & ECRII Investigators. (2002). So what do we know from all this? Synthesis points of research on preschool inclusion. In S. L. Odom (Ed.), *Widening the circle: Including children with disabilities in preschool programs* (pp. 154–174). New York: Teachers College Press.

Odom, S. L., & Wolery, M. (2003). A unified theory of practice in early intervention/early childhood special education: Evidence-based practices. *Journal of Special Education, 373,* 164–173.

Orkwis, R. (2003). *Universally designed instruction.* ERIC Clearinghouse on Disabilities and Gifted Education. Arlington, VA: ERIC/OSEP Special Project. Retrieved from http://www.ericdigests.org/2003-5/universally.htm

Ostrosky, M., McCollum, J., & SeonYeong, Y. (2007). Linking curriculum to children's social outcomes: Helping families support children's peer relationships. In E. Horn, C. Peterson, & L. Fox (Eds.), *Linking curriculum to child and family outcomes* (pp. 29–45). Missoula, MT: Division for Early Childhood.

Parks, G. (2000). The High/Scope Perry Preschool project. *Juvenile Justice Bulletin.* Retrieved from http://www.ncjrs.gov/pdffiles1/ojjdp/181725.pdf

Partnership for America's Economic Success. (2010). *The costs of disinvestment: Why states can't afford to cut smart early childhood programs.* Issue brief #13. PEW Center on the States. Retrieved from http://www.pewtrusts.org/uploadedFiles/wwwpewtrustsorg/Reports/Partnership_for_Americas_Economic_Success/Cost_of_Disinvestment_brief_final.pdf?n=1454

Peterson, G. B. (2004). A day of great illumination: B. F. Skinner's discovery of shaping. *Journal of the Experimental Analysis of Behavior, 82,* 317–328. Retrieved fromhttp://www.pubmedcentral.nih.gov/articlerender.fcgi?tool=pmcentrez&artid=1285014

Peterson, N. L. (1987). *Early intervention for handicapped and at-risk children; An introduction to early childhood special education.* Denver, CO: Love.

Piaget, J. (1937/1954). *La construction du réel chez l'enfant/The construction of reality in the child.* New York: Basic Books.

Pretti-Frontczak, P., & Bricker, D. (2004). *An activity-based approach to early intervention* (3rd ed.). Baltimore: Paul H. Brookes.

Reynolds, T. (2008). Extended early childhood intervention and school achievement: Age 13 findings from the Chicago longitudinal study. Retrieved from http://ideas.repec.org/p/wop/wispod/1095-96.html

Sandall, S. R., Giacomini, J., Smith, B. J., & Hemmeter, M. L. (2006). *DEC Recommended Practices toolkit*. Missoula, MT: Division for Early Childhood.

Sandall, S. R., Hemmeter, M. L., Smith, B. J., & McLean, M. E. (2005). *DEC recommended practices: A comprehensive guide for practical application in early intervention/early childhood special education*. Longmont, CO: Sopris West.

Schwartz, I., Sandall, S. R., Odom, S. L., Horn, E., & Beckman, P. J. (2002). "I know it when I see it": In search of a common definition of inclusion. In S. L. Odom (Ed.), *Widening the circle: Including children with disabilities in preschool programs* (pp. 10–24). New York: Teachers College Press.

Snow, K. (2009). *People first language*. Retrieved from http://www.disabilityisnatural.com/images/PDF/pfl09.pdf

Stewart, R. M., Martella, R. C., Marchand-Martella, N. E., & Benner, G. J. (2005). Three-tier models of reading and behavior. *Journal of Early and Intensive Behavior Intervention, 2*(3), 115–124.

Stowe, M. J., & Turnbull, H. R. (2001). Legal considerations of inclusion for infants and toddlers and preschool-aged children. In M. J. Guralnick (Ed.), *Early childhood inclusion: Focus on change* (pp. 69–100). Baltimore: Paul H. Brookes.

Strain, P. S., Bovey, E. H., II, Wilson, K., & Roybal, R. (2009). LEAP preschool: Lessons learned over 28 years of inclusive services for young children with autism. In *Young Exceptional Children Monograph Series No. 11: Quality Inclusive services in a diverse society*. Missoula, MT: Division for Early Childhood.

Trivette, C. M., & Dunst, C. J. (2005). DEC recommended practices: Family-based practices. In S. Sandall, M. E. McLean, & B. J. Smith (Eds.), *DEC recommended practices in early intervention/early childhood special education* (pp. 107–126). Longmont, CO: Sopris West.

VanDerHeyden, A. M., & Snyder, P. (2006). Integrating frameworks from early childhood intervention and school psychology to accelerate growth for all young children. *School Psychology Review, 35*, 519–534.

Wolery, M. (2005). DEC recommended practices: Child-focused practices. In S. Sandall, M. E. McLean, & B. J. Smith (Eds.), *DEC recommended practices in early intervention/early childhood special education* (pp. 71–106). Longmont, CO: Sopris West.

Young, R., Shields, L., & Chandler, L. K. (2009). Questions and answers on response to intervention: The emerging early childhood (EC) RtI movement: Promoting early schooling successes for three-to-five-year-olds. Council of Administrators of Special Education (CASE) *Journal of Special Education Leadership, 51*(1), 5–7.

Chapter 3

Services for Children with Special Needs in Head Start and Early Head Start

Amanda C. Quesenberry and Patricia Morris Clark

"AND HOW ARE THE CHILDREN?"

The hallmark of a strong and stable society can be seen in how it treats its children. This is epitomized through a traditional Masai greeting acknowledging the high value that the seminomadic African tribe places on their children. Because the Masai understand the well-being of their society depends upon the health of their children, even the fiercest warriors without children ask the question, "And How Are the Children?" The traditional answer is, "All the children are well" (O'Neill, 1991). The future of every great society depends on fostering the safety, health, and welfare of its children.

Although the United States is arguably the most powerful nation in the world, do we prioritize the needs of our youngest to ensure their health, safety, education, and overall well-being? Some would argue that attempting to meet the needs of our children is too expensive and is the responsibility of parents, not those of society. Ultimately though, who pays the cost when we as a society do not invest in the needs of our young children?

Research has shown that over time, investments in early care and education programs, especially those that target the needs of children with multiple risk factors such as special needs, families from low-income settings, households with one parent, etc. do, indeed, pay off (Lynch, 2005). Long-term studies of early childhood education programs like the Chicago Child-Parent Center Project, the Perry Preschool Project, and the Prenatal/Early Infancy Project show that everyone benefits when we invest in early childhood programs. Specifically, these studies found that when children participate in high-quality early childhood programs, they have greater academic success in school, are less likely to need special education services, have lower rates of dropout, are more likely to graduate from high school, obtain postsecondary education, become employed, make higher wages, and take part in less criminal acts (Karoly et al., 1998; Lynch, 2005; Masse & Barnett, 2002; Reynolds, Temple, Robertson, & Mann, 2002). In fact, the calculated benefit-cost analysis for each child participating in the Perry Preschool Project alone has been estimated at 17.01 to 1 (Schweinhart, 2004). That means that for every dollar spent on a child in that program, there was a return of over $17.00 in benefits to society. Given the overwhelming evidence that high-quality early childhood experiences for young children at risk are sound investments, it is hard to believe that we are still struggling to find adequate funding for programs such as Head Start, an early childhood program that serves nearly one million children living in poverty every year.

Head Start, the nation's only large-scale, comprehensive preschool program, has proven to be worth the investment over the past four decades. Services provided in Head Start are much more than those in a regular preschool program, including educational, medical, dental, nutritional, mental health, and family support to children and families living at or below poverty level and children with special needs. The main goal of Head Start has always been to lessen the effects of poverty on children and families who are at risk of delays (Zigler & Muenchow, 1992). Since the project was launched in 1965, over 25 million children have benefited from Head Start's comprehensive services (Administration of Children and Families [ACF], 2008a).

In the landmark book, *From Neurons to Neighborhoods*, Shonkoff and Phillips (2000) suggest that the first months and years of a child's life are critical to their later development. Environmental influences greatly impact brain development, especially in the first three years of life. They also explain that a child's health, development, and overall well-being are closely linked to the well-being of their parents. When children and families are living under stressful and perhaps dangerous conditions, this impacts the well-being of parents and children. Despite efforts to curb poverty and negative environmental influences, young children remain the poorest members of society in America, with 25.8 percent living in poverty (Children's Defense Fund, 2008). Research has shown that growing up in poverty significantly increases the odds that children will be exposed to environments and other circumstances that could negatively impact their overall well-being and later outcomes and school success (Brooks-Gunn & Duncan, 1997; Shonkoff & Phillips, 2000). In *From Neurons to Neighborhoods*, Shonkoff and Phillips call us to action by stating that:

> Striking disparities in what children know and can do are evident well before they enter kindergarten. These differences are strongly associated with social and economic circumstances and are predictive of subsequent academic performance. Redressing these disparities is critical, whose goals demand that children be prepared to begin school, achieve academic success, and ultimately sustain economic independence and engage constructively with others as adult citizens. (p. 5)

Fortunately, we know that there are programs that are successful in intervening to make a difference in the lives of children and families who face multiple risk factors. The most successful programs, however, are comprehensive and expensive (Shonkoff & Phillips, 2002).

Early childhood research has markedly increased over the past 40 years, especially in the areas of school readiness and quality early childhood programs. Long-term follow-up studies from other compensatory programs, including the HighScope Perry Preschool Project, Chicago Parent-Child Centers, and the Abecedarian Project, have provided documentation for the importance of high-quality early experiences in homes and classrooms. All three model programs involved children from low-income households who were primarily or entirely African American. They all had a parent education component and involved highly trained staff (Barnett, 2007). In an analysis of 10 major studies of preschool, Wat (2007) found that high-quality preschool sets the course for a lifetime of positive outcomes for children as well as families and entire communities. He also discovered that the teachers in these studies had bachelor's degrees or above and training in early childhood education, human development, or a related field.

According to a study conducted in 2003 by the National Institute for Early Education Research (NIEER), children attending high-quality preschools scored at least 31 percent higher in vocabulary assessments than their peers who did not attend preschool. Researchers have found that vocabulary scores have a high correlation with cognitive abilities and later success in reading (Barnett, Lamy, & Jung, 2005). Other studies have shown a higher graduation rate, by as much as 29 percent, for students who participated in high-quality preschool programs. Gilliam and Zigler (2004) found a 44 percent reduction in grade retentions and vast improvements in standardized test scores in reading and math for children attending high-quality preschool programs.

Head Start is the oldest federal preschool and is the last remaining project from President Johnson's War on Poverty launched in the mid-1960s. One reason for the program's success is its concentration on the family and individual needs of the parents. Besides assisting parents to go back to school, get a job, or learn new skills, Head Start has encouraged families to participate fully in their child's educational program (Zigler & Muenchow, 1992). Parents are encouraged not only to volunteer in their children's classrooms, but also to assist in operating the program (Reight-Parker, 2007).

In addition to parental involvement as a critical component of Head Start, community involvement and collaboration are also critical to the success of the Head Start model. One of the programs' greatest strengths and weaknesses lie in the flexibility in guidelines that allow each individual program to develop program delivery options and educational strategies based on the needs of the community (Zigler & Muenchow, 1992). The strength resides in the local program's ability to evolve over time, often changing the programmatic options available to meet the changing needs of the children and families in a service area. On the other hand, local flexibility can be perceived as a weakness because some feel that there is a lack of oversight at the state level.

Head Start began as an eight-week summer program for 3- to 5-year-olds who were primarily served in public school buildings and were typically operated by community action agencies or other local community organizations (Zigler & Muenchow, 1992). As more programs converted to the nine-month and half-day option, the need for space outside of public schools and more comprehensive curricula increased. Throughout the years, Head Start programs have continued to evolve to meet the needs of the children and families that they serve. Recently, additional funding and other considerations have been at the forefront as programs meet the needs of working parents and convert from part-day, part-year to full-day, full-year options. To be clear, major programmatic modifications cannot be made without approval; if a program decides it would like to modify their service delivery model, they must prove that the change would fulfill a substantial need in their community. Other branches of Head Start, including Early Head Start, Migrant and Seasonal, and American Indian Alaskan Native programs, also must follow these guidelines when making programmatic revisions. Of utmost importance is ensuring that the programmatic options that are available are meeting the needs of those within the community or service area.

This chapter will provide information related to services provided to children with special needs in Head Start and Early Head Start. The first portion of the chapter provides a historical view of Head Start and services for children with special needs from the 1960s through the present. The next section describes services provided for children with special needs in Head Start and Early Head Start. The following section will review research that has been done in Head Start and Early Head Start programs. Finally, the chapter ends with a discussion of future directions for Head Start and the field.

HISTORICAL PERSPECTIVES

The War on Poverty

The modern roots of early childhood intervention were born in the 1960s in an era of optimism, creativity, and broad public support for social services (Meisels & Shonkoff, 2000). Three important social issues coalesced under two presidents that would lay the foundation for early childhood education and intervention for the next 40 years. The three issues included: President John Kennedy's desire to prevent mental retardation, President Lyndon Johnson's quest to wipe out poverty, and a movement in the country to promote civil rights (Meisels & Shonkoff, 2000).

Given Kennedy's personal family history with mental retardation, this was an issue close to his heart. In 1961, Kennedy formed a commission to study issues surrounding mental retardation, including prevention and research, and in 1963, P.L. 88-156 was passed to provide funding through Title V of the Social Security Act for special projects for children with mental retardation. As a former teacher in a one-room schoolhouse in rural Texas, President Lyndon Johnson saw first-hand the effects of poverty and illness on children's learning. President Johnson shared views with the director of the Office of Economic Opportunity, Sargent Shriver. In 1964, the Economic Opportunity Act (EOA) of 1964 was passed by Congress and a year later, Head Start was born.

Project Head Start emerged in an era when many Americans believed poverty could be eliminated or, at least, the effects could be mediated with education (Meisels & Shonkoff, 2000). As a part of the

War on Poverty, President Johnson convened a panel of 14 early childhood and medical experts to create a comprehensive early childhood program, later to be known as Project Head Start, to combat impoverishment and the ensuing problems associated with it. It was thought that the circle of generational poverty contributed to mental retardation, and that by intervening with education and environmental changes, the cycle could be broken (Zigler & Valentine, 1979). The panel knew that children from low-income households can face immense barriers to success in school and later in life. All of these factors can put children behind before they can even begin school (Lybolt, Armstrong, Techmanski, & Gottfred, 2007). As one of the first compensatory programs in the 1960s, Head Start played a leading role in early childhood special education from the beginning without using the term "special education" (Garguilo & Kilgo, 2000). The compensatory education programs were created to offset the debilitating forces of poverty and "cultural deprivation" (Gearhart, Mullen, & Gearhart, 1993).

In its inception in 1965, Project Head Start was an eight-week summer pilot program directed toward the nation's poorest preschoolers. That summer, it served approximately 550,000 4- and 5-year-olds throughout the country (Garguilo & Kilgo, 2000). Teachers and other leaders quickly saw that eight weeks in the summer was not enough time to provide the "head start" they were hoping the children would get before entering kindergarten. Therefore, despite questions about whether or not there was enough funding or support to do so, Head Start changed to a nine-month program in most areas.

Head Start was designed to be a multifaceted program, offering children education, two meals a day, and psychological, social, medical, and dental care. Parents were encouraged to volunteer, create goals, learn about their children's development and nutrition, and continue their education or obtain a job. Families were referred to social services and resources as needed (Zigler & Muenchow, 1992). Although one of the founding principles for Head Start was to prevent mental retardation and raise IQ scores, in the early days of Head Start, no special efforts were made to serve children with special needs.

Throughout the remainder of the 1960s, Head Start rode a roller coaster of waxing and waning support. Two controversial and unique facets of Project Head Start were funding and administration. Unlike many other federal programs, Head Start was designed to be overseen by organizations in a community, many times a community action agency. By doing this, money was given directly to the local groups who were running the programs, bypassing the usual route through state government. Head Start administration also included parents and community members rather than state and local government or educational officials. Therefore, much of the power and funding in Head Start was given to minority groups. The Head Start funding and administrative structure remains controversial to this day (Zigler & Styfco, 2004).

Federal Support for Children with Special Needs

Although serving children with special needs was not a part of the original Head Start program design, President Johnson nevertheless encouraged Head Start programs to begin serving children with special needs. Then, in 1968, P.L. 90-538, the Handicapped Children's Early Education Assistance Act, was passed. This act provided funding for university education programs as well as early education experimental programs serving children with disabilities from birth through age 5 (Garguilo & Kilgo, 2000). Pilot and demonstration projects soon began to appear across the nation, which, in turn, produced home visitors to work with young children with special needs (Meisels & Shonkoff, 2000). Many Head Start sites offered training programs in home visiting, parent support, and quality early childhood education for children in underprivileged areas (Martin, 1989). These programs helped to meet the increasing demands for teachers who specialized in early childhood special education.

Then in 1972, P.L. 92-424, the Economic Opportunity Amendments (EOA), were passed, requiring all Head Start programs to serve children with identified special needs. This law laid the groundwork for other laws providing services to students with special needs (Zigler & Muenchow, 1992). Around the same time, Head Start began providing home visits to children in rural areas and in areas without public transportation through a program called Home Start (Garguilo & Kilgo, 2005). Similar to Head Start, this program focused on providing comprehensive services for families from low-income backgrounds and preschool children in the home setting.

The educational system in the United States would be forever changed with the passage of P.L. 94-142, the Education for All Handicapped Children Act, in 1975. This law required states to provide a free and appropriate public education (FAPE) for students over 6 years of age (Wright & Wright, 2003). Although states were not required to serve children under the age of 6, financial incentives were given to states to serve children from ages 3 to 5. At that time, little support was given to research or provide services for children under the age of 3.

Surviving Through Slashing of Social Service

The 1980s were dark years for federally funded children's programs. President Reagan campaigned on and carried through with promises to reduce the number of social services paid by the federal government. Basically, he believed that the state and local governments, rather than the federal government, should be providing direct services to citizens (Ginsberg & Miller-Cribbs, 2005). As a result, federal funding for many social service programs were cut drastically, or the programs were totally dismantled. Somehow, despite massive cuts to other federal programs, Head Start found its way into the Reagan administration's "safety net" of programs that continued to receive federal funds throughout his time in office.

In 1986, the Education for All Handicapped Children Act was amended to include more comprehensive and coordinated effort at the state level for children under the age of 3 and their families. Although this statute was not fully implemented until the early 1990s, it did provide further incentives to states to serve children ages 3 through 5 and established a foundation for services to be provided to children under the age of 3. Some argue that many of the provisions in P.L. 99-457 resulted from Head Start's success in serving young children with special needs (Zigler & Muenchow, 1992).

Public Support versus Individual Responsibility

The 1990s were the "glory days" for Head Start and early intervention. In 1990, when President George H. W. Bush entered office, he pledged full funding for Head Start, and soon after, the program received a budget increase of $2.4 billion. Throughout the decade, Head Start enjoyed bipartisan support. By 2000, funding levels had more than doubled, and the program was serving almost twice as many children. Part of the growth in funding and numbers came from the creation of Early Head Start.

Since the early days of Head Start in the 1960s, there were conversations about Head Start serving children under the age of 3. In the 1970s, Migrant Head Start programs began serving children under age 3, but the concept did not come to fruition until the 1990s (Lombardi & Bogle, 2004). On May 18, 1994, the Head Start Reauthorization Bill was signed, which included a "set-aside of Head Start funds to provide family-centered services for low-income families with very young children and for pregnant women" (Lombardi & Bogle, 2004, p. xiv). Over the summer of 1994, an Advisory Committee met a number of times to carefully plan the development and implementation of what became known as Early Head Start. Early Head Start espoused all of the founding principles of Head Start with a special focus on family involvement. In 1995, 68 Early Head Start programs were funded, with an appropriation of $106 million. Additional programs continued to be funded through the mid-2000s, with 741 programs in existence as of 2009.

The 1990s also brought welfare reform. In 1996, the Personal Responsibility and Work Opportunity Act was passed, which dramatically changed our nation's welfare system. This act eliminated the entitlement of federal aid to impoverished children and families, converting the system to a welfare-to-work format. Aid to Families with Dependent Children (AFDC) was changed to Temporary Assistance to Needy Families (TANF), offering a time-limited assistance to families for two years as parents found training and work.

Although this was meant to act as an incentive to some, it served as a hardship to parents with children with disabilities who were unable to find and pay for care for their children, especially after benefits ran out. Those who were impacted most were parents who had special needs themselves and their children who often had or were at risk for developmental delays. Children with disabilities and children at risk developmentally were affected the most as well as parents who had disabilities. Ohlson (1998) explained that the new system imposed harsh sanctions on families from low socioeconomic status who were already stressed by their situations. Besides reductions in funding for Social Security, Income Insurance, and redefined eligibility for Medicaid, funding was eliminated covering child care for parents participating in welfare-to-work or for those who were transitioning from welfare to school programs or to employment. Welfare reform also meant that thousands of parents who had been staying at home with their children were now required to go to work or school. For many families, child care became a patchwork of options that did not always include high-quality programs.

Even though some families were struggling to find high-quality child care options, early intervention received a major boost with the 1997 reauthorization of the Individuals with Disabilities Education Act (IDEA). For the first time ever, states were required to develop comprehensive and coordinated services for infants and toddlers with developmental delays. The act also mandated states to provide free and appropriate services to children ages 3 to 5 in the least restrictive environment. States were granted considerable freedom in program design and implementation, which led to a myriad of service delivery systems across the 50 states and territories.

Increased Accountability

We are nearing the end of another interesting decade in providing services to children at risk. The new millennium began with massive reforms to the American education system through the No Child Left Behind Act of 2001. No Child Left Behind impacted every level of education, including early childhood. In April 2002, President George W. Bush formally announced his plans regarding the early childhood programs in No Child Left Behind in a program called Good Start, Grow Smart (GSGS). GSGS outlines three major goals for early childhood programs: (1) strengthening Head Start, (2) partnering with states to improve early childhood education, and (3) providing information to teachers, caregivers, and parents (Department of Health and Human Services [DHHS] & Department of Education [DOE], 2006). As a result of GSGS, states were required to develop early learning standards for educating young children in the areas of language, literacy, and mathematics (National Association for the Education of Young Children [NAEYC], 2009). These standards were intended to provide a framework of indicators by which programs could judge the quality of the curriculum in their program, with the ultimate goal of implementing evidence-based practices to narrow achievement gaps often found among young preschool children (DHHS & DOE, 2006).

A significant focus of GSGS was to "strengthen Head Start." In the spring of 2003, the Head Start Act came up for reauthorization by Congress. For the next four years, Head Start programs stood in limbo as the House and Senate debated details of the Head Start Act. Finally, on December 12, 2007, President Bush signed P.L. 110-134, the Improving Head Start for School Readiness Act. This legislation ended the long and bitter debate over where Head Start would reside and if programs would continue testing all Head Start children with the National Reporting System. Head Start would remain a part of the Department of Health and Human Services, not in the Department of Education, and the act mandated that programs no longer administer or use data from the National Reporting System. Although the Head

Start Act of 2007 provides a number of new mandates for programs, just 14 days after signing it into law, President Bush signed an appropriations bill that significantly cut funding for Head Start rather than providing increases needed so programs could meet new requirements (Parrott, 2008).

Just as early care and education programs were feeling the major crunch of the economic downturn, in February 2009, President Obama signed P.L. 111-5 into law, the American Recovery and Reinvestment Act (ARRA). This bill included in the ARRA was a funding increase of $2.1 billion for Head Start, $1.1 billion of which is for Early Head Start expansion and $1 billion of which is to be allocated in accordance with the Head Start Act. In addition, as part of the FY 2009 appropriations process, Congress provided a $234.8 million funding increase for Head Start, of which up to 10 percent of awards was available for training and technical assistance for Early Head Start grants (Office of Head Start, 2009). In addition, over $2 billion was allotted to states through the Child Care Development Block Grants (CCDBG) to provide funding to improve quality in child care programs (National Association of Child Care Resource and Referral Agencies [NACCRRA], 2009). Early childhood special education programs gained nearly $1 billion, with Part B (Section 619) for preschool children receiving $400 million and Part C for infants and toddlers in early intervention receiving $500 million over two years (Samuels, 2009).

Many uncertainties lay ahead on the horizon for early childhood programs. Although record funding increases were born with the economic stimulus package, many states still face major budget challenges, which could cause cuts to early care and education programs. Debates on the reauthorization of IDEA and No Child Left Behind are sure to continue in the near future.

Advancements in the area of brain research with infants and young children offer even greater knowledge about the critical importance of early intervention for children with special needs or who are at risk, and preschool education to children's later cognitive, social, emotional, and physical development (Bowman, Donovan, & Burns, 2001; Shonkoff & Phillips, 2000; Whitehurst & Lonigan, 2001). This research, along with a rising number of children being cared for outside of the home, has placed early childhood education at the center of public and policy deliberations. This is especially true in regard to Head Start and public pre-K (Neuman, Copple, & Bredekamp, 2000; Pianta, Cox, & Snow, 2007; Scott-Little, Kagan, & Frelow, 2006;

Strickland & Riley-Ayers, 2007). As we discuss in the next section of this chapter, Head Start has long been a leader in the field for providing services to young children with special needs and for children who are at risk.

WHAT DO WE KNOW ABOUT SERVICES FOR CHILDREN WITH SPECIAL NEEDS IN HEAD START AND EARLY HEAD START?

Overview

Head Start was the first large-scale program to actively recruit, enroll, and serve young children with special needs (Zigler & Muenchow, 1992). Prior to 1972, most Head Start programs were not including children with special needs because there were no mandates or supports to do so. However, in 1972 with the passage of Public Law 92-424, the Economic Opportunity Amendments, all Head Start programs were required to reserve at least 10 percent of enrollment opportunities for children with special needs (Meisels & Shonkoff, 2000). At that time in our nation's history, very few programs were serving children with special needs in inclusive settings, and certainly none were including children on such a large scale (Zigler & Muenchow, 1992). Suddenly, a program that might be serving 379,000 children was now required to recruit and enroll 37,900 children with diagnosed special needs (ACF, 2008a). Local programs undertook this challenge, and by 1977, 13 percent of children enrolled in Head Start were children with diagnosed special needs (Health, Education, & Welfare [HEW] Report, 1978).

Because serving children with special needs in inclusive settings, such as Head Start classrooms, was a new concept, 14 Resource Access Projects (RAPs) were funded in 1976 by Head Start and the Office of Education's Bureau of Education for the Handicapped to support local programs in their efforts to serve young children with special needs (Zigler & Muenchow, 1992). These RAP programs were housed in universities and colleges across the country to provide training and technical assistance to teachers in Head Start programs. The staff at the RAP programs worked with professional organizations like the Division for Early Childhood (DEC) of the Council for Exceptional Children (CEC) to develop training manuals for Head Start teachers to support children with special needs enrolled in the program and their families (Meisels & Shonkoff, 2000; Zigler & Muenchow, 1992). Although RAP programs no longer exist, programs still work closely with regional training and technical assistance providers to ensure high-quality services are provided to children with special needs and their families.

Over time, Head Start has continued to provide inclusive services for young children with special needs. In 1995, Head Start expanded to begin providing services for infants, toddlers, and pregnant women through Early Head Start. Both Head Start and Early Head Start programs are also obligated to follow other federal laws of nondiscrimination, including the Americans with Disabilities Act (ADA) and the Individuals with Disabilities Education Act (IDEA). The Head Start Act (2007) requires that, beginning October 1, 2008, "not less than 10% of the total number of children actually enrolled by each Head Start agency and each delegate agency will be children with disabilities who are determined to be eligible for special education and related services, or early intervention services . . . by the state or local agency providing services under section 619 or part C of the Individuals with Disabilities Education Act [IDEA]" (p. 19).

All Head Start and Early Head Start programs are required to have a written Disabilities Service Plan that outlines how services are provided for children with special needs and their families (ACF, 1993). The purpose of this plan is to ensure "that all components of Head Start are appropriately involved in the integration of children with disabilities and their parents and that resources are used efficiently" (ACF, 1993, p. 257). Each Head Start and Early Head Start program must have a disabilities coordinator to make sure that the plan is updated annually and addresses all of the essential components of the plan, including (1) community involvement, (2) recruitment and enrollment of children with special needs, (3) the referral process, (4) identification and evaluation of children with suspected special needs, (5) planning and implementing services for children with special needs, and (6) transition of children from Head Start or Early Head Start into their next placement (OHS, 2008). Throughout the following sections, each of these areas will be discussed in further detail, citing examples of how Head Start and Early Head Start programs recruit, enroll, and serve children with special needs.

Community Involvement and Interagency Agreements

Oftentimes, services for children with special needs in early childhood programs can be disconnected and disorganized (Shonkoff & Phillips, 2000). For that reason, Head Start and Early Head Start programs are required to collaborate with local schools and organizations to provide appropriate services for children with special needs. Head Start programs must develop written interagency agreements with local education agencies (LEAs), and likewise, Early Head Start programs must partner with programs that provide early intervention (EI) services. LEAs and EI programs are ultimately responsible under IDEA to serve children with special needs in a given service area; however, Head Start and Early Head Start programs are required to partner with these programs to ensure that quality, seamless services are provided to the children enrolled in both programs in a timely manner.

Written interagency agreements between Head Start/Early Head Start programs and LEA/EI programs must include, but are not limited to:

> dates and times that are specific to (a) joint training of staff and parents, (b) procedures for referral for evaluations, (c) planning and implementation of Individualized Family Service Plans (IFSP) for children ages birth to three and Individualized Education Programs (IEP) for children three and over, (d) transition planning, (e) sharing resources, (f) Head Start's participation in Child Find efforts, and any other items agreed to by both parties. (OHS, 2008, p. 13)

Ultimately, the goal of all community partnerships in Head Start and Early Head Start programs is to guarantee that all agencies in a community or service area are working together to provide the highest level of comprehensive, developmentally and culturally appropriate services possible for the children and families who reside in a given area (ACF, 2008b).

Recruitment and Enrollment of Children with Special Needs

Because of the Head Start Act's requirements regarding the percentage of children with disabilities enrolled in Head Start and Early Head Start, programs must continuously and actively recruit children with special needs. Each program must have a recruitment plan that spells out efforts to recruit and enroll children with special needs, including children with significant special needs. When recruiting and enrolling children with special needs, a Head Start program

> must not deny placement on the basis of a disability or its severity to any child when: (a) the parents wish to enroll the child, (b) the child meets the Head Start age and income

eligibility criteria, (c) Head Start is an appropriate placement according to the child's IEP, and (d) the program has space to enroll more children, even though the program has made ten percent of its enrollment opportunities available to children with disabilities. (ACF, 1993, p. 275)

Screening, Referral, and Evaluation

One way to enroll children with special needs in the program is to recruit children with identified special needs. However, because Head Start and/or Early Head Start may be the first program-based care a child receives, some children are identified with special needs after they are enrolled in the program. Within the first 45 days of entry into a Head Start or Early Head Start program, each child must take part in a series of developmental screenings to detect any concerns that may warrant further evaluations to determine if a child has a special need. The written interagency agreement between each program and the LEA or EI program should outline processes for timely evaluations that meet mandates described in IDEA.

Planning and Implementing Services for Children with Special Needs

Once a child is determined to have a special need, or if a child is enrolled in the program with a diagnosed special need, it is the responsibility of the Head Start or Early Head Start program to ensure that each child is "included in the full range of services normally provided to all children and provisions for any modifications necessary to meet special needs of the children with disabilities" are made (ACF, 1993, p. 259). A number of models for providing services to children with special needs in Head Start and Early Head Start have been used to ensure that comprehensive, individualized services are provided to all children. Ideally, children with special needs who are enrolled in Head Start or Early Head Start would receive specialized services, such as occupational, physical, or speech therapy, during daily routines and activities. In some cases, a child may spend a part of their day in the Head Start or Early Head Start program and another portion in a different program that provides specialized services.

When including children with special needs, early childhood programs must take into consideration the individual needs of each child and family as well as local, state, and national guidelines for developmentally and culturally appropriate practices. National organizations such as the Division for Early Childhood (DEC) of the Council for Exceptional Children (CEC) and the National Association for the Education of Young Children (NAEYC) have guidelines for supporting children with special needs in inclusive settings. In 2009, DEC and NAEYC released a joint statement, including the following definition of early childhood inclusion:

> Early childhood inclusion embodies the values, policies, and practices that support the right of every infant and young child and his or her family, regardless of ability, to participate in a broad range of activities and contexts as full members of families, communities, and society. The desired results of inclusive experiences for children with and without disabilities and their families include a sense of belonging and membership, positive social relationships and friendships, and development and learning to reach their full potential. The defining features of inclusion that can be used to identify high-quality early childhood programs and services are access, participation, and supports. (Division for Early Childhood [DEC]/NAEYC, 2009)

This definition reflects the importance of collaborative and coordinated supports to promote inclusion in early childhood settings. A key aspect of services for all children in Head Start, including those with special needs, is individualized services. Individualization refers to "tailoring an approach that best engages and supports each child's and family's Head Start experience" (OHS, 2008, p. 29). When individualizing for children with special needs, Head Start staff should be part of the team that develops goals and objectives for each child's IEP or IFSP. In addition to setting goals, the team should work together to determine strategies to meet these goals in the program and at home and develop a system of ongoing assessment to track child progress toward goals over time. See Chapter 10 for more information about inclusive options for young children.

Including a child with special needs in a Head Start or Early Head Start program requires collaboration among the program, the family, and the LEA/EI and other agencies who may serve the child. Head Start and Early Head Start staff must work in tandem with the LEA or EI program to coordinate schedules and to ensure that each child receives therapy or other needed services in the least restrictive environment in a timely manner. Ongoing professional development and support is to be provided to teachers and teaching assistants to best meet the needs of each child. Programs must also collaborate to determine how transportation will be provided between agencies. Within Head Start and Early Head Start, staff members are required to modify the curriculum, the environment, and materials as needed to best support and accommodate the optimal development of each child.

Supporting Families of Children with Special Needs

Head Start has always recognized the importance of family involvement. When developing the Head Start program in the mid-1960s, Urie Bronfenbrenner, a member of the National Advisory Council for the National Institute of Child Health and Human Development during that time, insisted that for any program for young children to be effective, it would have to involve the child's family and community (Zigler & Muenchow, 1992). Since then, family involvement has been one of the hallmarks of the program. Today, family involvement is still a central part of services to children in Head Start and Early Head Start, and is especially crucial when including a child with special needs. Family services, disabilities services, and other staff should receive professional development on communicating with families to help them understand their child's special needs and to be an advocate for themselves and for their child. Of course, the level of involvement and support will vary depending on the needs and wishes of each family.

Each Head Start program is required to complete a Family Partnership Agreement to help them collaborate with families according to their unique circumstances and desires (ACF, 2008b). As a part of the Family Needs Assessment, family members are often asked to set goals for themselves and for their child over the coming year. This plan, along with the child's IEP or IFSP, should be used to guide services that are provided to the child and family.

Transition Planning for Children with Special Needs

Comprehensive planning is needed to support children with special needs and their families as they transition into and out of Early Head Start and/or Head Start programs. When a child is transitioning into the Head Start program, the disability coordinator must ensure that the child's teacher/home visitor and other pertinent program staff receive professional development on how to best meet the individualized needs of the child and family. There are also a number of supports that can be provided to the parents of children with special needs entering Head Start. Staff members should (1) provide materials and information on how to best support the development of their child at home, (2) describe the goals and objectives in their child's IEP/IFSP if unclear, (3) inform parents of their rights under IDEA, and (4) refer parents to support groups if agreed upon with parents (OHS, 2008). During the time a child is enrolled in Head Start or Early Head Start, the goal is for parents to increase their own skills, knowledge, and confidence so they are better able to access resources and advocate for their child(ren).

Transition planning for children with special needs who will be exiting the program requires collaboration among the Head Start program staff, the parents, the other agencies providing services for the child and family, and the receiving program. Support for children and families through the transition process should be individualized to meet the needs and requests of each family. In some cases, exiting programs will arrange to go on visits to new programs with parents while other exiting programs take a more hands-off approach by sending packets of information (with parental permission) to the child's new program. Most importantly, Head Start programs should provide resources, materials, and opportunities for parents to better understand the options that are available to them and their child and support them through the process of moving from one program to another.

Summary

For over four decades, Head Start has been at the forefront of providing services to children with special needs. Although all Head Start and Early Head Start programs must follow federal, state, and local mandates, each program must develop a plan for providing services based on the unique needs of the children and families who reside in their communities. While a child is enrolled in a Head Start or Early Head Start program, teachers and other program staff collaborate with other agencies, supplying services to each child and family to ensure that appropriate, individualized services are provided that support the family's wishes for their child as well as the goals and objectives in the child's IEP or IFSP. The ultimate goal is for the children to grow and develop as a result of their time in the program and for parents to better understand their rights and responsibilities as their child enters school or other future educational opportunities.

RESEARCH IN HEAD START AND EARLY HEAD START

As long as Head Start has existed, so too have questions about its effectiveness. Indeed, over the years, Head Start has been referred to as the nation's largest educational experiment and as a national laboratory (Zigler & Muenchow, 1992). From the very earliest days, research has been carried out to determine the effectiveness of the program. Most frequently, effectiveness has been determined by some measure of child and/or family outcomes.

After the first cohort of children went through the eight-week summer course in 1965, the Center for Urban Education conducted a study on the children who attended Head Start in New York City (Zigler & Muenchow, 1992). At first, the results seemed promising. The children who had attended Head Start scored higher on measures of school readiness than did a group of similar children who had not attended Head Start. Unfortunately, after several months in the public school, the two groups of children scored similarly on an achievement test. This was the first of many studies of Head Start in which the impact of time spent in Head Start appears to fade over time. In 1968–69, the first large-scale evaluation of Head Start was conducted by the Westinghouse Corporation and Ohio University. Despite arguments from many that it was too early to conduct a study of this magnitude on such a new program, the study went forward. The study found, as with the Center for Urban Education study, that regardless of early gains, long-term effects were not detected by grade 3 (Cicerelli, Evans, & Schiller, 1969). This report sparked a debate that continues today: Does the impact of Head Start fade over time, or are the public schools failing our children?

Since the Westinghouse Report was released, thousands of studies have been conducted in Head Start programs across the country by individual researchers, university groups, and federally funded evaluators. Head Start has undeniably become a national laboratory for educating young children. In recent years, several large-scale evaluations of Head Start and Early Head Start have been conducted with federal funds through the Office of Planning, Research and Evaluation (OPRE) housed within the Administration of Children and Families (ACF). The main goals of OPRE are spelled out in their mission statement:

> OPRE is responsible for advising the Assistant Secretary for Children and Families on increasing the effectiveness and efficiency

of programs to improve the economic and social well-being of children and families.

In collaboration with ACF program offices and others, OPRE is responsible for performance management for ACF, conducts research and policy analyses, and develops and oversees research and evaluation projects to assess program performance and inform policy and practice. The Office provides guidance, analysis, technical assistance, and oversight to ACF programs on: strategic planning; performance measurement; research and evaluation methods; statistical, policy, and program analysis; and synthesis and dissemination of research and demonstration findings. (Office of Planning, Research and Evaluation [OPRE], n.d.)

Two longitudinal studies have unearthed substantial data on the long-term impacts of Head Start for children and families. These two studies are the Family and Child Experiences Study and the Head Start Impact Study.

The Family and Child Experiences Study (FACES) gathers data from a nationally representative sample of Head Start programs, classrooms, teachers, parents, and children using a large battery of measures to better understand the quality and impacts of Head Start (ACF, 2006b). Measures used in FACES are gathered through classroom observation, parental interview, direct child assessment, and teacher-completed questionnaires. Data collection for FACES occurs in waves as information is gathered from programs over time. The first cohort of FACES began in 1997, the second in 2000, the third in 2003, and the last cohort in 2006. Most recently, the summary report for the 2003 cohort was released, sharing findings related to the children, families, and classrooms in 63 Head Start programs across the country.

FACES 2003 findings indicate that children in Head Start enter the program with below-average skills in mathematics and early literacy. However, over the program year, children in the program make significant gains in early mathematics, early writing, and in expansion of vocabulary skills (ACF, 2006b). Children also showed considerable growth in letter recognition, recognizing an average of four letters at the beginning of the year and 10 before leaving the program. Finally, FACES findings also showed that most children in the cohort showed gains in levels of social skills demonstrated throughout the program year, especially in the area of cooperative classroom behavior.

The FACES 2003 report (ACF, 2006b) showed that the average family participating in the FACES 2003 study consisted of four members with a median household income of $13,200 per year. One-third of Head Start children live with two parents who are married, and a similar percentage of families speak languages other than English in the home. Over 26 different languages are spoken by families of children in Head Start. A majority of families taking part in the FACES study (74%) indicated that they read to their child three or more times per week. The study also found that children whose parents read to them every day had higher vocabulary scores than did children whose parents read to them less often. Further, findings reveal that parental involvement in school is related to the improved child outcomes in a number of academic and social indicators.

Regarding classroom quality, FACES 2003 findings indicated that overall Head Start classroom quality is good, scoring an average of 4.8 on a 7-point scale on the Early Childhood Environmental Rating Scale (ECERS). Ratings on the ECERS also showed that 80 percent of teachers encouraged the development of positive interactions with mutual respect between children and adults and that 70 percent of teachers facilitated positive interactions among children and their peers. Ratings also demonstrated that 75 percent of teachers had a high level of integration of children with special needs in the classroom as indicated in the *Provisions for Children with Disabilities* section on the ECERS. Findings indicated that "In the spring of 2004, 19% of Head Start children had a special need identified . . . and that teachers reported that children received a variety of services to meet their needs" (ACF, 2006b).

Another longitudinal study of the impact of Head Start over time is the National Head Start Impact Study. This congressionally mandated study was conducted in 84 nationally representative Head Start agencies with approximately 5,000 children, using parental interviews, direct child assessments, classroom observational assessments, and teacher ratings of children (ACF, 2005). As applications were accepted for these 3- and 4-year-olds, the children were randomly assigned either to a group of children who would receive Head Start services, or to a "non-Head Start" comparison group in which their parents could enroll them in any community-based preschool other than Head Start. Data collection began in 2002 and continued on through 2006, when the children in the study entered the first grade. In addition, a third-grade follow-up was conducted last year to track progress for these students over time. The major goals of the Impact study were "to determine on a national basis how Head Start affects the school readiness of children participating in the program as compared to children not enrolled in Head Start and to determine under which conditions Head Start works best and for which children" (ACF, 2005, para. 2).

A summary of findings after the first year of the Impact Study indicate that both 3- and 4-year olds in the Head Start group showed moderately significant positive impacts in several cognitive constructs, including pre-reading, pre-writing, vocabulary, and parental reports of their child's literacy skills. When looking at parenting practices, the study found that parents of the children in the 3-year-old group had small statistically significant positive impacts on parenting skills, including increased use of educational activities in the home and a decreased use of physical discipline with their children (ACF, 2005).

Although it is a much younger program, a number of large-scale longitudinal studies have also been conducted in Early Head Start. Most notably, the congressionally mandated Early Head Start Research and Evaluation Project (EHSREP) was launched in 1996, one year after the first Early Head Start programs were funded. This large-scale study included a thorough examination of the implementation of Early Head Start and the impact on child and family outcomes in 17 nationally representative programs (ACF, 2006c). In this study, over 3,000 children were randomly assigned to either a group that would receive Early Head Start services or a comparison group who could participate in any program other than Early Head Start. A series of measures, including direct child assessments, parent reports of child development, parental observations, and parent interviews, were assessed periodically over the time that children were in either the Early Head Start program or comparison group.

Findings from this study demonstrated that children who participated in Early Head Start scored higher on cognitive, language, and social emotional measures than children in the non–Early Head Start comparison group. Regarding family outcomes, the strongest positive impacts were found in African American families who enrolled during pregnancy and had low-to-moderate demographic risks. Only families at the highest level of demographic risks showed no positive gains in parenting skills. In addition to overall results for children and families participating in the ESHREP, several findings had specific relevance to children with special needs. The study found that children who participated in Early Head Start had fewer delays in language and cognitive functions than children in the comparison group. Also, children who were in Early Head Start were much more likely to receive Part C services for diagnosed developmental delays (ACF, 2006c).

As a part of the EHSREP, a follow-up study was conducted with the children and families two years after participation. After leaving Early Head Start, many children moved on to some form of preschool or a prekindergarten program. Of the children who participated in the Early Head Start program, 47 percent were enrolled in formal pre-school programs at ages 3 and 4. This compared to 42 percent of children in the comparison group. The follow-up data showed that many of the positive impacts on child and family outcomes shown at the end of Early Head Start were still present two years later. The main areas of continued favorable impacts were in children's social emotional development and approaches to learning, parents' daily reading to their children, the overall home environment, and parent-child teaching activities (ACF, 2006c). African American parents whose children were enrolled in Early Head Start continued to demonstrate the most positive impacts from participating in the program. A fifth-grade follow-up study is currently underway with these children and families.

A number of other studies on the implementation and impact of Early Head Start are also in progress. Baby FACES (Family and Child Experiences Study), a longitudinal study with a cohort design, began in 2007 and will continue through 2012 (ACF, n.d.). This study builds on the findings from the EHSREP and uses a similar design as the Head Start FACES study. Another study building on these findings is the Survey of Early Head Start programs. This was the first of several descriptive studies to be conducted on the state of Early Head Start programs and how the program has changed over time to meet the needs of children and families. Research questions for this study included: (1) What are the characteristics of Early Head Start programs? (2) Who is served by Early Head Start programs? (3) What services do Early Head Start programs provide? (4) How are Early Head Start programs managed and staffed? (5) Do key program subgroups differ in their characteristics? If so, how? (ACF, 2006a, pp. xix–xx).

From their beginnings, both Head Start and Early Head Start have been examined closely to determine the impact the program has on outcomes for children and families. Large-scale studies like FACES, Baby FACES, the Head Start Impact Study, and the Early Head Start Research and Evaluation Project provide vital information on how Head Start and Early Head Start programs are continuously improving to meet the needs of the children and families in their programs. Over time, it will be critical to continue asking questions like these and others to get the most accurate depiction of how these programs are meeting the needs of the nation's neediest children and families.

FUTURE DIRECTIONS

Standing on Shaky Ground

Attempting to predict future directions is an extremely formidable task given the extremely uncertain times in which we are living. In an address to the joint session of Congress on February 24, 2009, President Barack Obama stated, "I know that for many Americans watching right now, the state of our economy is a concern that rises above all others. And rightly so . . . The impact of this recession is real, and it is everywhere" (Obama, 2009). As a result of the economic crisis, many state and local programs have been forced to slash budgets, which in turn have impacted services provided to the most disadvantaged among us. However, at the same time that many local and state budgets are diminishing, federal money has been flowing out to programs by way of the American Recovery and Reinvestment Act (ARRA).

President Obama signed P.L. 111-5 into law, the American Recovery and Reinvestment Act (ARRA), on February 17, 2009. The ARRA appropriated a total of $5.1 billion for the Administration for Children and Families (ACF), apportioned among the Child Care and Development Block Grant, Head Start, Early Head Start, and the Community Services Block Grant. This funding offered the opportunity for Head Start to collaborate with child care through cross training, implementing wraparound services, and other activities to benefit both programs by maximizing the dollars spent and helping families (OHS, 2009). Of this total figure, $2.3 billion was allocated to the Child Care and Development Block Grant to make up for shortfalls in state child care assistance programs for low-income families.

After years of budget cuts, increased federal appropriations came as welcome news for the Head Start community, especially in light of deep state and local budget cuts. Increases in Head Start funding through the ARRA appropriations provided opportunities to Head Start programs to convert part-day enrollment slots to full-day programs, which better accommodate working parents. As a result of increases in funding in Head Start and Early Head Start, record numbers of grant applications were submitted to the Office of Head Start in the summer of 2009 from organizations seeking money for newly funded Early Head Start programs as well as program expansion within current grantees.

Standing Firm on Our Promises to Young Children and Families

As a field, we have come a long way over the past 40 years. Every day, we learn new techniques and strategies to use when working with young children with special needs and their families. Even though we know more now than ever about how to best support the varying needs of children and families, we still face the challenge of bringing together multiple systems at the local, state, and federal levels to coordinate services and provide them in a timely manner. Moving forward, we must reflect on where we have been and take the lessons we have learned with us as we create supportive environments for young children and families. Inclusive programs for children at risk, like Head Start and Early Head Start, have long recognized the value of collaboration with community agencies, the importance of continuous professional development for staff members, and the crucial involvement of family in creating a successful program.

One successful collaborative model used to increase recruitment and enrollment of infants and toddlers with significant special needs in Early Head Start was the SpecialQuest professional development program. The first phase of this project, which was co-funded by the Office of Head Start and the Hilton Foundation, took place from 1997 through 2002, with the second phase occurring from 2003 through 2007. In this team-based model, Early Head Start programs were invited to attend a one-week professional development opportunity each year with a team of individuals from their service area.

In the final report from the first phase of SpecialQuest, 36 percent of participating Early Head Start programs reported enrolling children with special needs in at least 10 percent of their available slots (California Institute of Human Services [CIHS], 2002). Amazingly, at the end of SpecialQuest, 70 percent of participating programs had filled at least 10 percent of their slots with children with special needs. From 1997 through 2007, children and families in over 500 communities were positively impacted as a result of the SpecialQuest training program (CIHS, 2007). SpecialQuest provided a forum for these individuals from a community to work together to create inclusive environments for infants and toddlers with special needs.

Other collaborations that have been increasing Head Start teacher salaries as well as pushing higher education are the Head Start and public pre-K partnerships. Because of Head Start's track record working with children with disabilities and those who are at risk, public schools are increasingly seeking partnerships with Head Start. In these ventures, preschool classrooms offer a co-teaching model with Head Start and public school teachers working side by side and sharing the load. This offers benefits for everyone involved as scarce resources are combined from IDEA, Head Start, public school, professional development funding, and other sources of local, state, and federal dollars.

As we look to the future, it is imperative that we reduce the gap between research and practice by providing quality professional development opportunities for early childhood educators. This can be done by increasing opportunities for teachers to gain degrees and professional certification. In the 2007 reauthorization of the Head Start Act, new requirements were included for teacher qualifications. The act states that:

> [N]ot later than September 30, 2013, at least 50% of Head Start teachers nation-wide in center-based programs have (i) a baccalaureate or advanced degree in early childhood education; or (ii) a baccalaureate or advanced degree and coursework equivalent to a major relating to early childhood education, with experience teaching preschool-age children. (Head Start Act, 2007, p. 110)

In addition, the Head Start Act specifies that:

> [N]ot later than September 30, 2010, all teachers providing direct services to children and families participating in Early Head Start programs located in Early Head Start centers have a minimum of a child development associate credential and have been trained (or have equivalent coursework) in early childhood development. (Head Start Act, p. 93)

New requirements like these will mean that thousands of early childhood teachers will be entering early childhood education programs in the coming years. In addition to educating existing teachers, it is estimated that approximately 10,000 new Head Start and Early Head Start teachers will be needed as a result of program expansion funding from the ARRA. Finding and educating this many early childhood teachers in the time provided will be a real challenge.

To help prepare teachers for the anticipated 10,000 new positions available through ARRA, the Department of Education provided Teacher Quality Partnership (TQP) grants. The purpose of these grants included improving student achievement and the quality of new and prospective teachers by enhancing teacher preparation and professional development. To qualify for funding, partnerships had to develop among school districts, early childhood education, and higher education, especially in areas of high need (National Archives and Records Administration, 2009).

CONCLUSION

Over time, Head Start has remained true to its roots of providing a comprehensive program considering the whole child, including education, health, and nutrition, and working with families and encouraging their support. In this chapter, we have discussed the history of this program, the services provided to children and families, and the costs of these services, as well as evidence through research to tell us if these services make a difference in the lives of young children and their families. We began this chapter by discussing the real costs of not investing in quality care and education programs for children with multiple risk factors in our society. For those of us in the field of early childhood, on a daily basis we see the impacts on children and families who get "lost" in the system and do not get the supports and services they need. There is no question that our efforts are worth the investment; however, to leaders at local, state, and federal levels, these payoffs might not be as readily evident.

Some of these positive impacts can be measured by looking at tangible factors like academic success or school retention. However, others are less tangible and may take decades to come to fruition. What we do know now is that high-quality early intervention and education programs bring dividends to the children, families, communities, and the nation that far outweigh the costs associated with such programs (Lynch, 2005). The future of our society depends upon fostering the health and well-being of our children for tomorrow's world because "today's children become tomorrow's citizens, workers, and parents. When we invest wisely in children and families, the next generation will pay that back through a lifetime of productivity and responsible citizenship" (National Scientific Council on the Developing Child, 2007, p. 1). When we fail to invest in the next generation, providing them the foundation needed for them to thrive, we put our future at risk. In 10 years, when we are asked, "How are the children?" we must answer, "All the children are well" (O'Neill, 1991).

REFERENCES

Administration for Children and Families. (1993). *Head Start performance standards and other regulations.*

Administration for Children and Families. (2005). Head Start impact study first year findings. Office of Planning, Research and Evaluation.

Administration for Children and Families. (2006a). Findings from the Early Head Start programs: Communities, programs and families. Office of Planning, Research and Evaluation.

Administration for Children and Families. (2006b). Friendly FACES. Office of Planning, Research and Evaluation.

Administration for Children and Families. (2006c). Research to practice: Preliminary findings from the Early Head Start prekindergarten follow up. Early Head Start Research and Evaluation Project. Office of Planning, Research and Evaluation.

Administration for Children and Families. (2008a). *Head Start fact sheets.* Retrieved from http://eclkc.ohs.acf.hhs.gov/hslc/About%20Head%20Start/dHead StartProgr.htm

Administration for Children and Families. (2008b). *Head Start performance standards and other regulations,* Amended.

Administration for Children and Families. (n.d.). Overview of the Early Head Start family and child experiences study (Baby FACES). Office of Planning Research and Evaluation. Retrieved from http://www.acf.hhs.gov/programs/opre/ehs/descriptive_study/descriptive_overview.html#overview

Barnett, W., Lamy, C., & Jung, K. (2005). *The effects of state prekindergarten programs on young children's school readiness in five states.* New Brunswick, NJ: NIEER, Rutgers.

Barnett, W. S. (2007). Getting the measure of the mileage of preschool care. *Prevention Action.* Retrieved from http://www.preventionaction.org/research

Bowman, B., Donovan, M., & Burns, M. (2001). *Eager to learn.* Washington DC: National Academy Press.

Brooks-Gunn, J. & Duncan, G. J. (1997). Children and poverty. *The Future of Children, 7,* 55–71.

California Institute on Human Services. (2002). Hilton/Early Head Start training program 2002 final evaluation report. Sonoma State University.

California Institute on Human Services. (2007). Five-year final report 2002–2007. Sonoma State University.

Children's Defense Fund. (2008). *Children in the United States fact sheet.* Retrieved from http://www.childrensdefense.org/child-research-data-publications/data/state-data-repository/cits/children-in-the-states-2008-all.pdf

Cicerelli, V. G., Evans, J. W., & Schiller, J. S. (1969). The impact of Head Start: An evaluation of the effects of Head Start on children's cognitive and affective development. *Report to the United States Office of Economic Opportunity by Westinghouse Learning Corporation and Ohio University*. Washington, DC: Government Printing Office.

Department of Health and Human Services & Department of Education. (2006). Good Start, Grow Smart: A guide to Good Start, Grow Smart and other federal early learning initiatives. Retrieved from http://www.acf.hhs.gov/programs/ccb/initiatives/gsgs/fedpubs/GSGSBooklet.pdf

Division of Early Childhood of the Council for Exceptional Children & the National Association for the Education of Young Children (DEC/NAEYC). (2009). *Early childhood inclusion. Joint position statement*. Retrieved from http://www.naeyc.org/files/naeyc/file/positions/DEC_NAEYC_EC_updatedKS.pdf

Garguilo, R. M., & Kilgo, J. L. (2000). *Young children with special needs*. Albany, NY: Delmar Thomson Learning.

Garguilo, R. M., & Kilgo, J. L. (2005). *Young children with special needs* (2nd ed.). Clifton Park, NY: Delmar Thomson Learning.

Gearhart, B., Mullen, R., & Gearhart, C. (1993). *Exceptional individuals*. Pacific Grove, CA: Brooks/Cole.

Gilliam, W., & Zigler, E. (2004). *State efforts to evaluate the effects of prekindergarten: 1977–2003*. New Haven, CT: Yale University.

Ginsberg, L. & Miller-Cribbs, J. (2005). *Understanding social problems, policies, and programs* (4th ed.) Columbia: University of South Carolina Press.

Head Start Act. (2007). 42 U.S.C. 9801 *et seq*.

Health, Education, and Welfare (HEW) Report. (1978). *Report of preschool education, 10*.

Karoly, L., Greenwood, P., Everingham, S., Hoube, J., Kilburn, R., Rydell, C. P., et al. (1998). *Investing in our children: What we know and don't know about the costs and benefits of early childhood interventions*. Washington, DC: Rand Corporation.

Lombardi, J., & Bogle, M. (2004). *Beacon of Hope: The promise of Early Head Start for America's youngest children*. Washington, DC: Zero to Three.

Lybolt, J., Armstrong, J., Techmanski, K., & Gottfred, C. (2007). *Building language throughout the year: The preschool early literacy curriculum*. Baltimore: Paul H. Brookes.

Lynch, R. G. (2005). Early childhood investment yields big payoff. *WestEd Policy Perspectives*. Retrieved from http://www.wested.org/online_pubs/pp-05-02.pdf

Martin, E. W. (1989). Lessons from implementing P.L. 99-142. In J. Gallagher, P. L. Trohanis, & R. M. Clifford (Eds.), *Policy implementation & P.L. 99-457* (pp. 19–32). Baltimore: Paul H. Brookes.

Masse, L., & Barnett, W. S. (2002). *A benefit cost analysis of the Abecedarian early childhood intervention*. New Brunswick, NJ: National Institute for Early Education Research, Rutgers University.

Meisels, S. J., & Shonkoff, J. P. (2000). Early childhood intervention: A continuing evolution. In J. P. Shonkoff and S. J. Meisels (Eds.), *Handbook of early childhood intervention* (2nd ed., pp. 3–31). Cambridge: Cambridge University Press.

National Archives and Records Administration. (2009). Teacher quality partnership grant program. *Federal Register, 74*, 38592–38605.

National Association of Child Care Resource and Referral Agencies. (NACCRRA) (2009). *Economic stimulus briefing room.* Retrieved from http://www.naccrra.org/policy/economic-stimulus-briefing-room

National Association for the Education of Young Children. (2009). NAEYC position statement: Developmentally appropriate practice in early childhood programs serving children from birth through age 8. In C. Copple and S. Bredekamp (Eds.), *Developmentally Appropriate Practice in Early Childhood Programs* (3rd ed., pp. 1–31). Washington, DC: National Association for the Education of Young Children.

National Institute for Early Education Research. (2003). *Preschool Policy Matters: Investing in Head Start teachers.* New Brunswick, NJ: NIEER.

National Scientific Council on the Developing Child. (2007). *The science of early development: Closing the gap between what we know and what we do.* Boston: Center on the Developing Child, Harvard University.

Neuman, S., Copple, C., & Bredekamp, S. (2000). *Learning to read and write: Developmentally appropriate practices for young children.* Washington DC: NAEYC.

Obama, B. (2009). Remarks of President Barack Obama—as prepared for delivery, address to joint session of Congress, Tuesday, February 24th, 2009. Retrieved from http://www.whitehouse.gov/the_press_office/remarks-of-president-barack-obama-address-to-joint-session-of-congress

Office of Head Start. (2008). *Orientation guide for Head Start disabilities services coordinators.* Retrieved from http://eclkc.ohs.acf.hhs.gov/hslc/Professional%20Development/Staff%20Development/Disabilities/OrientationGuide.htm

Office of Head Start. (2009). Head Start funding increase. *Early Childhood Learning and Knowledge Center.* Retrieved from http://eclkc.ohs.acf.hhs.gov/hslc/Program%20Design%20and%20Management/Head%20Start%20Requirements/PIs/2009/resour_pri_006_040209.html

Office of Planning, Research and Evaluation. (n.d.). About OPRE. Retrieved from http://www.acf.hhs.gov/programs/opre/about_opre.html#mission

Ohlson, C. (1998). Welfare reform: Implications for young children with disabilities, their families, and service providers. *Journal of Early Intervention, 21,* 191–206.

O'Neill. P. T. (1991). *And How Are the Children?* Speech delivered at Unitarian Universalist Church, Framingham, MA.

Parrott, S. (2008). 2008 Omnibus appropriations bill cuts funding for Head Start: Bipartisan reauthorization bill enacted two weeks before omnibus was completed called for increased investment. Center on Budget and Policy Priorities. Retrieved from http://www.cbpp.org/files/2-5-08bud.pdf

Pianta, R., Cox, M., & Snow, K. (2007). *School readiness and the transition to kindergarten in the era of accountability.* Baltimore: Paul H. Brookes.

Reight-Parker, J. (2007). *Head Start in Maine.* Augusta, ME: Department of Health and Human Services.

Reynolds, A., Temple, J., Robertson, D., & Mann, E. (2002). Age 21 cost-benefit analysis of the Title I Chicago Parent Center. *Education Evaluation and Policy Analysis, 24,* 267–303.

Samuels, C. A. (2009). Stimulus providing big funding boost for early childhood. *Education Week, 28*(27), 8.

Schweinhart, L. (2004). *The High/Scope Perry Preschool study through age 40: Summary, conclusions, and frequently asked questions.* Ypsilanti, MI: HighScope Press.

Scott-Little, C., Kagan, S., & Frelow, V. (2006). Conceptualization of readiness and the content of early learning standards: The intersection of policy and research? *Early Childhood Research Quarterly, 21*, 153–173.

Shonkoff, J. P., & Phillips, D. A. (Eds.) (2000). *From neurons to neighborhoods: The science of early childhood development.* Washington, DC: National Academy Press.

Strickland, D., & Riley-Ayers, S. (2007). *Literacy leadership in early childhood: The essential guide.* New York: Teacher's College Press.

Wat, A. (2007). *Dollars and sense: A review of economic analyses of pre-k.* Washington, DC: Pre-K Now.

Whitehurst, G. J., & Lonigan, C. J. (2001). Emergent literacy: Development from prereaders to readers. In S. B. Neuman & D. K. Dickensen (Eds.), *Handbook of early literacy research* (pp. 11–29). New York: Guilford Press.

Wright, W. D., & Wright, P. D. (2003). *Wrightslaw: Special education law.* Hartfield, VA: Harbor House Law Press.

Zigler, E. F., & Muenchow, S. (1992). *Head Start: The inside story of America's most successful educational experiment.* New York: Basic Books.

Zigler, E. F., & Styfco, S. J. (2004). *The Head Start debates.* Baltimore: Paul H. Brookes.

Zigler, E. F., & Valentine, J. (Eds.). (1979). *Project Head Start: A legacy of the War on Poverty.* New York: Basic Books.

Chapter 4

Building a Comprehensive Assessment System in Early Intervention/Early Childhood Special Education

Cornelia Bruckner, Mary McLean, and Patricia Snyder

Assessment has been defined as "a generic term that refers to the process of gathering information for the purpose of making decisions" (McLean, Wolery, & Bailey, 2004, p. 13). Considering what decisions will be made as a result of assessment is an important first step in any discussion of assessment practices or strategies. According to Shepard, Kagan, and Wurtz (1998), "The intended use of an assessment—its

purpose—determines every other aspect of how the assessment is conducted" (p. 6). Practitioners in early intervention/early childhood special education (EI/ECSE) have a long history of conducting assessments to help inform decisions about eligibility for services, planning programs for intervention based on individualized goals and outcomes, and monitoring child progress toward those goals and outcomes. Recent innovations and issues in early care and education, general education, and special education, however, have resulted in changes in both the purposes and procedures for assessment in EI/ECSE. The purpose of this chapter is to provide an overview of traditional EI/ECSE assessment practices, identify recent innovations and issues that are influencing assessment practices for young children, and provide recommendations for facilitating an organized and comprehensive system for assessment as prompted by federal requirements.

TRADITIONAL ASSESSMENT FUNCTIONS IN EI/ECSE

Traditionally, five distinct functions or purposes of assessment have been identified in the EI/ECSE literature: (1) screening, (2) determining eligibility for early intervention or special education, (3) program planning, (4) monitoring child progress as a result of intervention, and (5) program evaluation or accountability (McLean, 2004). Federal and state laws, particularly the Individuals with Disabilities Education Act, have greatly influenced these functions of assessment for EI/ECSE. It should be noted that other federally or state-funded programs for young children, many of which also serve young children with disabilities, do not have the same requirements and, therefore, the primary purposes of assessment for those programs might be different. The brief review of each of the five functions of assessment below illustrates the various purposes for which assessment has traditionally been conducted.

Screening refers to a brief assessment designed to identify children who should be referred for further and more comprehensive assessment relative to development, behavior, hearing, vision, or health. Typically, data from screening is used to inform one of three decisions: (1) pass (screen "negative"), (2) do not pass (screen "positive"), or (3) need for follow-up screening or closer monitoring. The result of a "positive" screen often leads to a referral for further assessment to determine which children might need specialized equipment, services, or targeted instruction. For example, developmental screening is required within 45 days of enrollment for all children enrolled in Head Start. Some school districts provide developmental screening services to all young children residing within their catchment areas in an effort to identify those who need further assessment and who are in need of intervention as soon as possible. Some states offer periodic screening for all young children in the state who have been found to be at risk for developing a delay in their growth and development. Traditionally, screening of developmental, behavioral, or health status has been provided on a periodic basis.

Determination of eligibility for early intervention or early childhood special education is guided by federal law, specifically the Individuals with Disabilities Education Act (IDEA) (2004), which is further interpreted in state regulations. Federal law provides a general definition of which children are eligible for early infant/toddler services to age three (Part C of IDEA, Office of Special Education Programs & TA & D network, 2010b) and for early childhood special education preschool

Table 4.1 Categories of Eligibility for Infant/Toddler and Preschool Services under IDEA

Potential Categories of Eligibility for IDEA Part B, Section 619—Preschool	
Autism	Multiple Disabilities
Deaf-Blind	Orthopedic Impairment
Deaf	Specific Learning Disability
Developmental Delay	Speech or Language Impairment
Emotional Disturbance	Traumatic Brain Injury
Hearing Impairment	Visual Impairment/Blindness
Mental Retardation	
Potential Categories of Eligibility for IDEA Part C—Birth to Three	
Developmental Delay	
Diagnosed Condition	
At Risk	

services (Section 619 of Part B of IDEA, Office of Special Education Programs & TA & D network, 2010a). Three categories are delineated by federal law for Part C services, and 13 categories are delineated for Part B services (see Table 4.1 for a list of the categories for Part C and Part B, Section 619). States, in turn, are responsible for delineating more specific requirements for each category that conform to the federal definitions but provide specific guidelines for use by assessors to determine who is eligible and who is not eligible within their jurisdiction.

Variations in eligibility categories and eligibility determination systems exists across states, particularly with respect to whether and how the 13 Part B disability categories are applied (Danaher, Shackelford, & Harbin, 2004). For example, not all states include the category of developmental delay for preschool services. According to IDEA Part B, developmental delay can be a category for children between the ages of 3 and 9. Even among those states that do include a category of developmental delay, there is variation in the age range that is identified (Danaher, 2007). Most states require an assessment of the individual child's level of functioning relative to the typical functioning of same-aged peers as part of eligibility determination (Danaher, 2007; Shackelford, 2006). When developmental delay is used as an eligibility category either in Part C or for preschool children, eligibility criteria decisions typically are informed by a cutoff score designated either by standard deviation units below the mean or percent of delay in months by comparing an age equivalent score to chronological age. *Norm-referenced instruments* that consider a child's score relative to the score of a representative sample of children of the same age have traditionally been used for determining eligibility for early intervention or special education services.

Program planning assessment serves the purpose of informing decisions about the goals or outcomes to be specified on the individualized education program (IEP) for preschool children or the individualized family service plan (IFSP) for infants and toddlers, as well as special services to be provided and the service delivery format. Young children with disabilities should have access to and participate in the general preschool curriculum. Assessments used for program planning should help inform decisions about the individualized instruction or supports that a young child with disabilities needs to access and participate in the general preschool curriculum (Grisham-Brown, Hemmeter, & Pretti-Frontczak, 2005). Norm-referenced instruments typically are not designed for the purpose of informing decisions about individualized intervention goals or outcomes. *Criterion-referenced instruments*, however, help inform decisions about whether a child has met an established criterion level of performance in relation to skills that are deemed relevant and important. Criterion-referenced assessments provide data useful for informing decisions about "success or failure to meet some previously determined objective rather than providing information about the child's performance relative to other children his age" (Bailey, 2004, p. 34). Curriculum-based assessments (CBA), also referred to as curriculum-referenced assessments, are a specific type of criterion-referenced assessments that are directly aligned with a curriculum (Slentz & Hyatt, 2008). Curriculum-based assessments are used widely for informing decisions about program planning. Additional information about the child's disability-related needs as well as information about child and family routines and family or teacher priorities for intervention will also inform program planning decisions for a child, resulting in an individualized plan for intervention as designated by the IEP or IFSP.

Assessment for the purpose of *monitoring child progress* is also required by the Individuals with Disabilities Education Act. Several sources of data can be gathered and evaluated to inform progress-monitoring decisions. Goals and outcomes written on the IEP and IFSP must be written so that they are measurable. Child progress toward reaching the goals and outcomes must be reviewed with parents every six months for infants and toddlers, and every year for preschool children. This review serves as the basis for identifying changes that should be made in intervention goals, strategies, or services. Data from curriculum-based assessments, when administered repeatedly on a specified schedule (e.g., two to four times a year), can be used to inform decisions about progress related to curricular content. In recent years, the practice of gathering data more frequently on children's progress to inform decisions about their progress toward generalized outcomes has also been identified as important within a system of data-based decision making (Carta, Greenwood, Walker, & Buzhardt, 2010). A system referred to as curriculum-based measurement (CBM) that includes measures that are brief, targeted, and administered frequently are used to inform decisions about children's progress on key skill indicators that are associated with generalized outcomes. For example, Carta et al. describe a CBM measure related to a generalized movement outcome and how data from this measure might be used to inform decisions about child progress in relation to key skill indicators such as horizontal and vertical movements, throwing/rolling, and catching/trapping. CBM is useful for informing progress-monitoring decisions because it provides time-series information on the progress (level and slope of change) that individual children or groups of children are making. This approach to formative evaluation of child progress has also been referred to as "critical skills mastery" and is characterized by the assessment of specific skills that are sequenced according to difficulty within domains (Deno, 1986).

Program evaluation has been defined as the process of "systematically collecting, synthesizing, and interpreting information about programs for the purpose of assisting with decision making" (Snyder & Sheehan, 1996, p. 359). *Accountability* is a type of program evaluation and has been defined as the "systematic collection, analysis, and use of information to hold schools, educators, and others responsible for the performance of students and the education system" (Education Commission of the States, 1998, p. 3). Assessment for the purpose of accountability has been mandated by the most recent reauthorization of IDEA (2004). Prior to IDEA 2004, program evaluation in EI/ECSE was typically based on the requirements of funding agencies and often focused on assessing "process" variables such as hours of service, staff qualifications, or the ratio of the number of staff to the number of children served. The K–12 educational system, however, gradually came under increasing pressure to demonstrate results in the form of increased student achievement, and a similar requirement for demonstrating results for young children is in place for infants, toddlers, and preschoolers with disabilities under IDEA (Division for Early Childhood [DEC], 2007). At this time, however, a requirement for submitting child outcomes data for the purpose of accountability is not required by Head Start, by most state-funded early care and education programs, or by kindergarten or early elementary programs in the public schools.

Regardless of the purpose, the assessment process results in information that can be summarized and used to make decisions. The most common way to use information from assessment to make decisions is to evaluate scores or score patterns within a child (across subscales or time), across a group of children, or referenced to some external criteria (e.g., the performance of a norming group or academic standards). To compare information across subscales or groups of children, scores must be reported in a common metric. In the preceding sections, we talked about several metrics, including: met/not met as a criterion for evaluating progress on IEP goals, and progress toward generalized outcomes measured by reviewing change in scores within a child over time and referencing to expected performance. Many different metrics can be designed and used to summarize information and make decisions based on assessment results. In the next section, we will review some of the most common metrics and discuss the benefits and drawbacks of each.

METRICS FOR SUMMARIZING INFORMATION FROM ASSESSMENTS

When data are gathered through assessment, most frequently the data are based on a set of responses to individual items. The items often represent several different areas of development or constructs (e.g., motor, communication, social skills). Test developers combine items measuring similar constructs into sets. Each item in a set is considered to be an independent measure of the construct, and often the optimal measure of the construct is obtained by combining item responses across the item set. There are many different ways to combine a set of items, including adding them all together or computing the average item response. Test publishers often specify a preferred method for combining item responses, and this method is often linked to normative data. Those who administer assessments, interpret scores, and make decisions based on these scores need to understand how the test publisher or other users of the assessment have combined item responses, and they should use the same methods to score assessments.

Within EI/ECSE, a set of common metrics is used with many assessments. Any metric is based on item responses, and the quality of item responses determines the quality of the metric. As more items are included in an item set, the effects of a poorly designed item is diminished (Cronbach, 1951). Many metrics start with a raw score or the sum of the items within a set. The following section will describe two different types of metrics that can be derived from raw scores.

Transformed Scores

Raw scores can be transformed into metrics that provide the user with more information about a child's performance relative to the entire item set or relative to their previous performance on the same item set. The most common metrics of transformed scores are percent correct, average item response, and growth scores. *Percent correct* is the percentage of the items within the item set with correct responses. This metric ranges from zero to 100 percent and gives the user an idea of how close the child is to responding correctly to all the items. The benefit of this metric is that it is easily explained and interpreted by nontechnical users. The *average item response* is the sum of all item responses within the set divided by the highest possible score for the item set. The range of this metric is dependent on the range of the items. For example, for an item set where items can have a response between 0 and 5 and there are five items, the highest possible score would be 25, and the average item response would be determined by summing the response for all five items and dividing by 25. The average item score would range from 0 to 5. The benefit of this metric is that it is similar to the metric of the items. To the degree that the user understands how a child's ability is defined across different rating points in the item, she can interpret the average score.

Growth scores refer to a set of metrics that compare a child's performance to their own performance across time. For example, to determine whether a child is gaining new skills in preschool, many systems administer assessments at the beginning and the end of the school year and then compare scores between the two time points. To compare the scores, the change in raw scores or the sum of item responses at the end of the school year minus the sum of item responses at the beginning of the school year can be compared. Similarly, the change in average score or the average score at the end of the school year minus the average score at the beginning of the school year can be compared. The benefit of these growth metrics is that they can be easily combined across children or classrooms. All of the metrics just described share an important weakness: they do not take into account what is expected performance or growth. Without including information about expected performance, it is difficult to judge if the scores indicate sufficient acquisition or mastery of skills associated with the construct. To help inform decisions about a child's performance relative to expectations, referenced scores can be computed.

Referenced scores are scores that have been mapped to the performance of a reference sample or set of standards. It is critically important that users of these types of scores understand the characteristics of the sample or standards that were used for this mapping (American Education Research Association [AERA], American Psychological Association [APA], National Council on Measurement in Education [NCME], 1999). These referenced scores are only useful if the sample or standards used to derive them permit meaningful inferences and comparisons. Inferences and comparisons are meaningful if the characteristics of the sample or standards are relevant to your current context (e.g., the standards are based on constructs that you are currently teaching in your class, the children in the norming sample are representative of the children that you are assessing). Three types of referenced scores will be described: age equivalent scores, standard scores, and criterion referenced scores.

Age equivalent scores are typically a transformation of raw scores. Data are collected on a representative sample of children of different ages. The performance of children within different age groups is computed from this sample, and the expected raw score by age group is defined. The average performance is typically estimated using the median raw score of the norm group; however, it is often necessary to use statistical modeling to smooth the medians across age groups. An example of an assessment where the performance of a norming sample is used to create age equivalent scores is the Battelle Developmental Inventory, Second Edition (BDI-2; Newborg, 2005a, 2005b). For the BDI-2, data were collected on 2,500 children that represented the entire age range of the instrument and were representative of national demographics based on census regions. To calculate the age at which a raw score is typical, the observed median raw scores for each subdomain and each age group was plotted across ages and smoothed when necessary (Newborg, 2005a, 2005b). This information is typically presented as a table listing raw scores by the age or age range when that raw score is typically achieved. When item responses within an item set are totaled for an individual child, the child's raw score is located in the table described above and an age or age range is linked to that score. The benefit of this metric is that it is easily interpreted by users given the score is reported in months or years, which is an intuitive metric.

Standard scores are used to describe a child's functioning relative to a group of children that would be expected to be performing at the same level as the target child. For example, standard scores would compare the performance of a 3-year-old child to the performance of a representative sample of other 3-year-old children. Standard scores use the mean and the standard deviation of the representative sample to describe the expected performance and spread of performance within a group of children. It is important to note that the use of standard scores assumes that the distribution of raw scores in the comparison group was a normal distribution. Standard scores are often presented in a metric with a mean of 100 and a standard deviation of 15, although other forms of standard scores exist (e.g., standard score of 40 with standard deviation of 10). This makes it easy for users with an understanding of means and standard deviations to interpret standard scores. For example, if a child has a standard score of 70, it is understood that the child is performing two standard deviations $(100 - [15 + 15] = 70)$ below the mean of the comparison group.

Criterion-referenced scores are scores that are referenced to a set of criteria. These scores are seen most frequently in standards-based assessment where it is being determined whether a child is meeting a set of standards or benchmarks appropriate for his age. The logic used to derive these scores is similar to that used for creating standard scores; however, instead of using the performance of a representative sample to determine the raw score expected for a group of children, the behavioral criterion defined by an external standard is used. It is important to note that these external standards are typically both empirical and theoretical. This is a benefit to the extent that the theory behind the external criteria is predictive of outcomes. Criterion-referenced scores are typically presented as either a pass/fail metric where a child meets or fails to meet a criterion or a range of scores that describe distinct proficiency levels—for example, at or above basic, at or above proficient, and at advanced (AERA, APA, NCME, 1999).

THE CHANGING LANDSCAPE OF ASSESSMENT PRACTICES

Recent influences in general education, special education, and early childhood care and education assessment practices have impacted assessment in EI/ECSE. Programs serving infants, toddlers, and preschoolers with disabilities feel the impact of these influences through changes in federal, state, and local requirements, through changes in the identification of recommended practice by professional organizations, and through new developments in published materials. Increased assessment requirements in an era of decreased funding for services have made it important to develop carefully and strategically an overall plan for quality assessment. Service providers might find that they must respond to very specific yet different assessment requirements for the various agencies that fund their programs. Increased pressure on providers to satisfy a myriad of assessment requirements has prompted assessors to question that cardinal rule of assessment that assessment instruments should be used only for the purpose for which they were developed. For example, Bricker, Squires, and Clifford (2010) recently discussed the need to expand the use of the ASQ screening tool to include eligibility-determination, program-planning, and progress-monitoring functions and the responsibilities that would accompany such decisions.

At the same time, research and changing models in general education and special education have resulted in new approaches to assessment that call into question the traditional purposes of assessment. For example, response-to-intervention models being used in preschool (e.g., Recognition and Response; Buysee & Wesley, 2006) has resulted in the need to redefine the purposes and recommended procedures for screening. The early work of the Early Childhood Research Institute on Measuring Growth and Development, which developed the Individual Growth and Development Indicators (IGDIs) (Greenwood et al., 2008) and the current work of the Center for Response to Intervention in Early Childhood (http://www.crtiec.org) have also influenced contemporary assessment practices related to screening and data-based decision making, including progress monitoring. Other issues and innovations that are influencing assessment practices for young children are also important to consider.

Role of Assessment in Standards-Based and Accountability Contexts

Stakeholders in early childhood education and early childhood special education attach clear accountability expectations to the programs that they participate in and fund (National Association for the Education of Young Children [NAEYC], 2003). Policy makers want to know the answers to questions such as "Do children who receive special education services perform better in elementary school than similar children that do not receive those services?" "Do children who receive early intervention meet educational standards in third grade?" To answer these and other questions, assessment systems that span birth through adulthood are needed. The challenges to implementing these systems are formidable, but solutions are a priority of both state and federal agencies (e.g., Race to the Top; U.S. Department of Education, 2009).

Standards-based education and accountability initiatives are shaping the types and frequency of assessments for children who are receiving services in early childhood settings. More and more programs are held accountable for the progress of children that receive their services. This progress is measured in different ways in different areas and for different types of children. To determine if children make sufficient progress, their progress must be measured and compared to a set of valid expectations. Some common metrics for looking at child progress include developmental status after receiving services (e.g., kindergarten readiness) and growth between the beginning and end of services. Expectations can be related to state standards for early childhood or amount of progress relative to similar children. Child progress information then needs to be summarized at the program level in a metric that can be used to judge the sufficiency of child progress in the program relative to some criterion or standard. States that are implementing standards-based early childhood education will need to know the number of children that are meeting the state standards. Accountability initiatives will often use a different metric, like the number of children that entered below age expectations that "close the gap." One important impact of standards-based and accountability assessment is the need for tests in early childhood that can be used to compare a child's functioning to age-level expectations. Assessments that have been used to meet this new purpose include those typically used for eligibility assessment, and fewer used for program planning. It is important to keep in mind recommended practices in assessment in EI/ECSE as large scale standards-based and accountability assessment are developed.

Impact of Standards-Based Education

In 2004, 41 states had early learning standards (Scott-Little & Kagan, 2004). Linking assessment to state standards ensures that children's learning is aligned to state expectations about what young children should know or be able to do. Assessment systems that measure children's progress toward standards can be used to monitor implementation of standards-based early education. This supports equality of educational expectations across regions in a state or across different classrooms. Many different approaches have been used to link assessment to standards for K–12. Currently, two primary approaches are used to assess children's learning as it aligns to state expectations. One method is to develop an assessment that is aligned to the state standards. This allows precise measurement of the achievement of standards using a method that is easily understood by consumers. The challenge to developing this type of instrument is putting together an instrument development team with the appropriate content and measurement expertise. Also, assessments that are directly aligned to standards will need to be revised as standards are revised, which can be an expensive process. A second method that can be used to measure children's learning as it aligns to state standards is to select an existing assessment or set of assessments that meet standards of best practices and cover the constructs included in the standards. The items from these assessments will be aligned to standards by reviewing the behaviors measured by the items and comparing them to the behaviors in the standards. This method allows states to use assessments that teachers and programs are familiar with and may already be using for a new purpose. One drawback of this method is the difficulty of computing one metric across several assessments.

Accountability Requirements

Beginning in 2006, all states were required by the Office of Special Education Programs to report on the progress that children birth to age 5 who participate in EI/ECSE attain across three child outcomes including: positive social emotional skills (including positive social relationships), acquisition and use of knowledge and skills (including early language/communication [and early literacy]), and use of appropriate behaviors to meet needs. For each of these outcomes, states report the percentage of children in each of five categories of progress, ranging from "did not improve functioning" to "maintained functioning at a level comparable to same-aged peers." When this requirement was released, many states had to rapidly mount a child outcomes measurement system. Currently, the Child Outcomes Summary Form (COSF; Early Childhood Outcomes Center, 2006) is used to summarize status and progress on the three outcomes described earlier by most states, including 41 (73%) states for Part C measurement and 36 (61%) for Part B

619 measurement (Office of Special Education Programs & TA&D network, 2010a, 2010b). The COSF is a judgment-based rating scale that is completed by the IEP of IFSP team based on information from other assessments.

Other states use the scores from commercially available assessments or state-developed tools to directly measure outcomes without using the COSF. For states that are using other tools, items from the assessments are aligned to the three OSEP outcomes, and these items are combined into three item sets representing each of the three OSEP outcomes. States using the COSF also refer to the crosswalks between items and OSEP outcomes as a tool for interpreting assessment information (Early Childhood Outcomes Center, 2006). These item sets are scored and referenced to some standard based on either the performance of a norm group or a set of external standards for performance, like early learning standards. The most frequently used assessments for Part B 619 are the Creative Curriculum Developmental Continuum used by 22 states and the BDI-2 used by 20 states (Office of Special Education Programs & TA&D network, 2010). The most frequently used assessments for Part C are Hawaii Early Learning Profile (HELP), used by 31 states, and the Assessment and Evaluation and Programming System for Infants and Children (AEPS), used by 23 states.

Increasing Diversity in Children and Families

The population of children and families in the United States who receive early childhood education or EI/ECSE services is increasingly diverse. The 2008 Kid's Count Data for the State of California, for example, shows that 50 percent of children birth through age 5 in the state of California are Hispanic or Latino (http://datacenter.kidscount.org). Children in early childhood programs mirror the racial, ethnic, cultural, linguistic, and socioeconomic diversity of the society in which they live. Early childhood programs are more likely than school-age programs to have children who have not yet learned to speak English and perhaps also to serve families who do not speak English. In some cities and parts of the country, the number of different languages that are spoken by children entering early childhood programs and their families creates a particular challenge for obtaining valid assessment information. Assessors need to be aware of the issues involved in assessing children who are culturally and linguistically diverse, and they also need to be aware of how to access the resources needed to obtain valid assessment information.

Specifying a Language for Assessment

Children who are learning a second language are a heterogeneous group. The degree of proficiency achieved in each language will depend on when and how extensively the child has been exposed to each of the languages. Some children in early childhood programs may have very little skill in English; others may have some skill in English but more skill in their home language. Still others may receptively understand some English but produce very little of it. In planning for appropriate assessment procedures, it is important to consider each child individually and to gather information prior to the assessment that will allow planning for the most individually appropriate assessment procedures.

The Individuals with Disabilities Education Act (IDEA) is clear about the procedures that are to be followed for evaluation to determine eligibility for special education services. Children are to be assessed in their dominant language. The dominant language is the language the child prefers to speak and speaks most proficiently at the time of the assessment (Roseberry-McKibben, 1994). According to IDEA, children who are English language learners (ELLs) who have been referred for evaluation to determine eligibility for special education services should first be assessed to determine their dominant language. Determining the dominant language is, however, frequently a complex undertaking that may require the skills of a speech and language pathologist working in conjunction with others. For young children, this process may require observation of the child in an environment where he or she is comfortable and likely to be uninhibited about speaking. In addition, it may be necessary to interview caregivers and family members about the child's typical language outside of the early childhood setting.

The effect of acquiring a second language on a child's cognitive, language, and social development can be complex. It is generally believed that learning a second language may enhance cognitive and social development (Ben-Zeev, 1977). However, it is also believed that the process of learning a second language may actually result in an interaction between the two languages that could reduce the child's proficiency in both languages at least temporarily (Schiff-Myers, 1992). As a result, it is recommended that children be assessed in both their home language and also in the second language so that information will be available from both conditions (California Department of Education, Special Education Division, 2007; Quinones-Eatman, 2001; Tabors, 2008).

Assessment Methods

A position statement developed by the Division for Early Childhood (DEC) for the purpose of providing recommendations for curriculum, assessment, and program evaluation specifies that assessment methods for young children should be "culturally and linguistically responsive" to limit bias in assessment (DEC, 2007, p. 11). Identifying appropriate assessment instruments and strategies for children from cultural and linguistic environments that differ from the mainstream society can be a challenge, but certainly must be addressed. Most instruments that are norm-referenced have not included children from culturally or linguistically diverse backgrounds in the norming population. As a result, bias is introduced into the outcome of the assessment. The assessor should consult the examiner's manual of the instrument being used to determine how appropriate it is for a particular child relative to culture and to language. If the child being assessed is different from the children included in the norming population, then the instrument scores should not be reported.

The use of observational rather than adult-directed assessment strategies would seem to be appropriate for reducing bias in assessment (Tabors, 2008). Most indicators that are included in criterion- or curriculum-referenced assessments have been derived from constructs of child development that were identified from research involving children growing up in mainstream society who speak English. While bias is perhaps less of a threat, it is still the case that the items or benchmarks being used to guide authentic assessment may not be a match culturally for the child. Similarly, observation of the child's language in authentic situations will need to be inclusive of both the home language and English to be most accurate and informative.

Recognition of the Importance of Assessment Procedures That Are Ecologically Valid

The field of EI/ECSE has been strongly influenced by an ecological model of human development, which considers the influence of the environment and various systems within the environment when planning intervention services for young children with disabilities and their families (Bailey & Wolery, 1992). The influence of the ecological model has been no less impactful on assessment practices for young children. In the past 25 years, assessment practices for young children have been transformed from highly structured, adult-directed assessment to assessment practices that rely on observational assessment of children in familiar environments over time (Bagnato, Neisworth, & Pretti-Frontczak, 2010). This change to ecologically valid assessment practices is evident in the standards and position statements of the major professional organizations, including the Division for Early Childhood (DEC) of the Council for Exceptional Children (DEC, 2007; Sandall, Hemmeter, Smith, & McLean, 2005) and the National Association for the Education of Young Children (NAEYC) (NAEYC, 2003).

Assessment that is based on observation of the child over time in the typical environment with familiar caregivers while engaged in real-life activities is referred to as "authentic assessment." As defined by Bagnato and Yeh-Ho (2006), "authentic assessment refers to the systematic recording of developmental observations over time about the naturally occurring behaviors and functional competencies of young children in daily routines by familiar and knowledgeable caregivers" (p. 16). The difficulties involved in the use of conventional norm-referenced tests with young children with disabilities (Neisworth & Bagnato, 2004) along with the realization that authentic assessment yields immediately useful and valid information for planning and evaluating intervention has led to a significant shift toward the use of authentic assessment strategies (Bagnato, 2007; Meisels, 2006). This shift has increased the need to ensure that assessors and service providers are knowledgeable and skilled in the behaviors required to conduct authentic assessments of children over time in typical environments and to gather information from parents and other care providers to be used in conjunction with ongoing observations.

Parents and Primary Caregivers as Part of the Assessment Team

Parents and primary caregivers observe and interact with young children over time and across a variety of settings. They are uniquely situated to observe continuity and discontinuity in child development and behavior across time, settings, and people. Although practitioners often acknowledge that, "parents [or primary caregivers] know a child best," assessment practices in EI/ECSE often contradict this adage. The roles parents and primary caregivers should or would like to assume in assessment often are not consistently enacted or explicitly discussed.

Gathering information from families and primary caregivers about child development and behavior is essential for making *ecologically valid* assessment decisions. As noted by Suen, Lu, Neisworth, and Bagnato (1993), given different perspectives and contexts in which development and behavior is observed, assessment data contributed by families or primary caregivers should be considered independent rather than interchangeable with data provided by others who are less familiar with the child. Convergent data between families or primary caregivers and others less familiar with the child might suggest consistency in child development and behavior across people and settings. Data that are not convergent should not be viewed as problematic; rather, they should set the occasion for focused discussions by families and practitioners about what types of decisions will be made based on the information that has been gathered and the assessment questions to be addressed.

Gathering information from families and primary caregivers is especially important when an assessor has limited contact with a child. For example, if the child attends an early childhood program and receives only related special education services, such as speech therapy, then the primary IEP service provider might find it useful to ask both the family and the general education teacher for their observations about the child's development and behavior. Asking parents to share their observations is also particularly useful for those skills the child might not demonstrate routinely in the early education or care setting. For example, a teacher or therapist is not likely to observe a child's self-care skills during bathing.

Ecologically Valid Assessment

Given variability in child development and behavior across time, people, and settings, parental and primary caregiver perspectives are likely to differ from assessment data gathered at a static point in time, by adults unfamiliar with the child, and in situations that might not be familiar to the child. As Uri Bronfenbrenner noted when characterizing the use of analogue or laboratory settings to study child development, child assessment conducted under these conditions represents "the science of strange behavior of children in strange situations with strange adults for the briefest possible period of time" (Bronfenbrenner, 1977, p. 513). Assessments conducted only under these conditions are not considered ecologically valid because they do not contribute information about child development and behavior beyond the immediate situation.

More than 20 years ago, Bailey (1989) characterized key components of ecologically valid assessment. He suggested that ecologically valid assessments are those that (1) involve parents as significant partners in assessment processes; (2) focus heavily on naturalistic observation of child behavior during everyday routines and activities and how these behaviors are integrated for functional use; (3) are nondiscriminatory by considering a child's learning history, cultural background, and family values; and (4) consider subsequent environments in which the child will participate and identify behaviors and skills likely to be needed by the child in these environments. These components are consistent with contemporary recommended assessment practices in EI/ECSE (Bagnato & Neisworth, 2005; DEC, 2007). Nevertheless, we have yet to implement fully ecologically valid assessment practices in EI/ECSE.

The Role of Families in Assessment

Despite the identified benefits of having data gathered from parents or primary caregivers inform assessment decisions, practitioners frequently question whether information provided by parents or primary caregivers about child development and behavior is reliable and valid. Reliability reflects the extent to which information is consistent, or free from error, including consistent across time or observers. Validity refers to the types of meaningful inferences that can be made from information or data provided. For example, language samples gathered from young children in authentic settings might permit meaningful (valid) inferences about a child's communication skills.

Two terms have historically dominated the empirical literature focused on examining the reliability and validity of parental perspectives about child development and behavior: overestimation and underestimation. The term *parental overestimation* initially appeared in empirical studies conducted from the early 1950s through the 1990s that examined parent and professional congruence (meaning consistency or agreement) about child developmental and behavioral status. Many of these studies reported that parents overestimated their child's developmental status or behavior when compared to estimates obtained from professionals (see Dinnebeil & Rule [1994] and Snyder, Thompson, & Sexton [1993] for a review of this research). These studies suffered from procedural or methodological limitations, however, and did not permit definitive conclusions about parental overestimation. For example, in many studies, different instruments were used by parents and professionals to report perspectives about child development or behavior. Parents often completed judgment-based rating scales designed to gather information about child development or behavior, while professionals administered a standardized test directly to the child. These variations in the instruments and approaches used to gather information introduced confounds that led researchers to suggest that parental overestimation might be an artifact of the methods used.

In the 1980s, Beckman (1984) and Gradel, Thompson, and Sheehan (1981) suggested that it might be equally likely that professionals *underestimate* child status, particularly when professionals only gather information at a single point in time in a standardized testing situation. In fact, Snyder et al. (1993) found that 73 pairs of primary caregivers and parents had very high levels of consistency and agreement about child development and behavior when they completed the same instruments in the same way and had repeated opportunities to observe the 73 children in the study sample over time. These findings suggest that not only are family observations reliable and valid, but they are an essential part of a comprehensive assessment process.

Do Family Observations Have to Agree with Professional Observations?

Although congruence (i.e., consistency or agreement) in observations might be important in some situations, contemporary perspectives in early childhood assessment suggest that both parents and professionals have important information to share about children. As Suen, Logan, Neisworth, and Bagnato (1995) noted, professional observations are reliable snapshots of children's behavior in certain settings (e.g., classrooms), whereas parental perspectives are based on a full-length feature film that provides rich information to enhance professional observations. Thus, rather than focusing on parental overestimation or professional underestimation, the value of each perspective for gaining a more complete and convergent picture of the child across people, settings, and time should be recognized.

IMPLICATIONS FOR BUILDING COMPREHENSIVE AND INCLUSIVE ASSESSMENT SYSTEMS

The previous sections of this chapter have focused on the changing landscape of assessment in EI/ECSE. The populations being assessed and the methods being used to conduct and understand assessments are changing and will continue to change. For the first time, as a result of federal accountability initiatives, states are faced with the challenge and the opportunity of building statewide systems of assessment in EI/ECSE to address accountability requirements. Building such a system provides states with the opportunity to consider assessment in general and also to attempt to develop an appropriate and useful system for purposes other than accountability. With budget cuts leading to reduced funding available to programs, any assessment system must be efficient and must provide information that can be used to information decision making at multiple levels from program planning to presenting progress data to the legislature. This final section will describe key components to consider in the development of assessment systems that are both efficient and useful.

The first step to developing a high-quality assessment system is to determine the purpose of the system and communicate that purpose to others (Early Childhood Outcomes Center, 2009). The purpose should include statements about why data are being collected and how data will be used. The purpose should also define who will use the data and for what purposes (e.g., providers will use assessment data to monitor progress on state standards; state agency will use the data to report on child outcomes to the legislature). The importance of collecting information about all components of the service delivery system should be considered. Decisions will be made about which components are critical, and other components may be phased in over time. Stakeholders are critical to determining priorities for the data elements, frequency of data collection, and service components to be included in the assessment system. Stakeholders can help set these priorities because they understand how the data elements manifest in the system and how the system will impact the service delivery system. Once the purpose has been developed, it should be made available to local administrators, providers, and the general public (e.g., on the Web, in family brochures, in training manuals), and comments should be systematically collected. Sharing the purpose will provide opportunities for people to react to the system, allowing adaptations to be made before the expensive work of systems development is underway.

Once the purpose and scope of the assessment system has been determined, it is important to decide on the data collection and transmission approach that best fits the assessment system and currently implemented data collection efforts and implement this approach (Early Childhood Outcomes Center, 2009). Recommended practices in assessing young children should be considered. To ensure that data are of high quality and not compromised by misunderstood procedures, policies and procedures must be clear and readily accessible to the people implementing the assessment system. Often this additional assessment requirement will be placed on staff that is already overburdened. To minimize the burden of tracking data collection and submission timelines on staff, it is important to make processes available that facilitate efficient and complete data collection (e.g., weekly reminders about deadlines, administrative reports that pinpoint data issues that must be resolved before data can be reported). To minimize the burden on staff and the children being assessed, it is important to ensure there is no duplication in collection of data elements and that timelines for all systems are aligned. Before a set of assessments and timelines are defined, those that are currently implemented across the settings where children are served should be reviewed (e.g., children served by preschool special education and Head Start). Existing assessment systems should be considered and incorporated as much as possible. As with all procedures, data collection and transmission procedures should be reviewed as needed based on needs of the field or state agency.

The final piece is to develop a comprehensive communication plan for interpreting, reporting, and disseminating data to relevant audiences, including families (Early Childhood Outcomes Center, 2009). This communication plan should include the potential audiences, tasks, timeline, frequency, and draft formats for reports. Representative stakeholders (e.g., families, providers, administrators) should be included in the process of review and interpretation of reports. It is important to prioritize reporting needs. It is often the case that once data become available, many different types of stakeholders become interested in having access to the data. The original purpose of the assessment system should be a guide in prioritizing reporting needs. For example, if it is important that the assessment system provides information that is helpful to teachers for program planning, reports that summarize individual child and classroom status and progress will be prioritized.

Although the process seems daunting, a well-planned and intentionally implemented assessment system will be well worth the effort. A system that allows stakeholders to quickly access summarized data relevant to the questions they want to answer will facilitate the use of information to improve services. A helpful tool that has been developed for implementing this process is the Early Childhood Outcome Center's Outcomes Measurement System Framework and Self Assessment (Early Childhood Outcomes Center, 2009). This includes a self-assessment that can be used to rate the level of implementation of 18 Quality Indicators identified as important for high-quality assessment and use of information by experts and stakeholders.

Selecting Appropriate Assessments for EI/ECSE

To aid readers in making decisions about assessments, we have developed the following checklist. It includes considerations that are described in more detail throughout the chapter. The reader should consider each item and how it will affect the end result of the assessment.

1) *What is the purpose of assessment?* Consider why you are conducting this assessment, there could be multiple purposes.
2) *What is the unit of assessment?* Given your purpose, what is the appropriate unit for assessment? For example, if the purpose is to examine program quality, classrooms may be the unit; if the purpose is to examine child progress in response to a new curriculum, children may be the unit.
3) *Who will complete the assessment?* Decide who within your network of resources is available to complete the assessment (e.g., care providers, parents, teachers, outside evaluators).
   a. Consider how this additional assessment work can be integrated with the responsibilities already held by the assessor.
   b. How long will it take to have the assessment administered with fidelity? Consider the match between the skills of the assessor and the training requirements of different assessments.
4) *What is the financial burden of the assessment?* Consider the costs of the assessment relative to benefits and compare to less expensive alternatives.
   a. Will you need to purchase test booklets?
   b. Will you need to pay for online subscriptions?
   c. What is the cost of training? Can it be done by program staff, or do outside experts need to conduct the training?
5) *Characteristics of the assessment unit*: Consider the natural variation present in the assessment unit. (For example, do the children that will be assessed speak multiple languages? Do the programs have differing levels of parent involvement?)
   a. Consider the appropriateness of the assessment across cultures including the effect of home language on scoring.
   b. Consider the flexibility of the assessment across settings.
6) *Alignment of assessment to best practices*: Does the assessment meet standards for best practices in EI/ECSE?
7) *How will information be summarized?* Consider how you will need to report the results of your assessment process, and make sure

that the scores from the assessment can be summarized in a way that is meaningful.

a. What audiences will need to use the information?

b. Does the assessment provide reports in a format understandable to lay people?

c. How will the information be combined? Ensure that the same information is gathered in the same way across all units that will be combined.

d. How will information be interpreted? Do you have the information you need to answer the questions you laid out in your vision for the assessment?

CONCLUSION

Assessment of young children with disabilities provides important information for parents, teachers, care providers, and stakeholders in EI/ECSE. Assessment is a tool that can used to inform decision making when it is conducted appropriately. In the design and implementation of an assessment system, users should consider the purposes for the system, the diversity of the population to be assessed, the alignment of administration procedures to best practices, and the impact of the process on the participants. In this chapter, we have highlighted current issues in assessment of young children with disabilities, including: new purposes for assessment, including families; assessing children who are culturally and linguistically diverse; accountability; and progress monitoring. We have presented information about current best practices in assessment for young children with disabilities.

Assessments are useful only if scores can be used for their intended purpose. Some purposes of early childhood assessment that were discussed in this chapter include (1) screening, (2) determining eligibility for early intervention or special education, (3) program planning, (4) monitoring child progress during intervention, and (5) program evaluation or accountability. Strategies were presented that make assessment systems more efficient, including include designing assessment systems that include all young children (including families in the assessment planning and implementation process), using assessments that are collaborative and developmentally appropriate, and regularly monitoring data quality. Information from well-implemented assessment systems provide information that can aid in making decisions that improve the lives of children and families.

References

American Educational Research Association (AERA), American Psychological Association (APA), and the National Council on Measurement in Education (NCME). (1999). *Standards for educational and psychological testing*. Washington, DC: AERA.

Bagnato, S. J. (2007). *Authentic assessment for early childhood intervention*. New York: Guilford Press.

Bagnato, S., & Neisworth, J. (2005). Recommended practices in assessment. In S. Sandall, M. L. Hemmeter, B. J. Smith, & M. E. McLean (Eds.), *DEC recommended practices in early intervention and early childhood special education*. Longmont, CO: Sopris West.

Bagnato, S. J., Neisworth, J. T., & Pretti-Frontczak, K. (2010). *LINKing authentic assessment and early childhood intervention: Best measures for best practices* (4th ed.). Baltimore: Paul H. Brookes.

Bagnato, S., & Yeh-Ho, H. (2006). High-stakes testing of preschool children: Violation of professional standards for evidence-based practice. *International Journal of Korean Educational Policy, 3*(1), 23–43.

Bailey, D. (1989). Assessment and its importance in early intervention. In D. Bailey & M. Wolery (Eds.), *Assessing infants and preschoolers with handicaps* (pp. 1–21). Columbus, OH: Merrill.

Bailey, D. (2004). Tests and test development. In M. McLean, M. Wolery, & D. B. Bailey, Jr. (Eds.), *Assessing infants and preschoolers with special needs* (3rd ed., pp. 22–44). Upper Saddle River, NJ: Pearson, Merrill, Prentice Hall.

Bailey, D., & Wolery, M. (1992). An ecological framework for early intervention. In D. Bailey & M. Wolery (Eds.), *Teaching infants and preschoolers with disabilities* (2nd ed.). Englewood Cliffs, NJ: Merrill Prentice Hall.

Beckman, P. (1984). Perceptions of young children with handicaps: A comparison of mothers and program staff. *Mental Retardation, 22*, 176–181.

Ben-Zeev, S. (1977). The influence of bilingualism on cognitive strategy and cognitive development. *Child Development, 48*(3), 1009–1018.

Bricker, D., Squires, J., & Clifford, J. (2010). Developmental screening measures: Stretching the use of the ASQ for other assessment purposes. *Infants and Young Children, 23*(1), 14–22. doi:10.1097/IYC.0b013e3181c816cc

Bronfenbrenner, U. (1977). Toward an experimental ecology of human development. *American Psychologist, 32*(7), 513–530.

Buysee, V., & Wesley, P. (Eds.). (2006). *Evidence-based practice in the early childhood field*. Washington, DC: Zero to Three.

California Department of Education, Special Education Division. (2007). *Assessing children with disabilities who are English language learners: Guidance for the DRDP access and the PS DRDP-R for Children with IEPs*. Retrieved from the Desired Results *access* Project, http://www.draccess.org/pdf/guidancefordrdp/ELGuidance.pdf

Carta, J., Greenwood, C., Walker, D., & Buzhardt, J. (2010). *Using IGDIs: Monitoring progress and improving intervention for infants and young children*. Baltimore: Paul H. Brookes.

Cronbach, L. J. (1951). Coefficient alpha and the internal structure of tests. *Psychometrika, 16*(3), 297–334.

Danaher, J. (2007, May). Eligibility policies and practices for young children under Part B of IDEA. *NECTAC Notes, 24*. Chapel Hill, NC: Frank Porter Graham Child Development Institute, National Early Childhood Technical Assistance Center.

Danaher, J., Shackelford, J., & Harbin, G. (2004). Revisiting a comparison of eligibility policies for infant/toddler programs and preschool special education programs. *Topics in Early Childhood Special Education, 24*(2), 59–67. doi:10.1177/02711214040240020101

Deno, S. L. (1986). Formative evaluation of individual student programs: A new role for school psychologists. *School Psychology Review, 15*, 358–374.

Dinnebeil, L., & Rule, S. (1994). Congruence between parents' and professionals' judgments about the development of young children with disabilities: A review of the literature. *Topics in Early Childhood Special Education, 14*(1), 1–25. doi:10.1177/027112149401400105

Division for Early Childhood (DEC). (2007). *Promoting positive outcomes for children with disabilities: Recommendations for curriculum, assessment, and program evaluation*. Missoula, MT: Author.

Early Childhood Outcomes Center. (2006a). *Child outcomes summary form*. Retrieved from the Early Childhood Outcomes Center, http://www.fpg.unc.edu/~eco/assets/docs/Child%20Outcomes%20Summary%20Form_4-21-06-3.rtf

Early Childhood Outcomes Center. (2006b). *Introduction to the ECO "Crosswalks" of birth-to-five assessment instruments to early childhood outcomes*. Retrieved from the Early Childhood Outcomes Center, http://www.fpg.unc.edu/~eco/assets/pdfs/Crosswalk_intro.pdf

Early Childhood Outcomes Center. (2009). *Scale for assessing state implementation of a child outcomes measurement system*. Retrieved from the Early Childhood Outcomes Center, http://www.fpg.unc.edu/~eco/pages/frame_dev.cfm

Education Commission of the States. (1998). *Designing and implementing standards-based accountability systems*. Denver, CO: Author.

Gradel, K., Thompson, M. S., & Sheehan, R. (1981). Parental and professional agreement in early childhood assessment. *Topics in Early Childhood Special Education, 1*(2), 31–39. doi:10.1177/027112148100100208

Greenwood, C. R., Carta, J., Baggett, K., Buzhardt, J., Walker, D., & Terry, B. (2008). Best practices in integrating progress monitoring and response-to-intervention concepts into early childhood systems. In A. Thomas, J. Grimes, & J. Gruba (Eds.), *Best practices in school psychology: V* (pp. 519–534). Bethesda, MD: National Association of School Psychologists.

Grisham-Brown, J., Hemmeter, M. L., & Pretti-Frontczak, K. (2005). *Blended practices for teaching young children in inclusive settings*. Baltimore: Paul H. Brookes.

Individuals with Disabilities Education Act (IDEA) of 2004, 20 U.S.C. § 1401D.

McLean, M. (2004). Assessment and its importance in early intervention/early childhood special education. In M. McLean, M. Wolery, & D. Bailey (Eds.), *Assessing infants and preschoolers with special needs* (3rd ed., pp. 1–21). Upper Saddle River, NJ: Pearson, Merrill, Prentice Hall.

McLean, M., Wolery, M., & Bailey, D. (2004). *Assessing infants and preschoolers with special needs* (3rd ed.). Upper Saddle River, NJ: Pearson, Merrill, Prentice Hall.

Meisels, S. J. (2006). *Accountability in early childhood: No easy answers*. (Occasional Paper No. 6). Retrieved from the Herr Research Center for Children and Social

Policy, http://www.erikson.edu/downloads/cmsFile.ashx?VersionID=3750 &PropertyID=78

National Association for the Education of Young Children (NAEYC). (2003). Early childhood curriculum, assessment, and program evaluation: Building an effective, accountable system in programs for children birth to age 8. A joint position statement of the National Association for the Education of Young Children (NAEYC) and the National Association of Early Childhood Specialists in State Department of Education (NAECS/SDE). Retrieved from http://www .naeyc.org/files/naeyc/file/positions/pscape.pdf

Neisworth, J. T., & Bagnato, S. J. (2004). The mismeasure of young children: The authentic assessment alternative. *Infants and Young Children, 17*(3), 198–212.

Newborg, J. (2005a). *Battelle Developmental Inventory* (2nd ed.). Rolling Meadows, IL: Riverside.

Newborg, J. (2005b). *Battelle Developmental Inventory* (2nd ed.), *Examiners manual.* Rolling Meadows, IL: Riverside.

Office of Special Education Programs & TA & D network. (2010a). *Part B SPPAPR 2009 indicator analyses.* Retrieved from the Early Childhood Outcomes Center, http://leadershipmega-conf-reg.tadnet.org/uploads/file_assets/attachments/203/original_original_42635_PartB_Text.pdf?1280108682

Office of Special Education Programs & TA & D network. (2010b). *Part C SPPAPR 2009 Indicator Analyses.* Retrieved from the Early Childhood Outcomes Center, http://leadershipmega-conf-reg.tadnet.org/uploads/file_assets/attachments/460/original_Analysis_of_Part_C_Indicators_FINAL080910.pdf?1283446411

Quinones-Eatman, J. (2001). *Preschool second language acquisition: What we know and how we can effectively communicate with young second language learners.* Technical Report #5, Culturally and Linguistically Appropriate Services, Early Childhood Research Institute. Champaign: University of Illinois.

Roseberry-McKibben, C. (1994). Assessment and intervention for children with limited English proficiency and language disorders. *American Journal of Speech-Language Pathology, 3*(3), 77–88.

Sandall, S., Hemmeter, M. L., Smith, B., & McLean, M. (Eds.). (2005). *DEC recommended practices: A comprehensive guide for practical application in early intervention/early childhood special education.*Missoula, MT: Division for Early Childhood.

Schiff-Myers, N. B. (1992). Considering arrested language development and language loss in the assessment of second language learners. *Language, Speech and Hearing Services in Schools, 23*(1), 28–33.

Scott-Little, C., & Kagan, S. L. (2004). *Reconsidering early care and education issues: Implications for the field.* Presentation for the National Association of Early Childhood Specialists in State Departments of Education, Anaheim, CA.

Shackelford, J. (2006). *State and jurisdictional eligibility definitions for infants and toddlers with disability under IDEA.* National Early Childhood Technical Assistance Center, *NECTAC Notes,* Volume 21, pp. 1-16. Chapel Hill: The University of North Carolina.

Shepard, L. A., Kagan, S. L., & Wurtz, E. (Eds.). (1998). *Principles and recommendations for early childhood assessments.* Washington, DC: National Educational Goals Panel.

Slentz, K. L., & Hyatt, K. (2008). Best practices in applying curriculum-based assessment in early childhood. In A. Thomas, J. Grimes, & J. Gruba (Eds.), *Best practices in school psychology: V* (pp. 519–534). Washington, DC: National Association of School Psychology.

Snyder, P. A., Thompson, B., & Sexton, D. (1993, January). *Congruence in maternal and professional early intervention assessments of young children with disabilities.* Paper presented at the annual meeting of the Southwest Educational Research Association (SERA), Austin. (Outstanding SERA paper for 1993, also presented in session [#25.17] for distinguished papers from regional research associations, American Educational Research Association, Atlanta, April 14, 1993.) ED 354 274

Snyder, S., & Sheehan, R. (1996). Program evaluation in early childhood special education. In S. L. Odom & M. E. McLean (Eds.), *Early intervention for infants and young children with disabilities and their families: Recommended practices* (pp. 359–378). Austin, TX: PRO-ED.

Suen, H. K., Logan, C. R., Neisworth, J., & Bagnato, S. (1995). Parent-professional congruence: Is it necessary? *Journal of Early Intervention, 19,* 243–252. doi:10.1177/105381519501900307

Suen, H. K., Lu, C. H., Neisworth, J. T., & Bagnato, S. J. (1993). Measurement of team decision-making through generalizability theory. *Journal of Psychoeducational Assessment, 11*(2), 120–132.

Tabors, P. O. (2008). *One child, two languages: A guide for preschool educators of children learning English as a second language* (2nd ed.). Baltimore: Paul H. Brookes.

U.S. Department of Education. (2009). *Race to the Top program: Executive summary* (white paper). Retrieved from U.S. Department of Education, http://www2.ed.gov/programs/racetothetop/executive-summary.pdf

Chapter 5

Sensory Processing: Tools for Supporting Young Children in Everyday Life

Winnie Dunn

There are many ways to support children and families so they thrive, develop, and get the most out of their lives together. Each approach that is based on evidence adds tools to the collection of strategies available to those who provide supports for children and families. Recently, sensory processing concepts have been getting an increasing amount of attention from professionals, researchers, and families. This increased interest has emerged from several sources. First, when we listen to families' stories, their children's reactions to sensory events (e.g., sounds, tastes, smells, touching) are woven through their stories. This style of reporting got the attention of professionals, who, trying to be responsive to a family's distress (e.g., "She will only eat soft foods with no texture; how will she get her nutrition?" or "He won't let me rock him") began considering ways to address sensory features of challenges in everyday life.

At the same time, advances in neuroscience and technology have enabled both basic science and applied science researchers to ask questions that target relationships between behavior and nervous-system activity. Knowing this relationship helps gain insights about why certain behaviors might exist or why certain interventions are helpful or not helpful (if the brain works a certain way, then interventions that are compatible with the brain's processing are likely to be more effective). Another factor influencing researchers was the environmental press of children moving from institutions to communities, then homes; this shift introduced complex reactions. When children were in institutions (or even separate classrooms or clinics for children with disabilities), we had more control over their sensory experiences. In community settings, the unpredictability of sounds, touch, etc., can trigger reactions that one does not observe in more controlled settings.

Therefore, a variety of events affecting behavioral responses to stimuli influence occupational therapists that have provided the research and practice leadership. Their work is now influencing interdisciplinary knowledge development to create greater understanding of the meaning of children's behaviors and a wider array of options for effective and innovative interdisciplinary approaches to serving children and families.

This chapter begins with an introduction to contemporary concepts of sensory processing, including a review of the research that supports these concepts. The next section provides a historical context for the development of sensory processing knowledge along with comparisons of traditional and contemporary practices that have a sensory processing emphasis. Finally, the last sections illustrate application of sensory processing concepts in early intervention and early childhood (EI/EC) services and provide examples of using sensory processing knowledge in home, school, and community contexts.

CONTEMPORARY CONCEPTS OF SENSORY PROCESSING

The contemporary principles of sensory processing are illustrated in Dunn's Model of Sensory Processing, seen in Figure 5.1 (Dunn, 1997). Anchoring this model are two underlying constructs: thresholds and

Neurological Threshold	Self-Regulation Continuum	
Continuum	Passive	Active
High	Registration	Seeking
Low	Sensitivity	Avoiding

Figure 5.1   Dunn's Model of Sensory Processing. Dunn, W. (1997). "The impact of sensory processing abilities on the daily lives of young children and families: A conceptual model." *Infants and Young Children, 9(4)*, 23–35. Used with permission.

self-regulation. The first construct is "neurological thresholds," which refers to the way the nervous system operates.

The entire nervous system reacts based on a balancing of excitatory and inhibitory inputs (Kandell, Schwartz, & Jessell, 2000). Each person has specific set points, or thresholds, that indicate a particular level at which a response occurs. Some people respond very quickly to sensory stimuli, while others have slower or delayed responses to the same stimuli. When responses are quick and frequent, we say that the person has "low thresholds" (i.e., it does not take very much input to activate the system); when responses are slow, we say the person has "high thresholds" (i.e., it takes a lot of input to activate the system).

The second underlying construct is "self-regulation," which refers to the way a person handles incoming sensory input. People tend to manage their own states by doing things to maintain a comfortable feeling. On one end of this continuum, people tend to let things happen around them and react (a passive approach to self-regulation), while at the other end of this continuum, people tend to engage in behaviors to control the input they receive (an active approach to self-regulation).

When we intersect these two constructs, four patterns emerge (see Figure 5.1). Seeking includes high thresholds and an active self-regulation strategy. Avoiding includes low thresholds and an active self-regulation strategy. Sensitivity represents low thresholds and a passive self-regulation strategy. Registration combines high thresholds and a passive self-regulation strategy. Each pattern represents a unique way of responding to sensory experiences in everyday life.

"Seekers" enjoy sensory input and find ways to get more. Their high thresholds mean they need a lot of input to get their thresholds to activate, and so they use active strategies to get enough input to meet their threshold needs. Seekers might make noises while playing; change positions a lot during an activity; like hats and accessories; select noisy, active, or intense play schemas; or love physical play.

"Avoiders" want as little sensory input as possible. They have very low thresholds, so it does not take much to feel overwhelmed. Avoiders find ways to minimize sensory input as their "active self-regulation" strategy. They might play in corners of the room or in another room when possible, have only a few clothing items that are okay to wear, withdraw (or cry) at family gatherings, or have very few preferred foods.

"Sensors" are very particular about their experiences. They notice many things that other people do not notice, which makes them precise, but noticing a lot can also be overwhelming. They are likely to have specific ways they want to get dressed or eat their food, play with a toy in only certain ways, be crabby with other children during play (because they need things to be in a certain pattern to stay within their thresholds), or notice sounds from another room that others do not hear.

People with "Registration" characteristics are called "Bystanders" because they fail to detect things that others are noticing. With high thresholds, many stimuli occur without their notice; this makes Bystanders very easygoing, but they might also forget materials in a group activity, miss the directions, seem more unkempt, or need to be called several times (and with touching) to get their attention.

As with all human characteristics, we explain these four patterns as if they are distinct categories, yet every person actually has some aspects of each pattern in their repertoire. A person might be a seeker for sounds, but an avoider for touch experiences. Knowing the person's patterns is the key to effective use of this model in practice (Dunn, 1999a, 2001).

Evidence Supporting the Concepts in Dunn's Model of Sensory Processing

Dunn's model of sensory processing emerged from research about how people respond to sensory experiences in their everyday lives (Brown & Dunn, 2002a; Dunn, 1999a, 2002b; Dunn & Brown, 1997; Dunn & Westman, 1997). Using the *Sensory Profile* assessments (Brown & Dunn, 2002; Dunn, 1999b, 2002, 2006a, 2006b) as the measure of a person's responsiveness to sensory experiences in everyday life, researchers report both patterns in the general population and in groups of people with disabilities.

The *Sensory Profile* assessments are parent/self reporting measures (i.e., children's parents report until they are 11 years old, then self-reporting occurs from age 11 through age 90). People respond to statements about sensory experiences in everyday life (e.g., "I like to walk barefoot in the grass") by saying how frequently the statement is true, using a five-point Likert-type scale (almost never to almost always).

Early studies involved a national sample of more than 1,000 children without disabilities. Occupational therapists had been asking families about their children's responses to sensory experiences as a routine part of their therapy assessments and intervention planning. However, since therapy was directed at children who were having difficulty, we only knew that many children with disabilities reacted frequently to sensory experiences. We did not know whether their peers without disabilities had similar or different responses. Therefore, these initial studies explored how peers without disabilities responded to the same sensory experiences to create a baseline performance expectation so we would know whether a child in therapy was reacting differently from peers.

Dunn (1999a) reported that children's responses were not only characterized by sensory systems (e.g., visual, touch, sound, etc.), which was expected, but could also be characterized by a pattern of responses that reflected thresholds and regulation. From this initial work, hypotheses were developed that evolved into Dunn's Model of Sensory Processing. This model was tested in subsequent studies of infants and toddlers (Dunn, 2002), adolescents, adults, and older adults (Brown & Dunn, 2002). The four patterns of sensory processing continued to emerge from factor analyses of these new populations, thus providing supporting evidence about these concepts.

Other researchers have provided evidence about the concepts in Dunn's model by comparing findings with physiological responses (e.g., Corbett, Schupp, Levine, & Mendoza, 2009; McIntosh, Miller, Shyu, & Hagerman, 1999; Schaaf, Miller, Seawell, & O'Keefe, 2003). They report that there is a complex relationship between sensory processing patterns and other physiological responses that indicate the status of the nervous system. Other researchers have used EEG technology and report that children with challenges in sensory processing as evidenced by *Sensory Profile* reporting have less ability to control sensory input when compared to peers without difficulties and seem to have a different pattern for developing sensory control mechanisms (Davies, Chang, & Gavin, 2009; Davies & Gavin 2007). Findings such as these suggest that we can ask about daily experiences and obtain information that indicates the status of other physiological mechanisms.

Consistent with the normative findings from Dunn (1997) and with patterns expected from a bell-curve distribution, Ben-Sasson, Carter, and Briggs-Gowan (2009) found that 16 percent of children with typical development 7–11 years old were bothered by touch or auditory sensations. Children in this "overly responsive" group had more dysregulation and less adaptive social behaviors than the rest of the sample. Gere, Capps, Mitchell, & Grubbs (2009) found similar patterns of sensitivity in children who are gifted. They linked the sensitivity to two other common characteristics of children who are gifted, their superior problem-solving ability, and their challenges with social relationships.

There is a growing body of evidence linking food preferences, eating, and feeding challenges with sensory processing. Children with typical development who were identified as "picky eaters" based on eating habits and scores on the *Sensory Profile* also had poorer appetites, had a more limited food repertoire, gagged, and bit their lips/cheeks more often when compared to peers (Smith, Roux, Naidoo, & Venter, 2005). In a comparison of children with Autistic Spectrum Disorder (ASD) to their siblings, children with ASD had significantly more eating problems primarily related to narrow food choices (Nadon, Feldman, Dunn, & Gisel, in press). Janvier and Rugino (2004) analyzed the records of a multidisciplinary feeding team and found that children grouped into "sensory-based feeding disorder" (SBFD), "sensory motor feeding disorder" (SMFD), and "nonsensory feeding disorder" (NFD). The children with the SBFD and SMFD had limited tolerance for taste, texture, and temperature of foods; children with SBFD were intolerant of mealtime structure; and children with SMFD had oral motor difficulties, such as having trouble moving food around in the mouth.

Researchers have also compared children with autism, Asperger disorder, Attention Deficit Hyperactivity Disorder (ADHD), and Fragile X syndrome to each other and peers without disabilities (Ermer & Dunn, 1998; Kientz & Dunn, 1997; Rogers, Hepburn, & Wehner, 2003; Tomchek & Dunn, 2007; Watling, Dietz, & White, 2001). They report that children with these disabilities have more intense reactions to sensory experiences than their peers without disabilities. Additionally, the groups of children with disabilities have different patterns from each other, suggesting that there are unique sensory patterns across these groups as well. Studies conclude that children with ADHD have significantly different sensory processing when compared to peers without ADHD (Dove & Dunn, 2009; Dunn & Bennett, 2002; Mangeot et al., 2001; Yochman, Parush, & Ornoy, 2004).

Others have reported that sensory processing patterns such as sensory seeking, sensory avoiding, and low registration occur more frequently in mental illness including obsessive compulsive disorder and schizophrenia (Brown, Cromwell, Filion, Dunn, & Tollefson, 2002; Reike & Anderson, 2009). Liss, Timmel, Baxley, and Killingworth (2005) found that parents with more sensory sensitivity also had more anxiety and depression. Atchison (2007) reports that there are sensory processing differences in children who have experienced trauma as well. The differences illustrate that matters of sensory processing in children with these disabilities is a legitimate area for consideration for research and practice.

A different approach is to link sensory processing with other aspects of children's performance. Minshew and Hobson (2008) linked sensory sensitivities with errors on perceptual tasks. There also appear to be relationships between sensory processing patterns and repetitive and stereotypic behaviors (Gabriels et al., 2008; Joosten & Bundy, 2008; Joosten, Bundy, & Einfeld, 2009; Wiggins, Robins, Bakeman, & Adamson, 2009; Zandt, Prior, & Kryios, 2009). Jasmin et al. (2009) reported a significant relationship between a person's level of reactivity to environmental stimuli, the tendency to avoid sensory input, and performance on daily living skills (e.g., overreacting to sounds might interfere with one's ability to get ready in the morning), even when cognition was controlled. Lane, Young, Baker, and Angley (2009) found a significant relationship between over-reactivity to sensory input (e.g., being overly sensitive to sounds, touch, etc.) and the "Maladaptive Behavior" scale on the Vineland Adaptive Behavior Scale. Active physical activities were a preference for Israeli children with atypical sensory processing patterns (Engel-Yeger, 2008). Sleep quality is also associated with sensory hypersensitivity in children who are typically developing (Shani-Adir, Rozenman, Kessel, & Engel-Yeger, 2009; Shochat, Tzischinsky, & Engel-Yeger, 2009).

Many studies report that children with ASD exhibit behaviors that reflect more intense sensory processing than peers. In a meta-analysis of 14 studies, Ben-Sasson, Hen, et al. (2009) reported that children with ASD exhibit both under- and over-responsivity to sensory experiences. Other authors also report significant differences in sensory processing patterns in children (Ashburner, Ziviani, & Rodgers, 2008; Cheung and Siu, 2009; Kern, Garver, Carmody, et al., 2007; Kern, Garver, Grannemann, et al., 2007) and adults with ASD (Crane, Goddard, & Pring, 2009; Kern, Garver, Grannemann, et al., 2007).

Ben-Sasson et al. (2007) compared 101 toddlers with autism with 100 typically developing toddlers and an additional 101 toddlers matched for mental age. Toddlers with ASD had significantly higher frequency of both under responsiveness and avoiding behaviors. This combined pattern of under-responding and avoiding was also reported by Dunn (2002). In another study, Ben-Sasson et al. (2008) examined the relationship between sensory processing patterns and social emotional status. They found that the 170 toddlers with ASD clustered into three groups of sensory patterns: low frequency of sensory symptoms (26%), high frequency of sensory symptoms (29%), and a combined pattern (45%). Children in the second and third groups had more negative emotions, depression, and anxiety than children in the first group, even when controlling for severity of ASD. The authors recommend that professionals consider the contribution of sensory processing to other aspects of ASD. Although it may seem contradictory at first, this pattern is visible in children's behavior. When one observes children with autism, there is a pattern of not responding to stimuli in the environment, and then something can trigger the child to notice and respond. The response can be very dramatic, with either intense aggression or withdrawal, both avoiding responses that get the child away from what is perceived to be dangerous or unfamiliar. This combination of failing to notice and overreaction upon noticing creates little room for engaging with the environment for learning. Knowing and managing a child's sensory needs throughout the day can mediate this dilemma of having very little time in the "ready-to-learn" state.

Other authors have examined specific sensory processing systems in children with ASD. Kern, Garver, Carmody, et al. (2007) reported that persons with ASD responded more frequently to movement sensations than matched controls. Jones et al. (2009) reported that a subgroup of adolescents with ASD (20%) were very sensitive to auditory discrimination tasks. In interviews with parents of children with and without ASD, they said they were more likely to associate their children's behaviors with sensory responses; food experiences were most common negative reports.

SENSORY PROCESSING AS A UNIVERSAL HUMAN EXPERIENCE

A very important and unexpected finding grew out of the sensory processing conceptual research. It began as a means for verifying that the right questions were being asked about children's experiences with sensory input to detect differences that mattered in everyday life. If every 5-year-old child reacted to touch in a certain way, that reaction should not be considered a marker of a problem. However, it became clear that responses to sensory events were on a continuum. Even though children with certain disabilities had more intense reactions, there were also a small number of children (and adults) in the typical population that also had those reactions (Dunn, 2008b). For example,

Ben-Sasson, Carter, and Briggs-Gowan (2009) found that 16 percent of children with typical development between 7 and 11 years old were bothered by touch or auditory sensations. This is the expected estimate of children who would fall above the +1 standard deviation mark on the bell curve. Gere et al. (2009) found similar patterns of sensitivity in children who are gifted; this is a special group of children, but not a group we would consider "disabled." In fact, Gere et al. (2009) suggested that their sensitivity may be a reason why they have better problem-solving skills (i.e., they notice more details and relationships, so they have more options for solving problems). Therefore, it seems we must be more cautious about automatically concluding that there is a dysfunction or disorder based solely on one's patterns of sensory processing.

On the other hand, the challenges that matter to providers and researchers are those that interfere with the child's and family's everyday life. We all know someone among our family and friends who is sensitive to sound or touch, and most of the time these persons have found strategies for managing their circumstances so their sensitivity does not interfere with daily routines and general life satisfaction. When parents know their child is sensitive to sounds, parents might make sure there is a separate room as a play option when visiting family. This also means that we must consider the parent's, the teacher's, and the sibling's/playmate's sensory processing patterns as we apply this approach in our practices. Preschool teachers with different sensory processing patterns prioritized different child traits as the most "teachable pupils" (Coffelt, 2004), suggesting that an approach that considers the caregivers' sensory patterns along with the children's patterns might be most effective.

When we consider the body of work about sensory processing as evidence about the human experience rather than evidence only about disability, we also introduce new possibilities. Behaviors that might have been viewed as "dysfunctional" or "irritating" can now be viewed as "interesting" or "quirky" (Ali, 2007; Grinker, 2007) because more people understand how and why the behaviors occur, and they do not associate the behaviors with a disorder. Accessibility of buildings began as a way to include people with physical challenges; then all of us began to use these entry points (electronic doors, curb cuts) because they were easier for everyone. Perhaps if we make home, community, and school environments friendlier for all types of sensory processing patterns, there will be fewer triggers for those who have sensitivity or other patterns that might interfere.

HISTORICAL CONTEXT FOR SENSORY PROCESSING

Just as Arnold Gesell introduced the concept of looking at the evolution of children's developmental behaviors and milestones, A. Jean Ayres introduced the concept of using neuroscience knowledge to examine and interpret the meaning of certain behaviors in children with "minimal brain dysfunction." Early pioneers such as these opened the door to new ways of thinking and problem solving.

A sensory approach to considering the meaning of a child's behaviors evolved from the work of Ayres. She observed children who had "minimal brain dysfunction" and considered how to apply neuroscience knowledge to create new ways to provide therapy for these children (Ayres, 1972, 1979). Ayres's work involved gathering evidence from evaluating, observing, and serving children with differences in their responses to sensory experiences. Her research revealed groupings of behaviors that occurred more frequently than one would expect, and illustrated ways to address the life challenges a child faced with these different behavioral repertoires.

She used the term "sensory integration" to refer to these ideas and hypotheses in her research. Sometimes the term "sensory integration" is confusing when discussing these ideas with colleagues and parents, because sensory integration is also a term used in neuroscience to describe the principle about how the brain organizes sensory input. For neuroscientists, sensory integration is a neurological process of organizing sensory information from the body and environment (see Kandell et al., 2000). Ayres's research informed us about how children use information to respond appropriately to environmental demands (i.e., how they create "adaptive responses"). Her interventions tapped the children's motivation to play and interact; she also referred to this therapy approach as "sensory integration."

Ayres's work is built on three core concepts (Ayres, 1963, 1972, 1979; Clark, Mailloux, & Parham, 1985; Clark, Mailloux, Parham, & Bissell, 1992; Fisher, Murray, & Bundy, 1991; Kimball, 1999). First, a person's ability to take in and organize sensory input (i.e., sensory integration) is a foundation for being able to interact with the environment. Second, sensory integration provides the foundation for cognitive development and emotional regulation. Third, our daily routines are full of sensory experiences, and because they are useful patterns of behaviors (e.g., getting dressed, taking a bath), the sensory input within our routines supports cognitive and emotional development. A Sensory Integration approach is an application of sound neuroscience knowledge (see Kandell et al., 2000). Ayres did not create the neuroscience foundational knowledge; she built applied science hypotheses on them. Factor analytic studies revealed patterns of performance that are indicative of specific performance difficulties (Ayres, 1972; Ayres & Marr, 1991; Fisher et al., 1991). These early studies made it possible to understand the role of sensory experiences in behavior and performance.

Miller, Anzalone, Lane, Cermak, and Osten (2007) built on Ayres's work and proposed a taxonomy that they believe will enhance diagnostic specificity. Working with focus groups and the literature, they proposed three categories of "Sensory Processing Disorder." In their taxonomy, "Sensory Modulation Disorder" includes children who are over-responsive, under-responsive, or who seek/crave sensory input. "Sensory Based Motor Disorder" includes children who have challenges with posture and stability or who have difficulty planning movements (called "dyspraxia"). The third category, "Sensory Discrimination Disorder," refers to children who have difficulty identifying the similarities and differences needed to make more precise decisions about input and actions. This approach reflects an underlying belief that it is important to identify a "disorder," and that this precision (if it can be achieved) will lead to more useful research findings and development of effective interventions.

Not everyone believes that taking a "disorder" approach is best. Studies using the *Sensory Profile* assessments revealed that there are core concepts about sensory processing that apply to the general population, not just children with specific disabilities (Dunn, 2008a). This broader view is built on Ayres's research and illustrates how knowledge grows and is influenced by policy and service systems. We are serving children and families in very different contexts today than Ayres and her colleagues had available in hospitals and segregated schools, so we can also consider additional ways to extend our knowledge to be relevant to today's demands.

COMPARISON OF SENSORY APPROACHES IN THE LITERATURE

With all this debate, it is challenging for interdisciplinary colleagues and parents to figure out what to do about sensory approaches in their EI and EC programs. In occupational therapy, there is a "Practice Framework" that outlines the domain of concern in occupational therapy. This framework provides a structure for comparing a "sensory integration" approach with a "sensory processing" approach.

The emphasis of a *sensory integration approach* is on the child's skills, capacities, and challenges that are interfering with everyday life. Knowing a child's difficulties in sensory processing, a therapist would set out to change or fix these difficulties so the child could interact better. For example, if a child is very sensitive to movement, one might structure increasingly challenging movement activities so the child would improve his movement processing. The idea is that when the child's ability to respond to movement input is broader, then his ability to play and interact with the other children will also be better.

The emphasis of a *sensory processing approach* is on the child's contexts and activities in everyday life. In this approach, a therapist would consider how to adjust task demands, objects, room placement, and routines so that they supported the child's sensory processing strengths and minimized sensory processing challenges. The idea here is that when the context and activities are more "friendly" to the child's sensory processing patterns, then the child's ability to participate in everyday life activities at home and school will also increase.

SUMMARY REVIEWS OF SENSORY APPROACHES TO INTERVENTION

Baranek (2002) conducted a summary review of sensory and motor interventions for children with autism and provided nine recommendations for education based on her findings. She reported that because of the prevalence of sensory processing challenges for children with autism, professionals need to create environments that accommodate their unique sensory needs in the functional context of educational goals. Accommodations might take the form of changing performance expectations, modifying activities to reduce a potentially upsetting sensory experience, or bypassing challenging areas to increase participation success. Baranek also commented on the importance of children being part of their educational program as much as possible, and recommended applying intervention ideas within the context of inclusive education rather than in isolated, traditional treatment sessions. She also stated, "thus, best practice would suggest that functional activities integrated into daily routines within naturalistic contexts increase retention and generalization of skills" (p. 419). Baranek recommended a conservative approach to including specific individual sensory or motor treatments, suggesting a short-term approach with frequent progress monitoring to decide whether to continue or change approaches.

Pollock (2009) wrote an evidence brief about sensory integration, summarizing her review of the available literature. She reports about studies of what she calls "classical" sensory integration therapy (SIT; one-to-one intervention with a therapist in a clinical environment with special equipment); as research methodologies have become more rigorous, results have been less favorable to "classical SIT." She also states that there have been some positive effects when sensory processing approaches have been used to make sensory-based changes in the activities and contexts that support children's participation (e.g., to increase on-task behavior and decrease self-stimulatory behavior; see Fertel Daly, Bedell, & Hinojosa, 2001; Smith, Press, Koenig, & Kinnealey, 2005; VandenBerg, 2001). She summarized that this area continues to be debated and studied. She recommended that attention be given to adapting children's environments; educating families, teachers, and other team members; and creating clear, functional, and measurable goals that can be used to mark progress. Pollock also recommended that "classical SIT" be considered a trial to be evaluated for effectiveness with individual children until further evidence makes decisions more clear about this approach.

Both of these reviews recommend intervention approaches that are embedded in children's everyday lives. This approach is compatible with EI/EC literature about natural environment interventions (Dunst, Bruder, et al., 2001; Dunst, Hamby, Trivette, Raab, & Bruder, 2000; Dunst & Raab, 2004; Hanft & Pilkington Ovland, 2000), person- and family-centered care principles (Dempsey & Dunst, 2004; Dunst, 1997, 2002; Trivette, Dunst, Boyd, & Hamby, 1996) and capacity-building approaches (Rush, Shelden, & Hanft, 2003). Therefore, it is appropriate to examine how to integrate sensory processing evidence with other evidence-based approaches to more readily enhance outcomes for children whose sensory processing patterns interfere with participation.

APPLICATION OF SENSORY PROCESSING CONCEPTS FOR EI/EC PRACTICES

Sensory Processing Knowledge as Part of Interdisciplinary EI/EC Practices

The *Workgroup on Principles and Practices in Natural Environments* (2008) reviewed current interdisciplinary literature and identified key evidence-based principles for serving children and families in natural environments. They recommended that for children to have the best functional outcomes, services need to be provided in the exact places that children live, play, and learn and need to be embedded into the routines of their everyday lives. They indicated that providers need to focus on children and family strengths and interests and work to build the capacity of the family and other providers to support the child across developmental periods. Parents and children profit from guidance that is directed at improving everyday participation. For example, parents were successful at finding and providing opportunities for their young children with ASD after only six sessions of review and practice (Vismara, Colombi, & Rogers, 2009).

Effective interventions must be built on an accurate appraisal of what is interfering with participation. A sensory processing approach intersects with these principles by focusing specialized knowledge on children's and families' routines, strengths, and capacities. Sensory processing knowledge provides additional insights into what might be interfering with the child's ability to participate with the family and at school. For example, if a child is a picky eater, it might be because the child is expressing independence or trying to be defiant. It might also be that the child is sensitive to some of the sensory aspects of food, including the texture, temperature, flavor, or smell of the food (Smith, Roux, et al., 2005). When we know sensory processing patterns might be a factor, we have the chance to make sure that we interpret the child's behavior precisely.

For example, to examine the relationship between sensory processing patterns and daily life activities, researchers examined play patterns in 53 preschool children without disabilities. They wanted to determine whether there were differences in play schemas for children with different sensory processing patterns (Mische-Lawson & Dunn, 2008). They coded body positions and toys across several play periods (i.e., five-minute coded observation periods adding up to 30 minutes per child). Children with more "avoiding" patterns from the *Sensory Profile* also had significantly fewer body positions during play. Children with more "seeking" characteristics were more likely to play with miniature pretend toys or vehicles. They suggest that therapists may need to take children's sensory processing patterns into account when planning activities.

Preschool teachers may also approach their work differently based on their sensory processing patterns (Coffelt, 2004). Sixty-seven preschool teachers completed the Adolescent Adult Sensory Profile and the Teachability Questionnaire, which asks what student traits are most important for teaching in the classroom. Teachers with extreme "seeking" patterns expected students to exhibit a high degree of personal/social traits (e.g., friendly, sense of humor, empathetic) and had lower expectations for demonstration of school-appropriate behaviors (e.g., follows directions, enjoys schoolwork). Teachers with extreme "avoiding" patterns had lower expectations of students across all areas. The authors suggest that therapists might need to provide related services based on both the child's and teacher's sensory processing patterns.

SITUATING SENSORY PROCESSING KNOWLEDGE WITHIN CORE PRINCIPLES

Researchers have tested hypotheses about the application of sensory processing concepts within children's natural environments (Fertel Daly et al., 2001; Schilling & Schwartz, 2004; Schilling, Washington, Billingsley, & Deitz, 2003; Stephenson & Carter, 2009; VandenBerg, 2001). Summarizing the neuroscience literature, some of these authors explain the organizing features of certain kinds of sensory input. For example, sensation in the muscles and joints (called proprioception) and firm touch on the skin (called touch pressure input) are part of the discriminatory sensory system (Kandell et al., 2000). This means that these sensory inputs contribute to maps of the body, muscles, and joints in the brain; it also means that these sensory inputs do not add to levels of arousal that might be distracting to a person (Dunn, 1998).

With this background, researchers proposed that children who are distracted, or who have trouble focusing, might profit from increased "discriminatory" input to their skin, muscles, and joints during activities that require focused attention. One application of "discriminatory" touch pressure and proprioceptive input has been the use of a weighted vest. Researchers have applied different amounts of weight for different amounts of time to children with ADHD (VandenBerg, 2001) and ASD (Cox, Gast, Luscre, & Ayers, 2009; Deris, Hagelman, Schilling, & DiCarlo, 2006; Fertel Daly et al., 2001; Morrison, 2009). The single subject designs revealed that some children improved attention and work product or decreased self-stimulatory behaviors that interfered with participation. Critiques of these studies point out that not everyone improved with this intervention (Morrison, 2009; Stephenson & Carter, 2009); figuring out who profits from this intervention will increase precision of evidence-based practices.

Other authors have applied the same neuroscience principles to seating interventions for children with ADHD and ASD (Schilling, 2006; Schilling et al., 2003; Schilling & Schwartz, 2004). Sitting on a flexible surface, such as sitting on a ball chair (an exercise-type ball with a stand to steady it on the floor) provides natural opportunities for the child to make body adjustments without leaving one's seat. Comparing regular chairs to ball chairs, researchers reported that children were more attentive and productive when using the ball chairs. In one of the studies, the teacher indicated that she would like to continue using the ball chairs, and children without disabilities indicated that they could pay better attention when using the ball chairs.

The weighted vests and ball chair studies provide examples of interventions that reflect sensory processing concepts and are applied in the natural environment to support children's participation. Additional work of this nature will be needed to document which children, activities, and circumstances generate the best functional outcomes.

ILLUSTRATIONS OF SENSORY PROCESSING CONCEPTS APPLIED IN "CHILDREN'S ROUTINES"

Sasha's Parents Want Her to Play with Her Cousins

Sasha's parents want Sasha to play with her cousins who live nearby. Sasha is 20 months old, and the cousins are 18 and 30 months old. When the families get together to play, before long, Sasha becomes irritable and then gets more aggressive, and has to be separated from the other two children. Mom and dad are really frustrated about the situation because family ties are very important to them. Both sets of parents have been excited to have children of similar ages and to live nearby so they can foster these strong bonds throughout their children's childhood.

The parents get connected with the local Infant Toddler (I/T) Service System, and a provider visits their home. The I/T services decided that an occupational therapist would be the primary provider for this family after reviewing initial information. The occupational therapist visits the home to get to know the parents and Sasha, completes the

Asset-Based Context Matrix (ABC) (Wilson, Mott, & Batman, 2004) and plans a time to visit when the cousins are coming over. With the information from this initial visit, Sasha and her family qualify for services; the occupational therapist asks the early educator and the behavior specialist to participate on Sasha's team.

Since the parents' primary concern is Sasha interacting successfully with her cousins, the team focuses on all the possible reasons why these interactions are unsuccessful now. They generate developmental, behavioral, and sensory processing ideas based on the parents' descriptions, and the educator and behaviorist coach the occupational therapist about what to look for during her visit with the cousins and Sasha's play time. The occupational therapist also takes the Infant Toddler Sensory Profile (ITSP) (Dunn, 2002) so the parents can complete the questionnaire and provide additional information about possible reasons why Sasha is struggling to play with her cousins. Table 5.1 illustrates what the team might generate as hypotheses from different conceptual frameworks.

During the next visit, the occupational therapist observed the cousins playing together. Sasha was clearly excited to see her cousins, and they went to the play area together. They played with blocks, all contributing to a structure; the older child continued to monitor the block placements, "improving" the stability as they went. Sasha's first outburst occurred when the structure collapsed and the blocks

Table 5.1 Examples of Ideas Generated about Sasha's Behavior

Behavior of concern: Sasha gets irritable and aggressive when playing with cousins

Framework for thinking	Possible reason for behavior	What we might do to support Sasha's participation
Developmental	The play is too advanced for her developmental level	Adjust the play routines to include Sasha's competence and interests
Behavioral	She wants attention or control over the toys/ situation	Create options for her to choose; model sharing, taking turns
Sensory Processing	She is overwhelmed by sounds, or touch, or movements	Identify what sensory mechanisms are challenging and make adjustments in play routines to accommodate Sasha's needs

showered onto the three of them. The other two shrieked with delight; Sasha began to cry. The adults calmed her and the situation and redirected the children into more structured parallel play for the rest of the visit.

Reporting back to the team, it seemed that the play was developmentally appropriate for Sasha, and the occupational therapist reported that Sasha had offered some blocks to her cousin, suggesting she was learning to share. The blocks falling on her, and the sounds of the children and the blocks, seem to be the trigger for Sasha to get irritable. Combining this observation with the ITSP findings led the team to hypothesize that Sasha might need some adjustments based on her sensory processing needs. The ITSP revealed that Sasha was more "sensitive" than other children, and that touch and sounds were more challenging for her than movement, visual, taste, or smell.

At the next visit, the occupational therapist shared her observations about all the things Sasha did well and how well they had structured the situation for the children. They also discussed the findings from the ITSP and the hypothesis about Sasha's sensitivities with the parents. With this information, the parents offered some additional examples of Sasha being sensitive, including at the grocery store, getting dressed and bathed, and at the park. They generated ideas together about how to rearrange challenging situations to reduce how much sound and touch she has to manage. For example, they discussed what toys the cousins could play with that would not be as noisy as the blocks.

They also discussed her favorite clothing items and what made them Sasha's favorites. The parents realized that Sasha likes more formfitting clothing like tights and other stretchable pieces. She did not have trouble with diapers but was not transitioning to panties very well. They discussed finding alternatives that were firm and evenly fitted to her skin to reduce irritability that can occur with loosely fitting undergarments (which stimulate the light-touch receptors that trigger more arousal [see Dunn, 1998; Kandell et al., 2000]). Since the parents understood this new reason why Sasha might become irritable, they could look at all their life routines in a new way.

Across time, the parents became more aware of the situations and circumstances that were challenging for Sasha and immediately began to problem-solve how to adjust factors in Sasha's favor. As Sasha had more successful experiences, she became more flexible as well; her repertoire of adaptive strategies increased as her parents enabled her to have more successful participation.

Peter's Teachers and Parents Need Him to Be Successful at Preschool

Peter is 4 years old, and he attends a neighborhood preschool program. The teachers and parents are increasingly concerned about Peter's activity level during the day. As he has grown and become more mobile, it seems that he cannot find enough ways to move nor is there enough time to satiate his movement needs. His movement is starting to interfere with his ability to engage with age-appropriate toys, tabletop activities, and interacting with peers in both structured and free-play situations. The parents and teacher both enjoy Peter, and they are concerned that his cognitive and emotional development might be at risk if they do not learn how to support Peter properly. The preschool has an occupational therapist who serves as a consultant for the program, and they get parents' permission to ask for her guidance.

The occupational therapist comes to the school to meet the teacher and observe Peter. She also calls the mother prior to the visit to find out the parents' ideas about the situation. Since she serves as a consultant, the occupational therapist is familiar with the curriculum and overall routines of the preschool. They employ a strengths-based model, which identifies and builds on children's abilities and skills to support their participation in age-appropriate activities.

His teacher marvels at Peter's creativity with his body. She explains that she can suddenly see Peter hanging upside down from a table or laying on a counter with his upper body cascading over the edge to look into the shelves (rather than walking up to them and looking in like the other children). He has a hard time sticking with activities, even those that the teacher would say are his preferred activities, such as playing soccer outside. His mother reports that Peter "jettisons" everywhere when he is moving, and when he wants to watch TV, he always finds some interesting way to place his body, such as dangling over the arm of the couch to watch upside down. She also says that getting ready in the morning is a nightmare for her because Peter keeps leaving his room to "fly" or "hop" somewhere else.

The occupational therapist observes some of these same behaviors when she visits the preschool. She also retrieves the ABC Matrix (Wilson et al., 2004) the parents and teacher completed together at the beginning of the year. She leaves the Sensory Profile School Companion (SC), a version of the questionnaire for teachers to complete about their students, for the teacher to complete and sends the *Sensory Profile* (Dunn, 1999b, 2006a) home for the parents to complete. These standardized tests can provide validity evidence for the observations and interview data already collected.

The parents, teacher, and occupational therapist meet one afternoon when the parents are coming to get Peter from preschool. This fits their work schedules and provides an opportunity to talk when Peter is still in his after-school group activities. They begin by discussing all of Peter's endearing and helpful characteristics. He is curious and enthusiastic about life and is always ready to try new things. He learns quickly, except when moving interferes with his attention to tasks. Other children want to play with Peter and seek him out during activities. The teacher comments that even with all the movement that interferes, he still seems to hear what is going on; he can answer questions and repeat what someone else said. This surprised the teacher at first, because she could not imagine that Peter was listening in the group. Parents laugh because Peter will repeat directions from his grandma about slowing down and he will say "Slow down, Peter" as he changes to slow-motion moving momentarily.

The occupational therapist summarizes the SP and SC by showing the parents and teacher that they agree about Peter's sensory processing patterns (sometimes the SP and SC are somewhat different, reflecting the importance of the school and home contexts for supporting or interfering with performance; see Dunn [2006b, 2008a] for explanation and details about this measure). It was no surprise to the teacher and parents that Peter seeks movement input much more than other 4-year-olds.

The occupational therapist explained that Peter's particular pattern of seeking seems to emphasize sensory input to the receptors in the muscles and joints that respond to pushing and pulling (i.e., the proprioceptive system). When Peter hangs upside down, jumps, and hops, he is introducing intense input to his body; jumping presses the joints and muscles together, while hanging pulls them apart because of the force of gravity. His father says he plays tennis and gets those sensations when his feet hit the pavement and when he slams the ball across the net. His mother comments that she insists that dad play tennis because he is unbearable without it. The occupational therapist points out that dad playing tennis is his way of getting the proprioceptive input just like Peter is hanging and jumping right now.

As they discuss further, the teacher, parents, and occupational therapist brainstorm ways for Peter to get extra sensory input throughout the day and ways to adjust those situations so he can get the input he needs without disrupting his participation. Table 5.2 illustrates an

Table 5.2 Portion of Peter's Activity Analysis to Determine Sensory Processing Options

Time	What Peter is typically doing	What Peter currently does to get movement/ joint input that interferes with participation	Options for meeting sensory needs within these activities
7:30 a.m. (home)	Getting up Getting ready for school Eating breakfast	Gets up quickly when called Runs up and down the halls, fleeing from bedroom where clothes are	Set up clothing in different parts of the house so Peter has to move a lot to gather his underwear, socks, shoes, etc. Place clothing in less convenient areas (e.g., higher on shelves) so he has to stretch to get them, activating his muscles and joints within the "getting dressed" routine
8:30 a.m. (transition)	Driving to preschool	Looks out windows Pushes feet against front seat	Place a cooler or other solid object under Peters feet so he has something to push against while sitting in his car seat
9:00 a.m. (preschool)	Good morning routine Structured cognitive activity Snack Free play Creative expression	Very fidgety in chairs, on carpet squares, disrupting lessons Leads physical play with other children	Have Peter sit on a movable inflated cushion in his chair so he can "fidget" without getting up as often Provide a "standing" place for Peter during morning routine Give Peter the book or easel to hold (the extra weight of the objects provides proprioception by pulling the muscles/joints apart as he holds the objects)
Noon	Lunch	Tries to leave lunch area frequently Eats very little	Have Peter help with passing out drinks, etc., by holding the full tray (weight) and moving around the table to serve others Use the moving cushion on his chair while he is eating

activity analysis of a typical day with suggestions for the parents and teacher to try to keep Peter on track. As the year progressed, the teacher and parents began to understand Peter's sensory processing needs and how these either supported or interfered with Peter's participation at school and home. Each time the occupational therapist checked in with them, they had more stories about ways they had made adjustments to support Peter. For example, the parents signed him up for karate lessons. They observed that these lessons created a structure for Peter's sensory needs, so instead of looking chaotic and random, he began to "practice his karate" a lot. They also included a seat cushion in Peter's school routines when he entered public school; Peter began to notice that it was a helpful strategy for him in class as well.

These two case studies provide a brief version of how sensory processing knowledge can be embedded into the children's routines to enhance outcomes. As stated earlier, sensory processing is intertwined with other approaches to support children in their natural environments, making these interventions consistent with other current interdisciplinary evidence-based practices for EI/EC services.

Table 5.3 provides a few examples of strategies that can be used in everyday life activities to support children's participation using a sensory processing approach. You will notice familiarity in the activities because they are good activity options for young children in general. Detecting the sensory processing aspect of activities enhances professionals' ability to design individually tailored interventions that meet children's precise needs as they participate in their daily life activities and routines.

Table 5.3   Examples of Ways to Support Children's Participation Based on Sensory Processing Patterns

Ideas for supporting participation for children who SEEK sensation	Ideas for supporting participation for children who do not REGISTER sensation
• Use soaps with textures imbedded in them to increase sensation to the skin	• Provide toys that make sounds while playing with them so the child gets more input
• Place favorite toys in harder to get places to increase climbing, crawling, etc.	• Have child look for things as you shop or run errands to increase visual interest
• Paint one wall with chalkboard paint so the child has chances to touch the	• Encourage barefoot play on a variety of surfaces (carpet, tile, wood, grass)

(Continued)

Table 5.3   (Continued)

chalk, feel the texture of the wall when drawing on it • Add texture to handles and other toy surfaces so the child gets more touch input	to activate sensory input to the child's feet • Place mirrors at floor level to provide opportunity for visual feedback about play
Ideas for supporting participation for children who AVOID sensation	*Ideas for supporting participation for children who are SENSITIVE about sensation*
• Create play area with space away from other children to decrease sensory chaos during play • Use unscented products to clean toys to reduce the smell sensations for the child • Select undergarments with wide bands that fit evenly against the skin to decrease irritation that may come from thin elastic edges • Have seating available so young children don't have to be held all the time; holding children provides continuously changing input to the skin and may be overwhelming • Place plain sheets over toy shelves to reduce visual distractions	• Let the child pick own wash cloth to find one that the child can tolerate on the skin • Keep shades drawn and add light sparsely to reduce the light the child has to manage • Notice where vents blow in your home and direct them away from the child's seating or play areas to reduce the breeze on the child's skin • Limit the time you spend in large family gatherings because these situations are full of unpredictable sensory experiences that can overwhelm the child

Source: Excerpts from Dunn, W. (2008). *Living sensationally understanding your senses.* London: Jessica Kingsley Publications. Used with permission.

SUMMARY

Sensory processing is one of several perspectives for understanding and interpreting children's behaviors. Sensory processing can be overlooked because it is so intricately part of the overall human experience. Evidence reveals that there are four sensory processing patterns for people across the life span (seeking, avoiding, sensitivity, and registration); although everyone has certain patterns of sensory processing in their repertoire, children and adults with specific disabilities seem to experience a more intense version of these patterns in their everyday lives. The intensity of their sensory responses can interfere with their activities throughout the day. When professionals and families understand how sensory responses guide a child's experiences, more options emerge for supporting the child's participation.

Evidence does not currently support the use of segregated sessions for classical sensory integration therapy. Rather, interdisciplinary literature guides us to think about how to embed sensory processing strategies into children's and families' routines to support participation in settings where it matters and where the child gets more chances to practice. More research is needed to specify precisely which children, conditions and settings are best for the application of sensory processing knowledge in these imbedded routines.

REFERENCES

Ali, L. (2007). You and your quirky kid. *Newsweek*, September 17.

Ashburner, J., Ziviani, J., & Rodger, S. (2008). Sensory processing and classroom emotional, behavioral, and educational outcomes in children with autism spectrum disorder. *American Journal of Occupational Therapy, 62*(5), 564–573.

Atchison, B. J. (2007). Sensory modulation disorders among children with a history of trauma: A frame of reference for speech-language pathologists. *Language, Speech, and Hearing Services in Schools, 38*(2), 109–116.

Ayres, A. J. (1963). The development of perceptual motor abilities: a theoretical basis for treatment of dysfunction. *American Journal of Occupational Therapy, 17*, 221–225.

Ayres, A. J. (1972). *Sensory integration and learning disorders*. Los Angeles: Western Psychological Services.

Ayres, A. J. (1979). *Sensory integration and the child*. Los Angeles: Western Psychological Services.

Ayres, A. J., & Marr, D. (1991). Sensory integration and praxis tests. In A. Fisher, E. Murray, & A. Bundy, *Sensory integration theory and practice* (p. 203). Philadelphia, F. A. Davis.

Baranek, G. T. (2002). Efficacy of sensory and motor interventions for children with autism. *Journal of Autism and Developmental Disorders, 32*(5), 397–422.

Ben-Sasson, A., Carter, A. S., & Briggs-Gowan, M. J. (2009). Sensory over-responsivity in elementary school: Prevalence and social-emotional correlates. *Journal of Abnormal Child Psychology, 37*(5), 705–716.

Ben-Sasson, A., Cermak, S., Orsmond, G. I., Tager-Flusberg, H., Carter, A. S., Kadlec, M. B., & Dunn, W. (2007). Extreme sensory modulation behaviors in toddlers with autism spectrum disorders. *American Journal of Occupational Therapy, 61*(5), 584–592.

Ben-Sasson, A., Cermak, S. A., Orsmond, G. I., Tager-Flusberg, H., Kadlec, M. B., & Carter, A. S. (2008). Sensory clusters of toddlers with autism spectrum disorders: Differences in affective symptoms. *Journal of Child Psychology and Psychiatry, 49*(8), 817–825.

Ben-Sasson, A., Hen, L., Fluss, R. Cermak, S. A., Engel-Yeger, B., & Gal, E. (2009). A meta-analysis of sensory modulation symptoms in individuals with autism spectrum disorders. *Journal of Autism and Developmental Disorders, 39*(1), 1–11.

Brown, C., & Dunn, W. (2002). *The Adult Sensory Profile*. San Antonio, TX: Psychological Corporation.

Brown, T., Cromwell, R., Filion, D., Dunn, W., & Tollefson, N. (2002). Sensory processing in schizophrenia: Missing and avoiding information. *Schizophrenia Research 55*(1–2), 187–195.

Cheung, P., & Siu, A. (2009). A comparison of patterns of sensory processing in children with and without developmental disabilities. *Research in Developmental Disabilities*, August 6.

Clark, F., Mailloux, Z., & Parham, D. (1985). Sensory integration and children with learning disabilities. In P. Pratt & A. Allen (Eds.), *Occupational Therapy for Children* (p. 384). St. Louis, MO: Mosby.

Clark, F., Mailloux, Z., Parham, D., & Bissell, J. C. (1992). Sensory integration and children with learning disabilities. In P. Pratt & A. Allen (Eds.), *Occupational Therapy for Children* (pp. 457–507). St. Louis, MO: Mosby.

Coffelt, K. (2004). The relationship between sensory processing patterns and expectations of students' performance in preschool teachers. *Occupational Therapy Education*. Kansas City, MO: University of Kansas. Master of Science in Occupational Therapy.

Corbett, B., Schupp, C., Levine, S., & Mendoza, S. (2009). Comparing cortisol, stress and sensory sentivitity in children with autism. *Autism Research, 2*(1), 39–49.

Cox, A. L., Gast, D. L., Luscre, D., & Ayers, K. M. (2009). The effects of weighted vests on appropriate in-seat behaviors of elementary-age students with autism and severe to profound intellectual disabilities. *Focus on Autism and Other Developmental Disabilities, 24*(1), 17–26.

Crane, L., Goddard, L., & Pring, L. (2009). Sensory processing in adults with autism spectrum disorders. *Autism 13*(3), 215–228.

Davies, P., Chang, W., & Gavin, W. (2009). Maturation of sensory gating performance in children with and without sensory processing disorders. *International Journal of Psychophysiology, 72*, 187–197.

Davies, P., & Gavin, W. (2007). Validating the diagnosis of sensory processing disorders using EEG technology. *American Journal of Occupational Therapy, 61*(2), 176–189.

Dempsey, I., & Dunst, C. J. (2004). Helpgiving styles and parent empowerment in families with a young child with a disability. *Journal of Intellectual and Developmental Disability 29*(1), 40–51.

Deris, A. R., Hagelman, E. M., Schilling, K., & DiCarlo, C. F. (2006). Using a weighted or pressure vest for a child with autistic spectrum disorder. Retreived from http://www.eric.ed.gov/PDFS/ED490780.pdf

Dove, S., & Dunn, W. (2009). Sensory processing patterns in learning disabilities. *Occupational Therapy in Early Intervention, Preschool and Schools, 2*(1), 1–11.

Dunn, W. (1997). The impact of sensory processing abilities on the daily lives of young children and families: A conceptual model. *Infants and Young Children, 9*(4), 23–35.

Dunn, W. (1998). Implementing neuroscience principles to support habilitation and recovery. In C. Christiansen & C. Baum, *Occupational therapy: Achieving human performance needs in daily living*. Thorofare, NJ: Slack.

Dunn, W. (1999a). *The Sensory Profile*. San Antonio, TX: Psychological Corporation.

Dunn, W. (1999b). *The Sensory Profile Manual*. San Antonio, TX: Psychological Corporation.

Dunn, W. (2001). The sensations of everyday life: Theoretical, conceptual and pragmatic considerations. *American Journal of Occupational Therapy, 55*(6), 608–620.

Dunn, W. (2002). *The Infant Toddler Sensory Profile*. San Antonio, TX: Psychological Coorporation.

Dunn, W. (2006a). *Sensory Profile School Companion*. San Antonio, TX: Psychological Corporation.

Dunn, W. (2006b). *Sensory Profile Supplement*. San Antonio, TX: The Psychological Corporation.

Dunn, W. (2008a). Harnessing teacher's wisdom for evidence based practice: Standardization data from the Sensory Profile School Companion. *Journal of Occupational Therapy, Schools, and Early Intervention, 1*(3–4), 206–214.

Dunn, W. (2008b). *Living sensationally understanding your senses*. London: Jessica Kingsley Publications.

Dunn, W., & Bennett, D. (2002). Patterns of sensory processing in children with attention deficit hyperactivity disorder. *Occupational Therapy Journal of Research, 22*(1), 4–15.

Dunn, W., & Brown, C. (1997). Factor analysis on the Sensory Profile from a national sample of children without disabilities. *American Journal of Occupational Therapy, 51*(7), 490–495.

Dunn, W., & Westman, K. (1997). The sensory profile: The performance of a national sample of children without disabilities. *American Journal of Occupational Therapy, 51*(1), 25–34.

Dunst, C. J. (1997). Conceptual and empirical foundations of family-centered practice. In R. J. Illback, C. T. Cobb et al. (Eds.), *Integrated services for children and families: Opportunities for psychological practice* (pp. 75–91). Washington, DC: American Psychological Association.

Dunst, C. J. (2002). Family-centered practices: Birth through high school. *Journal of Special Education, 36*(3), 139–147.

Dunst, C. J., Bruder, M. B., Trivette, C. M., Hamby, D., Raab, M., & McLean, M. (2001). Characteristics and consequences of everyday natural learning opportunities. *Topics in Early Childhood Special Education, 21*(2), 68–92.

Dunst, C. J., Hamby, D., Trivette, C. M., Raab, M., & Bruder, M. B. (2000). Everyday family and community life and children's naturally occurring learning opportunities. *Journal of Early Intervention, 23*(3), 151–164.

Dunst, C. J., & Raab, M. (2004). Parents' and practitioners' perspectives of young children's everyday natural learning environments. *Psychological Reports, 94* (1), 251–256.

Engel-Yeger, B. (2008). Sensory processing patterns and daily activity preferences of Israeli children. *Canadian Journal of Occupational Therapy, 75*(4), 220–229.

Ermer, J., & Dunn, W. (1998). The sensory profile: A discriminant analysis of children with and without disabilities. *American Journal of Occupational Therapy, 52* (4), 283–290.

Fertel Daly, D., Bedell, G., & Hinojosa, J. (2001). Effects of a weighted vest on attention to task and self stimulatory behaviors in preschoolers with pervasive developmental disorders. *American Journal of Occupational Therapy, 55*(6), 629–640.

Fisher, A., Murray, E., & Bundy, A. (1991). *Sensory integration theory and practice.* Philadelphia, PA: F. A. Davis.

Gabriels, R., Agnew, J., Miller, L. J., Gralla, J., Pan, Z., Goldson, E., et al. (2008). Is there a relationship between restricted, repetitive, stereotyped behaviors and interests and abnormal sensory response in children with autism spectrum disorders? *Research in Autism Spectrum Disorders, 2*(4), 660–670.

Gere, D., Capps, S., Mitchell, D., & Grubbs, E. (2009). Sensory sensitivities of gifted children. *American Journal of Occupational Therapy, 63*(3), 288–295.

Grinker, R. (2007). *Unstrange minds: Remapping the world of autism.* Cambridge, MA: Basic Books.

Hanft, B., & Pilkington Ovland, K. (2000). Therapy in natural environments: The means or end goal for early intervention? *Infants and Young Children, 12*(4), 1–13.

Janvier, Y., & Rugino, T. (2004). Characteristics of sensory based feeding disorders and sensory motor feeding disorders in children. *Journal of Developmental and Behavioral Pediatrics, 25*(5), 381.

Jasmin, E., Couture, M., McKinley, P., Reid, G., Fombonne, E., & Gisel, E. (2009). Sensori-motor and daily living skills of preschool children with autism spectrum disorders. *Journal of Autism and Developmental Disorders, 39*(2), 231–241.

Jones, C., Happe, F., Baird, G., Simonoff, E., Marsden, A., Tregay, J. et al. (2009). Auditory discrimination and auditory sensory behaviours in autism spectrum disorders. *Neuropsychologia*, June 21.

Joosten, A., & Bundy, A. (2008). The motivation of stereotypic and repetitive behavior: Examination of construct validity of the motivation assessment scale. *Journal of Autism and Developmental Disorders, 38*(7), 1341–1348.

Joosten, A., Bundy, A., & Einfeld, S. (2009). Intrinsic and extrinsic motivation for stereotypic and repetitive behavior. *Journal of Autism and Developmental Disorders, 39*(3), 521–531.

Kandell, E., Schwartz, J., & Jessell, T. (2000). *Principles of neural science.* New York: McGraw Hill.

Kern, J. K., Garver, C. R., Carmody, T., Andrews, A. A., Trivedi, M. H., & Mehta, J. A. (2007). Examining sensory quadrants in autism. *Research in Autism Spectrum Disorders, 1*(2), 185–193.

Kern, J. K., Garver, C. R., Grannemann, B. D., Trivedi, M. H., Carmody, T., Andrews, A. A., & Mehta, J. A. (2007). Response to vestibular sensory events in autism. *Research in Autism Spectrum Disorders, 1*(1), 67–74.

Kientz, M. A., & Dunn, W. (1997). Comparison of the performance of children with and without autism on the Sensory Profile. *American Journal of Occupational Therapy, 51*(7), 530–537.

Kimball, J. (1999). Sensory integrative frame of reference. In P. Kramer & J. Hinojosa (Eds.), *Frames of reference for pediatric occupational therapy* (pp. 169–204). Baltimore: Williams & Wilkins.

Lane, A., Young, R., Baker, A. E., & Angley, M. T. (2009). Sensory processing subtypes in autism: Association with adaptive behavior. *Journal of Autism and Developmental Disorders, 40*(1), 112–122.

Liss, M., Timmel, L., Baxley, K., & Killingworth, P. (2005). Sensory processing sensitivity and its relation to parental bonding, anxiety and depression. *Personality and Individual Differences, 39*, 1429–1439.

Mangeot, S. D., Miller, L. J., McIntosh, D. N., McGrath-Clarke, J., Simon, J., Hagerman, R., & Goldson, E. (2001). Sensory modulation dysfunction in children with attention-deficit-hyperactivity disorder. *Developmental Medicine and Child Neurology, 43*(6), 399–406.

McIntosh, D., Miller, L., Shyu, V., & Hagerman, R. (1999). Sensory modulation disruption, electrodermal responses and functional behaviors. *Developmental Medicine and Child Neurology, 41*(9), 608–615.

Miller, L., Anzalone, M., Lane, S., Cermak, S., & Osten, E. (2007). Concept evolution in sensory integration: A proposed nosology for diagnosis. *American Journal of Occupational Therapy, 61*(2), 135–140.

Minshew, N., & Hobson, J. (2008). Sensory sensitivities and performance on sensory perceptual tasks in high functioning individuals with autism. *Journal of Autism and Developmental Disorders, 38*(8), 1485–1498.

Mische-Lawson, L., & Dunn, W. (2008). Children's sensory processing patterns and play preferences. *Annuls of Therapeutic Recreation, 17*, 1–14.

Morrison, E. (2009). A review of research on the use of weighted vests with children on the autism spectrum. *Education, 127*(3), 323–327.

Nadon, G., Feldman, D., Dunn, W., & Gisel, E. G. (in press). Mealtime problems in children with autism spectrum disorder and their typically developing siblings: A comparison study. *Autism*.

National Early Childhood Technical Assistance Center (NECTAC). (2008). Workgroup on principles and practices in natural environments. Retrieved from http://www.nectac.org/topics/families/families.asp

Pollock, N. (2009). Sensory integration: A review of the current state of the evidence. *OT Now, 11*(4), 6–10.

Reike, E., & Anderson, D. (2009). Adolescent/adult sensory profile and obsessive-compulsive disorder. *American Journal of Occupational Therapy, 63*(2), 138–145.

Rogers, S., Hepburn, S., & Wehner, E. (2003). Parent report of sensory symptoms in toddlers with autism and those with other developmental disorders. *Journal of Autism and Developmental Disorders, 33*(6), 631–642.

Rush, D., Shelden, M., & Hanft, B. (2003). Coaching families and colleagues: A process for collaboration in natural settings. *Infants and Young Children, 16*(1), 33–47.

Schaaf, R., Miller, L., Seawell, D., & O'Keefe, S. (2003). Children with disturbances in sensory processing: A pilot study examining the role of the parasympathetic nervous system. *American Journal of Occupational Therapy, 57*(4), 442–449.

Schilling, D. (2006, Spring). Alternative seating devices for children with ADHD: Effects on classroom behavior. *Pediatric Physical Therapy, 18*(1), 81.

Schilling, D., Washington, K., Billingsley, F. F., & Deitz, J. (2003). Classroom seating for children with attention deficit hyperactivity disorder: Therapy balls versus chairs. *American Journal of Occupational Therapy, 57*(5), 534–541.

Schilling, D. L., & Schwartz, I. L. (2004, August). Alternative seating for young children with autism spectrum disorder: Effects on classroom behavior. *Journal of Autism and Developmental Disorders, 34*(4), 423–432.

Shani-Adir, A., Rozenman, D., Kessel, A., & Engel-Yeger, B. (2009). The relationship between sensory hypersensitivity and sleep quality of children with atopic dermatitis. *Pediatric Dermatology, 26*(2), 143–149.

Shochat, T., Tzischinsky, O., & Engel-Yeger, B. (2009). Sensory hypersensitivity as a contributing facrot in the relation between sleep and behavioral disorders in normal school children. *Behavioral Sleep Medicine, 7*(1), 53–62.

Smith, A., Roux, S., Naidoo, N. T., & Venter, D. (2005). Food choices of tactile defensive children. *Nutrition, 21*(1), 14–19.

Smith, S., Press, B., Koenig, K., & Kinnealey, M. (2005). Effects of sensory integration intervention on self-stimulating and self-injurious behaviors. *American Journal of Occupational Therapy, 59*, 418–425.

Stephenson, J., & Carter, M. (2009). The use of weighted vests with children with autism spectrum disorders and other disabilities. *Journal of Autism and Developmental Disorders, 39*(1), 105–114.

Tomchek, S., & Dunn, W. (2007). Sensory processing in children with and without autism: A comparative study utilizing the Short Sensory Profile. *American Journal of Occupational Therapy, 61*(2), 190–200.

Trivette, C. M., Dunst, C. J., Boyd, K., & Hamby, E. (1996). Family-oriented program models, helpgiving practices, and parental control appraisals. *Exceptional Children, 62*(3), 237–248.

VandenBerg, N. (2001). The use of a weighted vest to increase on-task behavior in children with attention difficulties. *American Journal of Occupational Therapy, 55*(6), 621–628.

Vismara, L., Colombi, C., & Rogers, S. (2009). Can one hour per week of therapy lead to lasting changes in young children with autism? *Autism, 13*(1), 93–115.

Watling, R., Dietz, J., & White, O. (2001). Comparison of Sensory Profile scores of young children with and without autism spectrum disorders. *American Journal of Occupational Therapy, 55*(4), 416–423.

Wiggins, L., Robins, D., Bakeman, R., & Adamson, L. B. (2009). Brief report: Sensory abnormalities as distinguishing symptoms of autism spectrum disorders in young children. *Journal of Autism and Developmental Disorders, 39*(7), 1087–1091.

Wilson, L., Mott, D., & Batman, D. (2004). The asset-based context matrix: A tool for assessing children's learning opportunities and participation in natural environments. *Topics in Early Childhoold Special Education, 24*(2), 110–120.

Yochman, A., Parush, S., & Ornoy, A. (2004). Responses of preschool children with and without ADHD to sensory events in daily life. *American Journal of Occupational Therapy, 58*(3), 294–302.

Zandt, F., Prior, M., & Kryios, M. (2009). Similarities and differences between children and adolescents with autism spectrum disorder and those with obsessive compulsive disorder: Executive functioning and repetitive behaviour. *Autism, 13*, 43–57.

Chapter 6

Teaching English-Language Learners: Proven Strategies and Instructional Practices

Susan M. Moore and Clara Pérez-Méndez

THE CHILDREN IN OUR WORLD

Understanding our changing world in early care and education demands recognition of the growth of a multicultural plurality and the growth in linguistic diversity among our youngest children. It is fact that among all children in the United States, more than one in five speak a language other than English at home (Federal Interagency Forum on Child and Family Statistics, 2010). Early care and education providers need also note that the fastest-growing population in the United States is young children ages birth to 6 of foreign-born immigrants; 96 percent of these children are also U.S. citizens. Among children in immigrant families, it is estimated that 72 percent speak a language other than English at home (Capps, Michael, Ost, Reardon-Anderson & Passel, 2004). In 2007, about 16.4 million children, or more than one in five children in the United States, had at least one immigrant parent (Matthews & Ewen, 2010).

Although it is recognized and documented that the ability to speak two languages has many advantages in terms of cognitive, academic, social, and economic benefits (August & Hakuta, 1997; Bialystok, 2001; Genesee, Paradis, & Crago, 2004; Hakuta, 1986; Lindholm-Leary, 2005; Yoshida, 2008), it is also recognized that linguistic diversity can be a barrier to access and equity in early childhood education (Barrera, 1993; Barrera, Corso, & Macpherson, 2003; Moore & Pérez-Méndez, 2006). This complexity can be overwhelming to parents and family members who want what is best for their children. If no one in the household speaks English well, the family is likely to encounter difficulties, accessing child care or early education programs, talking with children's teachers, and accessing health and other early intervention services (Hammer, Lawrence, & Miccio, 2007; Moore & Pérez-Méndez, 2006; Shields & Behrman, 2004). Data indicate that among children in immigrant families, 26 percent live in linguistically isolated households where no one age 14 or older has a strong command of the English language (Shields & Behrman, 2004). Current research also provides evidence that it should no longer be assumed that just because a child is identified with a disability, they cannot benefit from learning more than one language (Genesee et al., 2004; Kohnert, 2008; Tabors, 2008). Growing evidence implies that maintaining home language regardless of disability may strengthen a child's ability to transfer to learning a second language, while enhancing connections to culture, heritage, and communication with family, and establishing a strong self-identity (Espinoza, 2008; Genesee et al., 2004; Kohnert, Yim, Nett, Kan, & Duran, 2005; Pérez-Méndez & Moore, 2004; Restrepo et al., 2010; Winsler, Diaz, Espinoza, & Rodriguez, 1999). Parents and family members need information to make informed decisions about the languages their children will learn (Pérez-Méndez & Moore, 2004).

A key challenge in early childhood is to support each and every child in their development of learning languages and developing literacy by addressing their learning needs, including in this effort the increasing number of children who speak languages other than English. At the same time, it is critical to identify and provide early intervention to those who also may have a disability. This requires careful and accurate identification of early language challenges that might signal or identify a language disability from those language differences associated with influencing factors of dual language learning. To distinguish a language difference from a disability, one must understand factors and patterns of second-language acquisition and typical bilingual behaviors (Kohnert, 2008; Moore & Pérez-Méndez, 2006; Tabors, 2008) as well as the sociocultural and historical factors (Sánchez, 1999a; Sánchez & Thorp, 2008) that can influence the learning of languages and development of literacy among young dual language learners.

A critical piece of this challenge is also to prevent as well as reverse a long-standing history of misidentification, overrepresentation, and underrepresentation of linguistically and culturally diverse learners in our school systems. In a seminal study, Dunn (1968) found that a significantly high proportion of minorities and/or children from lower SES backgrounds (60–80%) were identified as in need of special education services. Unfortunately, a disproportionate representation persists, despite the attention of the Office of Civil Rights and the U.S. Department of Education (Artiles, Rueda, Salazar, & Higareda, 2005; Artiles & Trent, 1994; Artiles, Trent, & Palmer, 2004; Gersten & Woodward, 1994; Guiberson, 2009; Ortiz & Yates, 1983). It is necessary to recognize the realities of our changing world and adopt a "cultural lens" (Sánchez, 1999a; Sánchez & Thorp, 2008) through which to view the cultural, linguistic, and ability diversity and strengths of our youngest children. This will enable early care and education providers to successfully share important information with families about current research in bilingualism and international adoption. It will also help providers implement culturally and linguistically responsive teaching strategies with each and every child during the early childhood years.

The purpose of this chapter is to highlight the changing demographics here in the United States, implications for practice, what we know from research, what are some of the myths and misconceptions regarding second language acquisition and/or English-language learners, and proven strategies that can help all diverse children and their families.

DEMOGRAPHICS: CURRENT AND FUTURE TRENDS

If current trends continue, the demographic profile of our earliest learners will change dramatically as we strive to address the developmental and early education needs of our early childhood population. The PEW Research Center (Passel & Cohn, 2008) projects the racial and ethnic mix of our population will look quite different in 2050, with a significant increase in the Hispanic and Asian populations. Projections are based on trends over the past 50 years, during which immigration patterns of both authorized and unauthorized groups have influenced the profile of our early childhood population. In 2005, new immigrants and their U.S.-born descendants accounted for 51 percent of the population increase. It is projected that from 2005 to 2050, 82 percent of the population increase will be related to new immigration.

An examination of the demographic changes currently underway across the United States provides a context and rationale for identifying key strategies that address the needs of the growing number of young children who may or may not have variations in abilities, and who are learning English as a second language. In 2000, it was predicted that the growth of populations from culturally and linguistically diverse backgrounds in the United States would supersede all prior growth in demographic statistics. At that time, it was estimated that one out of five children would be exposed to a language other than English in their homes during their early childhood years. In 2000, 47 million (18%) in the United States spoke a language other than English or another language in addition to English, including numerous students who were learning English as a second language (U.S. Census, 2000). In 2001, approximately 4.6 million students were learning English as a second language in U.S. schools, representing an increase of 105 percent since 1990, and it was estimated that 79 percent of these students spoke Spanish (Goldstein, 2004; Kindler, 2002).

In fact, in 2007, 21 percent of school-age children in the United States spoke a language other than English at home, and 5 percent of school-age children both spoke a language other than English at home and were reported to have difficulty speaking English. Sixteen percent of school-age Asian children and 18 percent of school-age Hispanic children both spoke another language at home and had difficulty with English. About 6 percent of school-age children not only spoke a language other than English at home, but lived in a linguistically isolated household. A linguistically isolated household is one in which all persons age 14 or over speak a language other than English at home and no person age 14 or over speaks English "very well." In 2008, 56 percent of U.S. children were white, non-Hispanic; 22 percent were Hispanic; 15 percent were black; 4 percent were Asian; and 5 percent were "all other races." The percentage of children who are Hispanic has increased faster than that of any other racial or ethnic group, growing from 9 percent of the child population in 1980 to 22 percent in 2008. By 2050, it is projected that one in four children in the United States will be of Hispanic origin (Federal Interagency Forum on Child and Family Statistics, 2010). It is important to consider that a high percentage of children who enter school from non-English-speaking homes speak Spanish. However, over 300 different languages are spoken or represented in the U.S. population, and nearly 6 percent of the U.S. population does not speak English (Capps et al., 2004; Hernandez, 2004). Adoption of children from foreign countries has also increased significantly. Over 126,000 visas were issued between 2001 and 2006, with close to 20,000 visas issued in 2006 alone (U.S. Department of State, 2009). Although numbers of internationally adopted children have not continued to markedly increase, implications for education do continue. The composition of our early childhood population reflects these changes. It is critical to address linguistic and cultural variables impacting our young dual-language learners and to understand the current and future demands upon early childhood educators and providers to successfully address their learning needs.

IMPLICATIONS FOR PRACTICE

Early childhood educators and specialists have long recognized the importance of understanding child development as the foundation for addressing the learning needs of all children. This implies our early childhood provider workforce must also understand the development and implications for learning for very young children from a variety of different cultures or who speak languages different from their own (Anderson, 2004; Barrera, 1993; Gay, 2002). Early childhood educators and specialists need to understand patterns of second-language acquisition (SLA), factors influencing dual-language learning (Genesee, 2008), as well as abilities to distinguish language differences from disorders (Genesee et al., 2004; Kohnert, 2008; Moore & Pérez-Méndez, 2003; Tabors, 2008). To do this, they must be familiar with current research about bilingualism and dual-language learners and consider all background variables when providing culturally responsive early learning opportunities. This involves sharpening of focus through use of a "cultural lens" to identify the strengths and resilience of each and every young learner in the context of their family, culture, language, and abilities (Sánchez & Thorp, 1998; Sánchez & Thorp, 2008; Westby, 1990, 2009). According to these authors, it is critical for educators to explore the meaning of culture and dimensions of cultural diversity for each and every child and family they work with. Educators and specialists are charged with linking authentic assessment to instruction and/or intervention as needed and can also be a conduit for families to information that informs decision making about language learning, school programs available, and community resources and support (Moore & Pérez-Méndez, 2003, 2006).

Changes in preservice and in-service personnel preparation of early care and education providers and specialists are needed to insure their development and ability to implement current research and evidence-based practices (Buysse, Castro, & Peisner-Feinberg, 2010; Maude, Catlett, Moore, Sánchez, & Thorp, 2006; Maude et al., 2010; NAEYC, 1995; Winton, McCollum, & Catlett, 2008). Most importantly, early education providers and specialists will best serve the youngest population of learners by developing an "additive disposition" toward linguistic diversity in their practice with both children and families (Gay, 2000, 2002). Genesee, Paradis, and Crago (2004) as well as Kohnert and Derr (2004) describe this as contexts where there is substantial support for continued development of a child's first language and maintenance as the child acquires a second language.

Gay (2000) underscores and expands this concept by calling for a "sea change" or paradigm shift from a deficit model of identifying children "at risk" for failure to a strengths-based view of children who come to a program rich in a cultural legacy and who are capable of becoming competent learners. This reframing of persistent viewpoints and attitudes, that speaking a language other than English is a "problem," and that these children are "at risk" for educational success, shifts the focus from changing the lives of children and families to "looking toward" how we respond as educators to this challenge. When reframed, an early childhood educator or specialist can focus on providing responsive teaching strategies by designing supportive environments, creating meaningful and engaging learning areas and activities, developing a plan and schedule that promotes child engagement and success, planning for transitions, maintaining clear expectations, and supporting and enhancing children's learning of languages, literacy, and their social-emotional development (Milagros-Santos, Cheatham, & Ostrosky, 2006; Tabors, 2008).

Establishing connections and partnerships with home by listening to families' stories (Sánchez, 1999; Westby, 1990, 2009), as well as information, priorities, and concerns about their children in the context of their cultural and/or linguistic backgrounds (Division for Early Childhood [DEC], 2002; Lynch & Hanson, 2003; Moore, Pérez-Méndez, & Boerger, 2006), will enhance trust and ongoing communication. In this context, information about current research regarding bilingualism and educational choices can be shared with parents and family members and considered when making decisions about what languages their children will learn.

WHO ARE THE CHILDREN?

José. At the age of 3, José came to his early childhood setting speaking Spanish as his first language. This was his first experience with English as he was the child of an immigrant family who spoke only Spanish in their home, although both parents were learning English as a second language. Although he had been born in the United States, up until this time he had been cared for by his grandmother who spoke only Spanish, so he had limited exposure to English. He appeared shy and withdrawn and had a difficult time separating from his mother during his first days and weeks in this new setting. His parents were confused as they wanted José to be a successful learner and do well in school. They considered speaking to José only in English as they thought he would learn it more quickly and be better prepared for first grade when the time came. However, they value their cultural heritage and did not want their son to lose connections with his culture and heritage as well as with his grandmother. They had to put him in preschool because she was elderly and was now having health concerns that prevented her from caring for him all day at home. Yet, his parents wanted him to learn English so he could be successful in his country of birth.

Kim. Kim came to his early childhood toddler group program based upon a referral from People's Clinic citing concern about his delays in language development. His family also had concerns as they reported he was not learning as fast as his older brothers and sisters. They reported he was not talking as well and he was very slow to learn new words in both Korean and English. They reported he was learning Korean as his first language, as they spoke this language at home, although he was exposed to some English because his older siblings were all learning English at school, and his father spoke English fluently. His parents thought he just might be slower to learn because he was "confused," since he really had no time to learn Korean before they came to the United States when he was 6 months old. They want him to be exposed to more English in an early childhood setting to see if he can learn English now that he is 2 years old. They are not sure if they will be returning to Korea after Kim's father completed his PhD program, yet expressed it is important to sustain their Korean language so their children could also maintain connections to their culture, extended family of grandparents, aunts, uncles, cousins, and friends who spoke Korean. They are concerned that this decision is interfering with Kim's acquisition of English and that he will have difficulty learning both languages.

Dara. Dara, a healthy and precocious child, was adopted by her American parents from China when she was two years old, but was reportedly having difficulty learning her Chinese language while still in her orphanage in China. Her parents brought her home where she quickly began to attempt to use English words because that was the only language spoken in the family. She discontinued using any Chinese words by the end of her first month in her new home. Her parents quickly sought out information and advice as her emerging English was often unintelligible to her parents and sister and to those who did not know her outside the family. She was obviously very bright and often made her intent known through gestures (such as head nods and shakes, pointing, and getting objects herself). She seemed quick to pick up English in terms of understanding but had significant difficulty being understood using her new language. Her parents were referred to an early intervention program (Part C), but she received services only for a short period of time before she turned 3 and was transitioned to district supports for preschool.

To learn more about the learning needs of these children in the classroom, their early childhood educators and specialists need to know what current research tells us about dual language learners and internationally adopted children. They need to understand the influencing factors that should be considered as they discover how these children are learning language(s) and apply this information to promoting each child's development in all areas.

WHAT WE KNOW FROM RESEARCH FINDINGS

Children who are bilingual possess a wide range of language proficiencies that are dynamic and change over time. This makes studying children who are bilingual more difficult than studying children who are monolingual (Bialystok, 2009; Espinoza, 2008; Genesee et al., 2004; Kohnert, 2008). Factors such as type of language learning, simultaneous or sequential; or age, amount of exposure, and interaction with a second language, can all influence patterns of learning a second language. Additional factors related to the biological and cognitive capacity, motivation, and personality of a young child can also influence how a child responds to learning a second language or more than one language, just as these factors can influence how a child learns a first language.

Given basic biological capacity, a social interactionist approach would suggest all children are capable of learning languages they are exposed to through responsive interactions and a language- and literacy-rich environment provided by parents, care providers, and teachers. However, various patterns may emerge based upon both internal and external influencing factors. External factors that also may impact a significant portion of young language learners include poverty, single-parent families, poor teaching, adoption at an older age, language barriers to accessing information, and/or early care and education. As noted, children learning more than one language or a second language present a wide range of language proficiencies that are dynamic and change over time. Children exposed to learning more than one language, as well as children who are adopted and thus no longer exposed to their first language, present complexities that demand thoughtful and intentional examination. As professionals, we need additional research to truly understand implications for educational reform (August & Hakuta, 1997; August & Shanahan, 2006; Genesee et al., 2004; Snow, 2006).

Research to date indicates factors such as type of acquisition, timing and age of exposure, and interaction in a second language, as well as internal factors that the child brings to the learning situation, influence the pattern of learning. External factors such as the sociocultural context for learning languages can also significantly influence the heterogeneity of patterns identified. For example, simultaneous learners, or those exposed to more than one language from birth, can demonstrate acquisition that results in different or similar developmental patterns and language behaviors as their monolingual peers (Patterson & Pearson, 2004; Pearson & Fernandez, 1993). Sequential learners of more than one language, those that are exposed to a new language after they have begun to learn their first language, also demonstrate a wider range of variability in rates and stages of language acquisition (Genesee et al., 2004; Kayser, 2008; Kohnert & Medina, 2009; Nicoladis & Genesee, 1997, Roseberry-McKibbin, 2003, Tabors & Snow, 2001).

Internal factors such as language aptitude, motivation, and strength of first language may all influence rate of learning a second language. External factors, such as exposure to comprehensible and intentional input through conversational interactions and participatory engagement of parents, is critical in learning a new language as well as maintaining language proficiency once achieved. Age of exposure, amount of use in first and second languages, language use with siblings, and other family members, language of play, and general language ability all can influence rate and variability (Nicoladis & Genesee, 1997). Other variables, such as adult language practices in the home, languages siblings use, language of instruction, access to languages (language community) and exposure to languages through media, need to be considered (Patterson & Pearson, 2004). However, it is critical to note that this information tells us more about what might be influencing emerging patterns in the development of languages and how to support the learning of language(s) versus focusing on the faulty interpretation that exposure to more than one language is a cause of language delay (Espinoza, 2008; Genesee, 2008; Restrepo, 1998). See Figure 6.1 for more information about internal and external influencing factors.

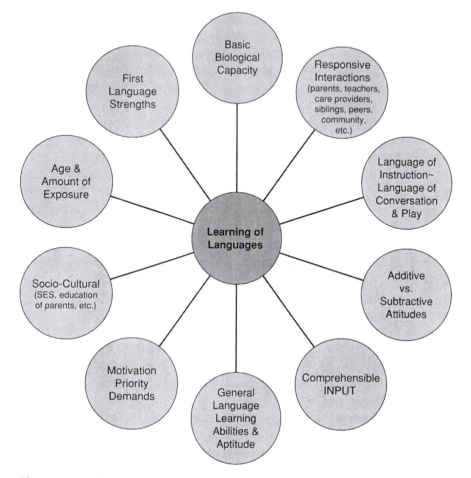

Figure 6.1   Internal and external: Influencing factors to learning of languages.

LEARNING MORE THAN ONE LANGUAGE IN EARLY CHILDHOOD

Many dual language learners in U.S. preschools or early care and education programs present themselves as sequential learners of English as their second language. Evidence suggests that anyone learning more than one language sequentially (after being exposed to their first language) follows certain stages/phases when meaningfully exposed to a second language (Krashen, 1982). These include silent receptive/comprehension, early production, speech emergence, intermediate fluency, and advanced fluency approaching proficiency. This basic continuum was later modified and applied to preschool children by Tabors (2008) based upon an ethnographic study of preschool-age children in a multilingual setting. Both of these authors, as well as many others (Cummins, 1989), describe the "silent period" or nonverbal phase followed by an early production phase and later productive language use similar to the increase in length and complexity of learning a first language. Cummins (1989), in particular, notes that oral language proficiency or basic interpersonal communication skills in a second language does not guarantee full linguistic proficiency in terms of listening, speaking, reading, and writing necessary for success in academic learning.

In the case of young sequential dual language learners, Tabors (2008) notes differences in how young children might adapt or cope with immediate exposure to a second language as the language of instruction in an early childhood setting. Some children are observed to continue to speak their first language for a short time until they realize they are not understood or it is "different." Other children might immediately become nonverbal while they listen and observe and try to "crack the code" of what is being said. Children who are motivated and feel comfortable "risking" may quickly imitate and use shortened phrases or words they hear to get results (e.g., "go home now," "my turn," "more please"). Children often begin use of "formulaic" speech and language (e.g., "I don't want to") that is a "prefabricated" chunk before they know the meaning of each word (Tabors, 2008). With time, exposure, and support, children are observed to demonstrate a syntactic understanding of the second language and move forward beyond the "chunks" to create and generate their own sentences that express their ideas and convey meaning. With more exposure and support, they become knowledgeable about more abstract vocabulary, and many eventually emerge as proficient in their second language. This resonates with the experience of many monolingual speakers who visit a different country and are immersed in a situation in which they cannot speak the language. Many might react by withdrawing, listening, and observing, yet eventually "risk" in an emergent way, speaking the unfamiliar language to become "conversational" in their new environment. Gradually, with use and exposure, proficiency continues to develop given consideration to the influencing factors that impact the learning of a second language.

With any second-language learner, certain bilingual behaviors emerge, such as first "language loss" associated with reduced exposure and interactions in the "first language." Language loss can be transitional during a period of inter-language, during which children may demonstrate semi-bilingualism; or it may be permanent if the first language is not supported and sustained, such as in the case of older children who are adopted into an English-speaking family and have no further exposure to their first language (Anderson, 2004; Wong Fillmore, 1991). It is critical to note that children who are adopted often present very distinct patterns from those children who continue to be exposed to more than one language and cannot be compared to those children who are truly becoming bilingual (Hwa-Froelich, 2007).

Many children who are learning a second language demonstrate cross-linguistic influence; transfer/interference from the first language may be exhibited as the second language is being learned. Findings suggest sequential learners bring conceptual, semantic, and morphological knowledge from their first language to learning a second language (August & Shanahan, 2006). More research is needed to completely understand and document exactly how the concepts of transfer and/ or interference support learning of languages. "Code switching" or "code mixing," the use of words from both languages in the same sentence, is commonly observed in bilingual speakers (Genesee, 2008; Genesee et al., 2004; Roseberry-McKibbin, 2003). In the case of a young sequential learner, these behaviors demonstrate a child's language-learning aptitude to discover how two different "codes" work. These behaviors are now considered typical and do not signal a delay, deficit, or disorder. Table 6.1 captures behaviors you might see consistent with continuity of second-language acquisition stages and phases of preschool-age sequential learners and responses by conversational partners and teachers that support ease of transition to higher levels and continued growth in second language acquisition.

MYTHS AND MISCONCEPTIONS

Will children learn a second language easily and effortlessly like "sponges," soaking up the new language through exposure alone?

Tabors and Snow (2001) suggest one of the most widespread and harmful myths impacting early care and education is that very young children will learn a second language automatically, quickly, and easily. It is assumed they do not need any special attention support, just exposure. Yet, the question remains, if left to their own learning

Table 6.1   Stages and Phases

The following stages with characteristic behaviors may be observed in young children who are dual-language learners. Suggested specific strategies for incorporation into classroom practices at the universal level are adapted from Tabors (2008) and Oster, McDonnell, and Jayaraman (2009). Recommended strategies are based upon keen observation of child behaviors and language level and are designed to support the child's ease with transition to high levels of second-language acquisition within a social context of predictable routines and engaging activities.
Stage: Home Language Use:

Observations: The child:

- Speaks to others in their home language yet slowly realizes he/she is not understood.
- May imitate nonverbal behaviors of others
- May experience rejection by peers
- Comprehension of English words is limited
- May develop nonverbal methods of communicating (gesture, leading, pantomiming)
- May exhibit signs of stress and appear withdrawn, overwhelmed, frustrated, and sad
- May begin to say "yes and no" or just shake head to indicate choices when asked

Response: Teachers and conversational partners can:

- Learn basic words in child's home language to help child comprehend and eventually engage in play and structured activities at nonverbal level
- Provide predictable classroom routines and use visual cues (pictures, props, real objects), especially as you introduce new words making input comprehensible
- Provide yes and no choices and initially reduce demands for verbal responses
- Spend extra one-on-one time to build trust and allow child to "take time" when overwhelmed, by creating a "safe haven" (e.g., book corner, quiet space, cozy corner)
- Use repetition in natural ways emphasizing key words
- Respond and encourage the child's home language speech attempts
- Facilitate the child's entry into play activities and serve as an interpreter for peers
- Focus on concepts that transcend culture, like family, food, animals, dance, etc.
- Respond to observed stress with comfort
- Design an environment that responds to and incorporates the culture of the child for all to share, such as familiar photos, books, toys, songs
- Engage and communicate with family members to learn more about the child

Silent Period/ Nonverbal:

(Continued)

Table 6.1   (Continued)

Observations: The child:

- Stops talking but may continue nonverbal communication attempts with gesture
- Demonstrates response to patterns and sounds of new language
- Responds to and demonstrates increased understanding of key vocabulary of new language
- Produces only a few utterances yet uses physical responses to make requests, protest, or initiate play with peers
- Relies heavily on contextual cues such as pictures and gestures of others and may appear to understand more of the new language as a result of imitating others and responding to contextual cues

Response: Teachers and conversational partners can:

- Use predictable routines to increase comfort level
- Continue to ask yes/no questions with minimal demand for verbal response
- Use props, real objects, and pictures to teach new words and concepts
- Repeat new words in various contexts
- Slow speech down to provide extra processing time
- Pre-read books in small group or one-on-one to introduce new vocabulary
- Continue communication with family to check on understanding and learn more about child's culture, routines, and likes and dislikes
- Provide prerecorded books in child's first language for use in the classroom
- Plan high-interest activities that build on child's prior knowledge
- Use secure, quiet places or activities that do not demand language use when child appears overwhelmed.

Telegraphic or Formulaic Language Use:

Observations: The child:

- Typically uses 1–2 word responses or short phrases ("I don't know"; "I need to go potty")
- Understands more vocabulary in new language
- With continued exposure to new language, will repeat words from conversations (but may not understand)
- Uses short phrases that include words from both languages (code switching)
- Continues to rely on contextual cues and familiar routines
- May often mispronounce words yet begins to discern segments
- May use emerging new language for socialization purposes

Response: Teachers and conversation partners can:

- Encourage and respond to all attempts to use new language
- Create safe environments to practice emerging skills
- Refrain from correcting but model correct usage
- Continue to make all input in new language comprehensible through use of contextual cues and daily or familiar routines
- Repeat words and phrases used

(Continued)

Table 6.1   (Continued)

- Reduce demands by providing additional processing time when asking questions and watch for behaviors that suggest stress or overload
- Ask questions that require one or two word responses and then model expansions of language use incorporating new vocabulary
- Encourage and set up "low-risk" social dialogues with peers and adults
- Facilitate peer support and interactions and connections to home

Productive Language Use

Observations: The child:

- Constructs short but grammatically correct sentences in the new language
- Sometimes demonstrates incorrect word use, word order, and pronunciation, especially as attempts longer utterances
- Learns new vocabulary every day; still relies on contextual cues to discern full meaning, but to a lesser extent
- Demonstrates stronger receptive language/comprehension of new language
- Can use words in social interactions and gradually improves use of academic language
- Continues to demonstrate increased proficiency as exposed to language and literacy rich environments and social interactions, but needs continued support to develop full academic language
- May become increasingly sensitive to mistakes

Response: Teachers and conversational partners can:

- Ask more open-ended questions to describe, compare, retell, predict.
- Continue to use comprehensible input to expand oral proficiency in new language
- Use and build on child's prior knowledge
- Describe more abstract and complex concepts in a meaningful context (e.g., before/after; same/different; etc.)
- Ask more cognitively demanding questions to engage child in high order thinking skills
- Provide opportunities for child to share knowledge and demonstrate level of growing proficiency in new language
- Maintain high expectations for age-appropriate performance and learning
- Maintain communication and connections with home to support activities that promote learning and enhance development

curve, are their needs being addressed in an optimal learning environment? Snow (2006) also notes that although there are a small number of studies that address bilingual children in the preschool period, those studies, for the most part, do not address questions related to the design of optimal learning environments that take into account the time and support to learn a second language. Many authors (Espinoza, 2008; Genesee et al., 2004; Moore & Pérez-Méndez, 2006; Sánchez & Thorp, 2008; Tabors, 2008) point out the need for starting

slowly with low demands for production of language when supporting young dual-language learners. Some children need supports to
overcome the "affective filter" of fear and anxiety that can accompany
stepping into an unfamiliar setting and not understanding the language
(s) being used. Sánchez (1999b) and Sánchez and Thorp (1998) further
elaborate that in settings where only one language is allowed to flourish
and home languages are explicitly or implicitly devalued, young children who are linguistically diverse often experience emotional reactions
as their home language is eliminated. They can be frustrated by the linguistic discontinuity between home and early education settings. Early
childhood educators and specialists need to use strategies that clearly
communicate that their setting is a safe, warm, and comforting environment, conducive to exploration and discovery that respects the languages and cultures represented by the children present. Strategies
such as learning a few words of the child's first language and open
respect and exposure to all children to both cultural and linguistic diversity in an authentic and meaningful way will often increase the feelings
of a "safe place" and enhance learning of a second language.

*Do children have to "give up" their first language to rapidly learn and
become proficient in a second language, especially when the second language
is the language of instruction?*

Snow (2006) provides evidence that young children can and will
learn a second language through supportive social interactions in an
additive environment that also recognizes that children do not have to
give up their first language to learn a second. Actually, there is emerging research that suggests eliminating first languages actually results
in lowered performance in overall learning and academics (Espinoza,
2008; Genesee, 2008; Sánchez & Thorp, 2008). More importantly, culture and language are considered the building blocks of self-identity
and connection to family. Elimination of language and often the associated cultural heritage, as critical components of growth and development in young children, may in fact lead to negative consequences of
discontinuity with language and learning, disconnection with family,
and disenfranchisement from community and heritage (Krashen,
1999; Nieto, 2000; Sánchez & Thorp, 2008; Tabors, 2008; Tatum, 2003;
Wong Fillmore, 1991).

*Will learning two languages during the early years overwhelm, confuse,
and/or delay a child's learning of English?*

Nicoladis and Genesee (1997) speak to this issue by explicitly noting
that nothing in scientifically based research would suggest the infant
brain is not capable of learning two languages. In fact, studies provide

evidence that young simultaneous learners of two languages can reach similar milestones in terms of perception, babbling first words, and growth in both understanding and ability to use two languages given an appropriately supportive environment (Kuhl, 2004; Patterson & Pearson, 2004; Pearson & Fernandez, 1993). Espinoza (2008) also contradicts this myth by citing examples from recent studies that suggest dual-language learners are not only capable of learning more than one language, but there are extended benefits in terms of brain plasticity that result (Mechelli et al., 2004). It is widely accepted that the benefits truly outweigh any short-term disadvantages as long as learning of both languages is fully supported. Learning of two languages does not cause a language delay.

Is there one or "a best way" to learn a second language?

Many believe the myth that the "best way" to learn a second language is to give up the first language while learning the second. In fact, this can compromise the learner, because "language loss" of the first language can produce contradictorily negative outcomes in terms of loss of self-esteem, connections to home and heritage, among other consequences (Wong Fillmore, 1991). Reviews of current research indicate that not only is giving up the first language neither necessary nor sufficient to learn another language, but it may be contraindicated in many situations resulting in lowered abilities in both languages (Genesee et al., 2004; Kohnert et al., 2005; Winsler et al., 1999). More recent research reviews indicate that "dual language programs" may be a preferred method of instruction (Espinoza, 2008; Lindholm-Leary, 2005). It is important to note that additional research is needed to determine results, amount of immersion, and conditions when one type of dual-language program is preferred over another. Specific types of dual-language programs, such as two-way immersion, integrate native English speakers and native speakers of another language and follow a systematic pattern of instruction in both languages. Barnett and colleagues (2007) compared a two-way immersion program to a monolingual English immersion program in preschool. Children in the two-way immersion program maintained growth patterns in both languages, whereas those in the monolingual English program gained only in English. It is important to note that there was no significant difference between groups in outcomes for English, but the two-way immersion group outperformed their counterparts in Spanish. Another variation involves heritage-language programs that mainly enroll students who are dominant in English but whose parents, grandparents, or other ancestors spoke the partner language. This model is prevalent for indigenous populations attempting to revitalize their language of heritage closely connected to tribal culture, life ways, and beliefs. It is important to recognize that sometimes there is no choice, and parents must place their children in schools with English instruction only. It is critical that early childhood educators increase awareness of patterns of language learning and address the learning needs of each and every child regardless of language of instruction.

REFRAMING MYTHS AND MISCONCEPTIONS

In analyzing the extant literature and emerging science related to dual-language learners, it is important to reframe prior myths and misperceptions into positive tenets that can drive evidence-based practice in early childhood education. Espinoza (2008) concludes there are several basic propositions that provide a foundation for encouraging the design of optimal early education learning environments that support dual-language learners. Recognizing that all children are capable of learning two languages, that language differences are in fact differences and not delays, and that bilingualism can be considered an asset are foundational concepts for changing early childhood practices. For too long, professionals have considered learning English as a second language as a "problem" that children bring to the classroom or, at the very least, that this signals a "risk" factor that negatively impacts learning. This belief may have more to do with other factors of influence such as poverty, or an unresponsive educational system with teachers who do not recognize the scientific findings related to the benefits of bilingualism and fail to understand how children can learn more than one language. Research claims young children can also benefit academically, socially, and emotionally from systematic support for the continued development of their first language, especially during the early years, from birth to age 8, when they are mastering sounds, structure, and functions of languages. This information is important to consider when determining evidence-based practices in early care and education for each and every child.

REFRAMING PRACTICE: FOCUS ON THE UNIVERSAL LEVEL

A "multitiered framework" or model of instruction and intervention has been used to describe how early care and education providers can design and scaffold learning opportunities for each and every child in their setting. The multitiered model has been used by many authors who use different terms in its application. Response to Intervention, or RtI (Burns, Appleton, & Stehouwer, 2005; Gersten et al., 2008), has been used to identify those children in kindergarten, first grade, and second grade who may demonstrate difficulties in learning to read. This model has been proposed and implemented to identify specific areas such as phonemic awareness, vocabulary, phonics, fluency, and comprehension (National Institute of Child Health and Development [NICHD], 2000) that can be improved by targeted intervention to allow children to succeed in establishing conventional reading abilities. The "pyramid model" (Hemmeter, Ostrosky, & Fox, 2006) and multitiered instruction have also been used to focus on prevention and early identification and direct implementation of strategies to address social and behavioral challenges in young children and students through positive behavior supports. These models have also been applied to early care and education (Coleman, Buysse, & Neitzel, 2006) to identify at an earlier age the pre-academic or learning challenges that many children face in establishing the foundations of language and literacy that impact later learning (see Figure 6.2).

As depicted in Figure 6.2, the *Universal Level* involves the foundation for early learning with active parent/family participation in which all children receive research-based, high-quality learning opportunities and curricula that incorporate ongoing universal screening, and progress monitoring. Expectations are taught; children gain world knowledge and learn developmentally appropriate information, including the foundations in language and literacy that support later conventional reading and writing. Interaction between child and adults as well as child to child are integrated into early leaning. The *Roadmap to Pre-K RTI: Applying Response to Intervention in Preschool Settings* (Coleman, Roth, & West, 2009), produced by the National Center for Learning Disabilities, reviews current practices regarding RTI for Pre-K. Across applications, data are used to inform teaching and individualize needs for each and every child. This includes universal strategies that specifically address the learning needs of young dual-language learners consistent with standards defined by state, federal, and professional organizations, such as the Division for Early Childhood of the Council for Exceptional Children (DEC/CEC) and the National Association for Education of Young Children (NAEYC).

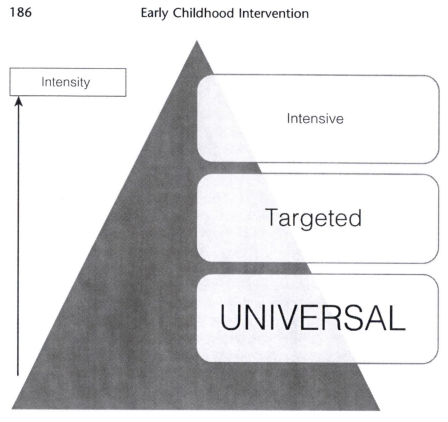

Figure 6.2   Tiered approach.

At the *Targeted Level*, children who are struggling in specific areas that might include academic, language, or social challenges, receive support for targeted challenges determined by data collected through observation. This involves staffing patterns that support the classroom teacher in problem solving and developing individualized learning goals and a plan for implementation. This might involve supplemental curriculum and instruction to the individual child or small groups of children. Assessing success of the instructional strategies, rate of child progress, and when to make changes in the individualized learning plan are integral to this process.

Need for Increased Intensity and Further Assessment

For those children who continue to struggle in specified areas, a staffing pattern that enables a specialized team to assist in the classroom with both intensive support for a child and for the classroom teacher, including the development, implementation, and evaluation of individualized instructional strategies. Data can then determine the need in some cases for referral for further in-depth assessment (e.g., Child Find; Mental Health Services). This three-tiered framework focuses on insuring that research-based and evidence-based practices in early education are integrated into all programs serving young children, including specific strategies designed to meet the needs of young dual-language learners at all three levels.

KEY STRATEGIES TO ENHANCE LEARNING OF YOUNG DUAL-LANGUAGE LEARNERS

Each and every child demonstrates variance in how they might respond as a simultaneous or sequential learner of more than one language. It is important to engage parent participation in determining how children, especially dual-language learners, can benefit from recommended practices and strategies at the universal level of a multi-tiered model. Refer to Table 6.1 for specifics regarding behaviors that might be observed in the preschool classroom or other early childhood setting with specific recommended practices to enhance growth and development of second-language learning.

José was reticent to leave his mother's side when he was dropped off at his preschool where English was the language of instruction. Even though his English-speaking teacher welcomed him with open arms, he initially withdrew from his teacher and the other children, most of whom spoke English. He would sit quietly, most often playing by himself, while observing all that went on around him. At snack time, he would respond by nodding if offered juice and crackers, and would sometimes point and gesture to indicate he wanted more, but was hesitant to engage or enjoy conversations with teachers or other children and would often gaze out the window with a solemn stare. When approached by other children to play, he would shake his head no and retreat to solitary play, while watching all that was going on around him. He would hold it together until his mother would reappear at the end of the session to pick him up and he would run into her arms speaking Spanish words with seeming relief. She would hold him and speak to the teacher about his day in English and often asked him questions about his day in Spanish. He would respond with whispered words and head nods and anxiously wait, sometimes with tears, until she was ready to leave. After a week of limited engagement and interaction, his teachers began to wonder if something was wrong with him. They tried over and over again to engage and include him in activities and play, but he would not respond. He seemed somewhat anxious, but was content to listen and to observe others; yet he played by himself. The other children began to ignore him and no longer attempted to include him in their play. His mother became increasingly distressed when told he was not joining in. Although he seemed content, he was not engaging in activities and play, but continued to watch and listen.

Are there specific strategies José's teachers could initiate that would help him adjust to his new preschool? What do they need to know? How can they find out? First, it would appear that they may need to know where José is in terms of both first- and second-language acquisition. Refer to Table 6.1. They know he has limited exposure to English in his home as both parents converse in Spanish, although they are learning English. However, his primary caregiver for three years has been his "abulita" (grandmother), who speaks only Spanish. It is necessary and helpful to learn more about his language learning in Spanish as well as his specific amount of exposure to English to better understand his behavior. Learning about the culture and the linguistic environments of each and every child in the classroom provides teachers with the information they need to create safe, comfortable settings for children "to risk" learning English as a second language. In reviewing the literature on stages and phases of learning a second language, his English-speaking teachers might assume he is "just in the silent/nonverbal period" and will "come around" with additional time and exposure to English in his classroom. However, there is danger in assuming this is the case until they explore with his parents all the factors that may be influencing his behaviors. During conversations with teachers, his parents share the fact that although José is a quiet and loving child, he speaks Spanish with all the family at home and will play with a young cousin his own age using Spanish to communicate. They feel he is developing Spanish typically for his age and will ask and answer simple questions, follow directions, tell his parents what he wants in sentences they understand, watch and understand TV in Spanish, and laugh and enjoy play with his dad, and he loves reading books with his mother at home. He tells his parents he does not like school because all the kids "talk funny."

Given this information from family (Restrepo, 1998), his teachers make more of an effort to engage José and actually use some Spanish words to converse with him. "Look at the house. House is casa in Spanish! You are so lucky to know Spanish. Tell me some other words in Spanish." The other children begin to also ask what a word means in Spanish and begin to understand that although José may be reticent to interact, he knows a lot of words in Spanish and understands more words in English each day. All the children bring pictures from home to make a book, *All About Me!* José's parents bring in pictures as well and this becomes a way for his teachers to learn more about him, the people in his life, and the words in Spanish to use when identifying his pictures and initiating conversations with him. His teachers "start slow" and do not demand that José produce the words in English, but they quickly learn he understands, through pointing upon request and imitating others, many more English words than they originally thought.

José becomes more comfortable taking the risk to imitate and even use some English words as his teachers make the effort to use gestures, pictures, objects, and actions to make sure "all input is comprehensible." He begins to enjoy activities like block building and playing cars alongside other children. He especially enjoys listening to stories like all the other children, especially when they are acted out with props and the new vocabulary is first introduced in a meaningful context. He demonstrates his comprehension of the narrative by taking a nonspeaking part in the story reenactment. His parents become more active in visiting and sharing songs and music they sing at home. Books in both Spanish and English appear in the cozy corner for children to look at and talk about. José begins to "warm up," becomes increasingly comfortable at school, and proceeds to learn more vocabulary words (August, Carlo, Dressler, & Snow, 2005), demonstrates increased comprehension of English, and eventually begins to use telegraphic phrases to request, protest, and respond during interactions with his peers. His parents and teachers work together in planning ways to enhance his learning of Spanish at home and his understanding and use of English in the classroom and in other situations with English-speaking peers. His parents also elect to attend a parent education and support program with other Spanish-speaking family members to enhance their understanding of early language and literacy development, bilingualism, and how they can enhance his development in both languages but continue to grow his first language at home through interactive story-book reading and focus on language during everyday routines, activities, and relationships (Moore & Pérez-Méndez, 2005b).

Kim's parents are concerned about his ability to learn two languages and need information and guidance from his teachers about how to proceed with their son's exposure to two languages. Although he appears to enjoy the play and interactive activities in his toddler group, he does not appear to be using either language as expected given exposure to both. His parents report he is beginning to use more words in Korean and actually strings two words together and produces simple phrases at home, but they are concerned that he refuses to imitate and attempt new words in English. His teachers observe that he seems happy to play alongside other children, yet very rarely interacts or responds to overtures by other children or adults in the classroom. His favorite activities are building with blocks by himself, playing in the "kitchen area" using elaborate sequences of stirring, pouring, and eating with pots, pans, and eating utensils that speak to emerging symbolic play, and he seems to enjoy looking through books. He will sit and watch others during story time but demonstrates minimal comprehension of what is going on in the book or story being read.

They wonder if they need some help and support to learn more about Kim's overall abilities, although they have no concerns about his motor development as he already uses crayons and pencils to make marks and "pictures," enjoys outdoor play, can complete simple puzzles with ease, and can move about with assurance, confidence, and with balance as he climbs stairs. They are clear that it seems his challenges are in language learning, but wonder if he is just moving through an expected nonverbal developmental stage of sequential language learning given his recent gain reported in Korean.

Given the wide range of variation reported in the literature for simultaneous learners of two languages, is Kim's current situation of concern? How can his teachers share information that will be helpful to his parents? What can they do in the inclusive toddler group program to learn more about Kim's abilities to understand and use language? It seems especially encouraging that Kim is using more Korean at home; however, more information as to his emerging development in Korean is needed to understand the level of his understanding and use of this language. After a conference with his parents, teachers learned they were using flash cards to attempt to elicit imitations of English vocabulary words and practice in using them.

What strategies might be more helpful in learning more about Kim's language abilities in both Korean and English? What could teachers do in the context of the toddler group to see if Kim is learning some English and understanding the meaning of English words? After several discussions, his teachers learned some Korean words that his parents reported he understood and used at home. They incorporated these words into their interactions with Kim during the day, especially words for greeting and food during snack and during his "kitchen play" partnered with words in English. Kim continues to enjoy play during his time in toddler group and seems to be responding well to the use of key vocabulary in Korean, as he smiles in recognition when his teachers use it. There is a focus on conversational "talk" using specific English vocabulary in meaningful contexts with pictures, props, and gestural cues (August et al., 2005). Ongoing communication with Kim's parents focused on meaningful contexts for learning new words during everyday routines, activities, and interactive book reading both in Korean at home with his mother and in English with his siblings and father. Kim began to attempt words in both languages. His parents, rather than demanding imitation of English words with flash cards, continued to converse with him in Korean and noted his growing abilities to use Korean at home. Kim reportedly is using some English words appropriately at home with his siblings (e.g., "hi" and "bye-bye") and is attempting some telegraphic language, including appropriate use of words and phrases in English both at home and school. He appears comfortable and confident in the classroom and is now very communicative, with use of gestures with vocal as well as verbal attempts to clarify his intent. He enjoys play and is engaging more often with peers. His teachers have decided to wait to request a referral for more assessment and to systematically implement their plan for increased exposure to English with high contextual cues and carefully record observed behaviors and progress in conjunction with ongoing communication with his parents. Within a year of preschool, with consistent exposure in both languages, Kim was demonstrating age-appropriate abilities in both languages.

Dara has a different story. She was adopted at 2 years of age from an orphanage in China by her parents who speak only English. She has an older sister, also adopted from China at 6 months, who is a proficient English speaker. Her sister is doing well in first grade and seemed to learn to speak in English and achieving developmental milestones well within normal expectations. Both of her parents are teachers. Once they brought Dara home, she began to attempt speaking only in English and even used English words to name them when they were first introduced to her in China. Yet, as she attempted more and more to speak in English, her speech was unintelligible to unfamiliar listeners. Her dad reported he could only understand certain words and not her attempts at simple sentences in English. Her mother said she had to ask her to repeat and often tried to distract her when she became frustrated with not being understood.

Dara's mother was able to understand more of her attempts than others, but realized Dara was having difficulty pronouncing English sounds. They sought help through the school district and ended up with a bilingual

Spanish-speaking speech and language pathologist as they were told her diffi-culty was related to bilingualism and difficulty learning a second language. Her child care teachers reported she was about 30 percent intelligible, and most peers did not attempt to engage her in play. At three and a half years of age, her parents were again concerned that there may be something going on besides learning English and sought a second opinion. They reported that within about a month of her adoption, Dara stopped attempting any Chinese words and also that providers in her orphanage had mentioned that she was difficult to understand in Chinese when she began speaking at about 22 months of age.

During the second evaluation, it was noted that although Dara was attempting to speak in English using word combinations and short sentences, she continued to have difficulty with motor programming of sequences sounds. She typically substituted many sounds for others and would drop all final consonants and syllables in words. She was observed to also transpose syllables as well as sounds in words, which continued to make her very diffi-cult to understand. She was an imaginative child, who loved to play dress up and dolls with her sister and would reenact complex scenarios in her play. She loved puzzles and was adept at completing them as well as learned all of her letters and primary numbers. She learned to write her name as well as other words. At preschool, she was noted to spend most free time engaged in complex puzzles, block designs, and building highly elaborate buildings. She freely talked a great deal and constantly inquired "Why?" in conversations.

She listened quietly to books and pointed to pictures accurately, and would attempt to name objects and pictures. She asked "why" questions consistently to keep the story going. Her receptive language and comprehension and cogni-tive skills were strengths. Dara's parents took advantage of intensive individ-ual and small-group speech therapy during the summer and noticed an increase in intelligibility of sound productions. As she became more intelli-gible and her speech became clearer, she engaged in longer and more complex sentence constructions during conversations, demonstrating her increased knowledge of English syntax and grammar. After nine months of intervention for speech, Dara was discontinued from services and reevaluated one year later, or four years post adoption. Although she continued to demonstrate some motor programming of complex sound sequences and persistent speech processes, this did not interfere with her overall intelligibility. Her parents reported significantly increased intelligibility at home and at school. Occasional syntactical rule system errors were noted in longer, more complex sentences during conversation; however, Dara seemed to self-monitor both her speech and expressive language. Abilities were judged to be within normal age expectations.

What does the research suggest regarding children who are adopted and are no longer exposed to interactions in their first language? First, children who are internationally adopted (IA) are bilingual only for a very short period of time if their parents do not speak the birth language. They become monolingual learners of a second language. Hwa-Froelich (2007) notes language development for these children significantly differs from multilingual children who remain exposed to birth languages. Research suggests children who are IA quickly lose any preestablished abilities in their first language within 3–12 months post adoption, and often "catch up" in speech and language within a few years. They acculturate to their new adoptive culture and learn language rapidly (Glennon, 2007a; Glennon & Masters, 2002; Hwa-Froelich, 2007). It is important to note that age of adoption influences subsequent patterns of language acquisition as well as variations demonstrated by children in institutionalized care versus foster care. According to Glennon (2007a, 2007b), toddlers like Dara, who were adopted at age 2, demonstrated expressive language development lagging behind receptive language at 12 months post adoption. Preliminary evidence from studies of children who are IA suggests initial assessments, within six months of adoption, when children demonstrate higher receptive abilities for this age group, can predict later successful expressive language development, with the majority demonstrating some delays but achieve scores falling within 1.25 SD of native-born children, one to two years later (Glennon, 2007a, 2007b; Hwa-Froelich, 2007). These data suggest young children who are IA and were adopted by 3 to 4 years of age can be assessed within six months to determine patterns of strength that can predict which children will do well and which will lag behind one year later. There are few reported large sample studies that have examined phonological development or articulation. However, preliminary evidence suggests very few children adopted from foreign countries display persistent articulation or phonological delays two years post adoption (Pollock, 1983, 2005; Roberts et al., 2005). Yet Dara was noted to demonstrate persistent phonological errors that interfered with intelligibility, suggesting intervention was needed. She responded positively and quickly to intensive intervention provided given high cognitive abilities, strengths in comprehension, and ability to self-correct her error patterns with ongoing support from her parents. She is now considered a high achiever by her teachers, who are amazed at her above-age-expectation performance in math, reading, and any activity that involves visual spatial strengths.

How did Dara's teachers handle her initial difficulty with speech production and unintelligibility? Specific attention to Dara's cognitive strengths and ongoing communication with her parents enabled Dara to demonstrate her abilities as a learner and to excel in multiple areas of learning. Given appropriate attention to struggles with speech intelligibility, they responded to her needs by reducing demands for expressive interactions until she demonstrated competency. They never lowered their expectations of Dara's abilities to succeed as a learner and often facilitated her emerging speech intelligibility, especially in play with peers, by providing age-appropriate modeling of expressive speech and language, focusing on her demonstrated strengths in comprehension, tracking her growth in expressive language, and sharing changes with parents and other providers. Dara was supported at the universal level in a high-quality preschool, with teachers who understood her communication profile within the context of her overall abilities and drew from her strengths to facilitate her success and growth as a learner.

LESSONS LEARNED FROM STORIES OF CHILDREN & FAMILIES

Teachers and specialists need to know and apply research-based practice. It is apparent that a myriad of factors can influence a child's growth, development, and learning during the preschool years to build the oral language, early literacy, and social emotional competence necessary for later success in education. Both internal factors that the child brings to the learning situation and external factors must be understood in the ecological context of the developing child and his or her family. It is even more apparent that educators and specialists need to be aware of the research about children who are learning more than one language or who are monolingual learners of a second language to address and support individualized learning needs. Knowledge of typical patterns of second-language acquisition and variations in behaviors based upon competing factors of influence must be examined and are often more helpful in determining a child's profile than standardized assessments, especially given the paucity of reliable and valid formal assessments available. Observations of a child's language and social emotional behaviors coupled with parent reporting may provide the starting point for educators and specialists to engage each and every child in the learning process. Evidence-based practices at the universal level involving research-based curriculum frameworks and ongoing progress monitoring of learning are requisite to appropriate early childhood education for all children, including those who are culturally, linguistically, and ability diverse. These differences can create a rich tapestry and wealth of learning opportunities that benefit each and every child.

Connections to home enhance learning. Authentic and relevant ongoing reciprocal communication promotes active parent participation (Dunst, Trivette, & Hamby, 2008). Establishing relationships with family will facilitate learning about the individual child's culture, life ways, values, and languages spoken in the home and reveal important ways to support the child's learning. Establishing communication with families who speak a language other than English may involve effective use of cultural mediators, interpreters, and translators (Moore & Pérez-Méndez, 2005a). This is key to understanding ways to support the child and develop communication paths that provide parents with evidence-based information as they make decisions about their young child's education and languages they will learn. Parents have the information about how their child is learning languages compared to other children in their home. This was found to be a significant predictive factor by Restrepo (1998) in distinguishing those children who were demonstrating language differences versus delays. Use of dynamic assessment strategies as described by Gutiérrez-Clellen and Pena (2001) can also be used to determine language difference from internally influenced language challenges. Early childhood educators will gain important understanding from listening to the families' stories (Sánchez, 1999b) versus relying on formal assessments of a child's prior knowledge of language. Use of cultural mediators or liaisons often facilitates open communication and the acquisition of critical information that can shed light on a child's development of both first and/or second languages. In family-centered, culturally competent practice (Moore & Pérez-Méndez, 2006) parents are assumed to be competent and know their child best. Parental priorities, concerns, resources, and life ways are to be respected while providing an enriched cultural perspective.

Learning about children in the context of their family also builds bridges to home in terms of ongoing parent-school partnerships that welcome families into settings and classrooms as volunteers, participants in learning, and key providers of continuity in a young child's life (Sánchez, 1999a). Intentional communication from the classroom (*Inside-Out*) to home in the preferred language of the family through e-mails, home visits, newsletters, conferences, family nights, etc., build upon family engagement (Moore & Pérez-Méndez, 2006). Welcoming family members into the classroom or educational setting (*Outside-In*) through visits and participation focused on sharing aspects of family culture, photos, songs, foods, books, and storytelling specific to the child also engage parents and family members in their child's education. Special events and everyday routines can be shared that build upon parents' comfort, understanding, participation, and ability to navigate educational systems and supports. Another indirect benefit of ongoing involvement of family in early education is "parent-to-parent" and community networking and opportunities to build friendships among families as well as children.

Linking assessment to responsive instruction equals effective practice. Early childhood providers can determine and hone responsive interaction skills and environments to meet the learning needs of each and every child in their setting, especially when they observe, assess, and monitor functioning levels across domains for every child with whom they work. At the universal level in a tiered framework, early childhood educators can learn about each child, who their families are, and determine learning abilities, interests, strengths, and areas for growth for each child. Universal screening and progress monitoring across developmental domains is a necessary component to enhance learning and link assessment to instructional supports. This includes an intentional effort to learn about the early oral language and literacy abilities, including assessments that facilitate knowledge of language abilities in one or two languages.

Assessment strategies including observation, knowledge of influencing factors, and the stages and abilities in both first- and second-language acquisition exhibited will provide valuable information from which to determine needs for further dynamic assessment (Gutiérrez-Clellen & Pena, 2001) and targeted interventions consistent with an RtI model adapted to early childhood programs (Buysse et al., 2010; Coleman et al., 2009; Sandall & Schwartz, 2008). This information can shape next steps and specific strategies that can facilitate growth of all children, including those from culturally, linguistically, and ability-diverse backgrounds. All children thrive in a language- and literacy-rich environment that first respects who they are as learners.

PROVEN STRATEGIES CAN ENHANCE LEARNING

It clearly is important that teachers first know all the children they work within the context of their family, culture, and life ways to develop environments and daily routines for learning that are responsive and individualized. Supporting children who are learning two languages and/or transitioning from one language to another demands that educators apply what they know from research. Research syntheses, as described by Buysse and her colleagues (2010), lead teachers to consider the importance of supporting the child's primary language as a critical component of language development and readiness for later academic learning. Emerging evidence cited earlier in this chapter indicates that learning more than one language does not cause delays, and in actuality, supports provided for the development of more than one language may facilitate and enhance cognitive and linguistic abilities in English (Buysse et al., 2010; Restrepo et al., 2010). A second conclusion by these authors and others (Coleman et al., 2009; Sandall & Schwartz, 2008) supports the use of the RtI framework in use of the "best available practices" designed to enhance learning for all children, rather than reliance upon any one single curriculum. The third conclusion, derived from current research, points to differentiated instruction and, in some instances, additional supports and accommodations (Buysse et al., 2010) based upon specifically assessed strengths and areas for growth. It is critically important to continue to question, observe, and document effectiveness of specific strategies with each and every child. Strategies that make all input comprehensible focus on correct use of language versus correcting children's attempts, thereby establishing clear expectations and peer interactions that benefit every child in an early childhood program. Also, tailoring strategies such as "wait time" for those children who need extra processing time, small group work, and deliberate intentional scaffolding of experiences may differentiate instruction that supports a particular child. It goes without saying that interactive storybook reading, storytelling, and exposure to high-quality children's literature are integral to any high-quality early childhood program (Justice, 2006; Moore & Pérez-Méndez, 2005a). Promising practices will apply depending upon the accurate observation and ongoing assessment of each and every child who is a dual language learner (Castro, Peisner-Feinberg, Buysse, & Gillanders, 2010).

FULL CIRCLE

It is widely recognized by many experts and professionals that a change from a subtractive attitude to an additive attitude that values diversity and differences is integral to a child's success as a learner. Reframing of prior subtractive perspectives regarding differences in culture, languages spoken, and diverse abilities is needed to realize the potential for each and every child. Research provides early childhood educators with a starting point to enhance learning of all children with specific information regarding proven strategies for curriculum frameworks that focus on individualized assessment and progress monitoring linked to effective instructional practices. Linking assessment, including growth and development in language(s), to instructional practices using a multitiered framework is necessary but not sufficient in addressing the specific learning needs of each and every child, unless embedded in a relationship-based approach with both children and families.

Connections to home resulting in strong parent-school partnerships based upon respect, trust, ongoing reciprocal communication, and valuing of diverse perspectives are an integral link in the circle of supports needed to promote successful learning. Our youngest and most vulnerable populations of learners need high-quality, research-based, culturally competent, and family- and child-centered practices derived from the best available evidence regarding effective strategies and differentiated learning. Additional research regarding child outcomes relative to effectiveness of instructional strategies and curriculum frameworks is certainly needed. However, early childhood educators and specialists are in a unique position to make a difference in the lives of young children in partnership with their families.

REFERENCES

Anderson, R. (2004). First language loss in Spanish-speaking children: Patterns of loss and implications for clinical practice. In B. Goldstein (Ed.), *Bilingual language development and disorders in Spanish–English speakers* (pp. 187–212). Baltimore: Paul H. Brookes.

Artiles, A. J., Rueda, R., Salazar, J. J., & Hegareda, I. (2005). Within group diversity in minority disproportionate representation: English language learners in urban school districts. *Exceptional Children, 71*, 283–300.

Artiles, A. J., & Trent, S. C. (1994). Overrepresentation of minority students in special education: A continued debate. *Journal of Special Education, 22*, 410–436.

Artiles, A. J., Trent, S. C., & Palmer, J. (2004). Culturally diverse students in special education: Legacies and prospects. In J. A. Banks & C. M. Banks (Eds.), *Handbook of research on multicultural education* (2nd ed., pp. 716–735). San Francisco: Jossey-Bass.

August, D., Carlo, M., Dressler, C., & Snow, C. (2005). The critical role of vocabulary development for English language learners. *Learning Disabilities Research and Practice, 20,* 50–57.

August, D., & Hakuta, K. (1997). *Improving schooling for language-minority children: A research agenda.* Washington, DC: National Research Council.

August, D., & Shanahan, T. (2006). *Developing literacy in second-language learners: Report of the national literacy panel on language–minority children and youth.* Mahwah, NJ: Laurence Erlbaum.

Barnett, S., Yarosz, D., Thomas, J., Jung, K., & Blanco, D. (2007). Two-way and monolingual English immersion in preschool education: An experimental comparison. *Early Childhood Research Quarterly, 22*(3), 277–293.

Barrera, I. (1993). Effective and appropriate instruction for all children: The challenges of cultural/linguistic diversity and young children with special needs. *Topics in Early Childhood Special Education, 13*(4), 461–487.

Barrera, I., Corso, R., & Macpherson, D. (2003). *Skilled dialogue: Strategies for responding to cultural diversity.* Baltimore: Paul Brookes.

Bialystok, E. (2001). *Bilingualism in development: Language, literacy & cognition.* Cambridge: Cambridge University Press.

Bialystok, E. (2009). Bilingualism: The good, the bad, and the indifferent. *Bilingualism: Language and Cognition, 12,* 3–11.

Burns, M. K., Appleton, J. J., & Stehouwer, J. D. (2005). Meta-analytic review of responsiveness-to-intervention research: Examining field-based and research-implemented models. Journal of Psychoeducational Assessment, 23, 381–394.

Buysse, V., Castro, D., & Peisner-Feinberg, E. (2010). Effects of personnel development program on classroom practices and outcomes for Latino dual language learners. *Early Childhood Research Quarterly, 25*(2), 194–206.

Capps, R., Michael, F., Ost, J., Reardon-Anderson, J., & Passel, J. (2004). *The Health and Well-Being of Young Children of Immigrants.* Washington, DC: Urban Institute.

Castro, D., Peisner-Feinberg, E., Buysse, V., & Gillanders, C. (2010). Language and literacy development of Latino dual language learners: Promising instructional practices. In O. N. Saracho & B. Spodek (Eds.). *Contemporary perspectives in early childhood education series.* Great Britain: Information Age Publishing.

Coleman, M. R., Buysse, V., & Neitzel, J. (2006). *Recognition and response: An early intervening system for young children at-risk for learning disabilities.* Chapel Hill: University of North Carolina, FPG Child Development Institute.

Coleman, R., Roth, F., & West, T. (2009). *Roadmap to Pre-K RTI: Applying response to intervention in preschool settings.* New York: National Center for Learning Disabilities.

Cummins, J. (1989). *Empowering minority students.* Sacramento: California Association for Bilingual Education.

Division for Early Childhood (DEC). (2002). DEC position on responsiveness to family cultures, values, and languages. Denver, CO: Author.

Dunn, L. M. (1968). Special education for the mildly retarded: Is much of it justifiable? *Exceptional Children, 23,* 5–21.

Dunst, C., Trivette, C., & Hamby, D. (2008). *Research synthesis and meta-analysis of studies of family centered practice.* Asheville, NC: Winterberry Press.

Espinosa, L. (2008). Challenging common myths about young English language learners. *Foundation for Child Development, 8*, 2–11.

Federal Interagency Forum on Child and Family Statistics. (2010). *America's children in brief: Key national indicators of well-being, 2010*. Forum on Child and Family Statistics. Retrieved September 2, 2010, from http://www.childstats.gov

Gay, G. (2000). *Culturally responsive teaching: Theory, research, and practice*. New York: Teachers College Press.

Gay, G. (2002). Preparing for culturally responsive teaching. *Journal of Teacher Education, 53*(2), 106–116.

Genesee, F., Paradis, J., & Crago, M. (2004). *Dual language development and disorders*. Baltimore: Paul H. Brookes.

Genesee, F. (2008). Early dual language learning. *Zero to Three, 9*, 17–23.

Gersten, R., Compton, D., Connor, C. M., Dimino, J., Santoro, L., Linan-Thompson, S., & Tilly, W. D. (2008). *Assisting students struggling with reading: Response to intervention and multi-tier interventions for reading in the primary grades. A practice guide*. (NCEE 2009-4045). Washington, DC: National Center for Education Evaluation and Regional Assistance, Institute of Education Sciences, U.S. Department of Education. Retrieved from http://ies.ed.gov/ncee/wwc/publications/practiceguides

Gersten, R., & Woodward, J. (1994). The language-minority student and special education: Issues, trends, and paradoxes. *Exceptional Children, 60*, 310–322.

Glennon, S. (2007a). Predicting language outcomes for internationally adopted children. *Journal of Speech, Language, and Hearing Research, 50*, 529–548.

Glennon, S. (2007b). International adoption: Speech and language mythbusters. *Communication Disorders and Sciences in Culturally and Linguistically Diverse Populations, 14*(3), 3–8.

Glennon, S., & Masters, G. (2002). Typical and atypical language development in infants and toddlers adopted from Eastern Europe. *American Journal of Speech Language Pathology, 11*, 417–433.

Goldstein, B. (2004). *Bilingual language development and disorders*. Baltimore: Paul H. Brookes.

Guiberson, M. (2009). Hispanic representation in special education: Patterns and implications. *Preventing School Failure, 53*(3), 167–175.

Gutiérrez-Clellen, V. F., & Pena E. (2001). Dynamic assessment of diverse children: A tutorial. *Language, Speech, and Hearing Services in Schools, 32*, 212–224.

Hakuta, K. (1986). *Mirror of language: The debate on bilingualism*. New York: Basic Books.

Hammer, C. S., Lawrence, F. R., & Miccio, A. W. (2007). Bilingual children's language abilities and early reading outcomes in head start and kindergarten. *Language, 38*(3), 237–248.

Hemmeter, M. L., Ostrosky, M., & Fox, L. (2006). Social and emotional foundations for early learning: A conceptual model for intervention. *School Psychology Review, 35*(4), 583–601.

Hernandez, D. J. (2004). Demographic change and the life circumstances of immigrant families. *Future of Children, 14*(2), 17–48.

Hwa-Froelich, D. A. (2007). Infants and toddlers adopted from abroad: Clinical practices. In *Communication disorders and sciences in culturally and linguistically diverse populations*. Rockville, MD: ASHA.

Justice, L. (2006). Evidence-based practice responsive to intervention and prevention of reading difficulties. *Language, Speech, and Hearing Services in Schools, 37*, 284–297.

Kayser, H. (2008). *Educating Latino preschool children.* San Diego, CA: Plural.

Kindler, A. L. (2002). Survey of the states' limited English proficient students and available educational programs and services: 2001–2002 summary report. Washington, DC: National Clearinghouse for English Language Acquisition and Language Instruction and Educational Programs.

Kohnert, K. (2008). *Language disorders in bilingual children and adults.* San Diego: Plural Publishing.

Kohnert, K., & Derr, A. (2004). Language intervention with bilingual children. In B. Goldstein (Ed.), *Bilingual language development and disorders in Spanish-English speakers* (pp. 315–343). Baltimore: Paul H. Brookes.

Kohnert, K., & Medina, A. (2009). Bilingual children and communication disorders: A 30-year research retrospective. *Seminars in Speech and Language, 30*, 219–233.

Kohnert, K., Yim, D., Nett, K., Kan, P. F., & Duran, L. (2005). Intervention with linguistically diverse preschool children: A focus on development of home language. *Language, Speech, and Hearing Services in Schools, 26*, 251–263.

Krashen, S. (1982). *Principles and practices in second language acquisition.* New York: Pergamon Press.

Krashen, S. (1999). *Condemned without a trial: Bogus arguments against bilingual education.* Portsmouth, NH: Heineman.

Kuhl, P. (2004). Early language acquisition: Cracking the speech code, *Neuroscience, 5*, 831–843.

Lindholm-Leary, K. J. (2005). The rich promise of two-way immersion. *Educational Leadership, 62*, 56–59.

Lynch, E. W., & Hanson, M. J. (2003). *Developing crosscultural competence: A guide for working with children and their families* (3rd ed.). Baltimore: Paul H. Brookes.

Matthews, H., & Ewen, D. (2010). *Early education programs and children of immigrants: Learning each other's language.* Washington, DC: Urban Institute.

Maude, S., Catlett, C., Moore, S., Sánchez, S., & Thorp, E. (2006). Educating and training students to work with culturally, linguistically, and ability-diverse young children and their families. *Zero to Three, 20*(3), 28–35.

Maude, S., Catlett, C., Moore, S., Sánchez, S., Thorp, E., & Corso, R. (2010). Infusing diversity constructs in preservice education: The impact of a systematic faculty development strategy. *Infants and Young Children, 23*(2), 105–121.

Mechelli, A., Crinion, J. T., Noppeney O'Doherty, J., Ashburner, J., Frackowiak, R., & Price, C. J. (2004). Structural plasticity in the bilingual brain. *Nature, 431*, 757.

Milagros-Santos, R. M., Cheatham, G., & Ostrosky, M. M. (2006). Enseñe me: Practical strategies for supporting the social and emotional development of young English language learners. *Language Learner, 1*(3), 5–9, 24.

Moore, S. M., & Pérez-Méndez, C. (2003). *Cultural contexts for early intervention.* Rockville, MD: American Speech-Language-Hearing Association.

Moore, S. M., & Pérez-Méndez, C. (2005a). *Beyond words: Effective use of cultural mediators, interpreters and translators.* Boulder, CO: Landlocked Films.

Moore, S. M., & Pérez-Méndez, C. (2005b). *The Story about El Grupo: A parent education and support group.* Boulder, CO: Landlocked Films.

Moore, S. M., & Pérez-Méndez, C. (2006). Working with linguistically diverse families in early intervention: Misconceptions and missed opportunities. *Seminars in Speech and Language, 27*, 187–198.

Moore, S. M., Pérez-Méndez, C., & Boerger, K. (2006) Meeting the needs of culturally and linguistically diverse families in early language and literacy intervention. In L. Justice (Ed.), *Clinical approaches to emergent literacy intervention*. San Diego, CA: Plural.

National Association for the Education of Young Children (NAEYC). (1995). *Responding to linguistic and cultural diversity recommendations for effective early childhood education: A position statement*. Washington, DC: Author.

National Institute of Child Health and Development. (2000). *Teaching children to read: An evidence-based assessment of the scientific research literature on reading and its implications for reading instruction* (NIH Publication No. 00-4769). Washington, DC: U.S. Government Printing Office.

Nicoladis, E., & Genesee, F. (1997). Language development in preschool bilingual children. *Journal of Speech-Language Pathology and Audiology, 21*, 258–270.

Nieto, S. (2000). *The light in their eyes: Creating multicultural learning communities*. New York: Teachers College Press.

Ortiz, A. A., & Yates, J. R. (1983). Incidence of exceptionality among Hispanics: Implications for manpower planning. *NABE Journal of Research and Practice, 7*, 41–54.

Oster, T., McDonnell, A., & Jayaraman, G. (2009, October). A synthesis of instructional strategies to support preschool children's English language acquisition. Paper presented at the 25th Annual International Conference on Young with Special Needs and their Families, Division for Early Childhood of the Council for Exceptional Children, Albuquerque, NM.

Paradis, J., Crago, M., Genesee, F., & Rice, M. (2003). Bilingual children with specific language impairment: How do they compare with their monolingual peers? *Journal of Speech, Language, and Hearing Research, 46*, 1–15.

Passel, J., & Cohn, D'V. (2008). *U.S. population projections: 2005–2050*. Washington, DC: PEW Research Center.

Patterson, J. L., & Pearson, B. Z. (2004). Bilingual lexical development: Influences, contexts, and processes. In B. A. Goldstein (Ed.), *Bilingual language development and disorders in Spanish-English speakers* (pp. 77–104). Baltimore: Paul H. Brookes.

Pearson, B. C., & Fernandez, S. C. (1993). Lexical development in bilingual infants and toddlers—Comparison to monolingual norms. *Language Learning, 43*, 93–120.

Pérez-Méndez, C., & Moore, S. M. (2004). *Culture and language: Respecting family choice*. Boulder, CO: Landlocked Films.

Pollock, K. E. (1983). Individual preferences: Case study of a phonologically delayed child. *Topics in Language Disorders, 3*, 1–25.

Pollock, K. E. (2005). Early language growth in children adopted from China: Preliminary normative data. *Seminars in Speech and Language, 26*(1), 22–32.

Restrepo, M. A. (1998). Identifiers of predominantly Spanish-speaking children with language impairment. *Journal of Speech, Language, and Hearing Research, 41*, 1398–1411.

Restrepo, M. A., Castilla, A., Schwanenflugel, S., Neuharth-Pritchett, P., Hamilton, C., & Arboleda, A. (2010). Effects of a supplemental Spanish oral language program on sentence length, complexity, and grammaticality in Spanish-speaking children attending English-only preschools. *Language, Speech, and Hearing Services in Schools, 41,* 3–13.

Roberts, J. A., Pollock, K. E., Krakow, R., Price, J., Fulmer, K. C., & Wang, P. (2005). Language development in pre-school age children adopted from China. *Journal of Speech, Language, and Hearing Research, 48*(1), 93–107.

Roseberry-McKibbin, C. (2003). *Assessment of bilingual learners: Language difference or disorder?* Rockville, MD: American Speech Language Hearing Association.

Sánchez, S. Y. (1999a). Issues of language and culture impacting the early care of young Latino children. *Child Care Bulletin, 24.* Retrieved from http://nccic.org/ccb/issue24.html

Sánchez, S. Y. (1999b). Learning from the stories of culturally and linguistically diverse families and communities. *Remedial and Special Education, 20,* 351–359.

Sánchez, S., & Thorp, E. (1998). Discovering the meanings of continuity. *Zero to Three, 18*(6), 2–6.

Sánchez, S., & Thorp, E. (2008). Teaching to transform: Infusing cultural and linguistic diversity. In P. Winton, J. McCollum, & C. Catlett (Eds.), *Practical approaches to early childhood professional development: Evidence, strategies, and resources* (pp. 81–97). Washington, DC: Zero to Three.

Sandall, S. R., & Schwartz, I. S. (2008). *Building blocks for teaching preschoolers with special needs* (2nd ed.). Baltimore: Paul H. Brookes.

Shields, M. K., & Behrmam, R. E. (2004). Children of immigrant families: Analysis and recommendations. *The Future of Children, 14*(2), 4–16.

Snow, C. (2006). Cross-cutting themes and future research directions. In D. August & T. Shanahan (Eds.), *Developing literacy in second language learners: Report of the national literacy panel on language-minority children and youth* (pp. 631–653). Mahwah, NJ: Lawrence Erlbaum.

Tabors, P. O. (2008). *One child: Two languages* (2nd ed.). Baltimore: Paul H. Brookes.

Tabors, P. O., & Snow, C. (2001). Young bilingual children and early literacy development. In S. Neuman & D. Dickinson (Eds.), *Handbook of early literacy research.* (Vol. 1, pp. 159–178) New York: Guilford.

Tatum, B. D. (2003). *Why are all the black kids sitting together in the cafeteria?* New York: Basic Books.

U.S. Census Bureau. (2000). *The Hispanic population: Census 2000 brief* (U.S. Census Bureau Publication No. C2KBR/01–3).Washington, DC: U.S. Government Printing Office.

U.S. Department of State. (2009) Statistics. Retrieved from http://www.adoption.state.gov

Westby, C. (1990). Ethnographic interviewing: Asking the right questions to the right people in the right ways. *Journal of Childhood Communication Disorders, 13*(1), 101–111.

Westby, C. (2009). Considerations when working successfully with culturally and linguistically diverse families in assessment and intervention of communication disorders. *Seminars in Speech and Language, 30*(4), 279–289.

Winsler, A., Diaz, R. M., Espinoza, L., & Rodriguez, J. L. (1999). When learning a second language does not mean losing the first: Bilingual language development in low-income, Spanish-speaking children attending bilingual preschool. *Child Development, 70,* 349–362.

Winton, P., McCollum, J. A., & Catlett, C. (2008). *Practical approaches to early child-hood professional development: Evidence, strategies, and resources.* Washington, DC: Zero to Three.

Wong Fillmore, L. (1991). When learning one language means losing the first. *Early Childhood Research Quarterly, 6*(3), 323–346.

Yoshida, H. (2008). The cognitive consequences of early bilingualism. *Zero to Three, 11,* 26–30.

Zentella, A. C. (2005). *Building on strength: Language and literacy in Latino families and communities.* New York: Teachers College Press.

Chapter 7

A Developmental and Family Systems Perspective on Mental Health in Young Children

Susan B. Campbell

During the toddler and preschool periods, positive adjustment in young children is defined by social and cognitive advances consistent with developmental level as reflected in positive relationships with parents, siblings, peers, and other important adults in the child's social network; the development of language and communication as well as basic concepts, consistent with school readiness; and the ability to adapt to reasonable changes in routines and expectations that are typically associated with family life, such as entry into child care or the birth of a sibling. In contrast, young children's adjustment difficulties may be expressed in many ways, including some combination of temper tantrums; limit-testing; defiance; aggression toward siblings, other children, and even adults; refusing to talk; sleep difficulties; fearful and clingy behavior; and/or withdrawal from social contact.

Children's problems also vary widely in their severity and persistence and thus in their implications for later development and adaptation. Many problems in young children tend to be age-related and transient, reflecting difficult developmental transitions, but more chronic and severe problems that interfere with children's acquisition of cognitive and social skills, impair relationships in the family and beyond, and are evident across situations are likely to require intervention that invariably must include work with the family or other primary caregivers (Campbell, 2002, 2006). Even when problems are age-related and transient, parents may benefit from help finding alternative parenting strategies that are likely to support children's adaptation (Gardner, Sonuga-Barke, & Sayal, 1999). Problems in young children may be a sign, then, of developmental challenge or change or a sign of family stress. The vignettes below illustrate some typical ways that young children respond to stressful events or changes.

When his mother returned to work because the family could not make ends meet on just one salary, 2-year-old Dylan entered child care at a family day-care home in his neighborhood. Dylan's mother tried hard to prepare him for the transition to this new setting and the experience of being away from her each day by talking to him about it and taking him for several visits to meet the caregiver and other children. Although Dylan was happy to visit, once he began attending on a regular basis, he became upset every morning, refusing to "go potty" or to cooperate with his mother while she was getting him dressed. When he arrived at child care, he initially refused to leave his mother's side, becoming tearful and clingy, although the caregiver, who was very sensitive and experienced, was able to interest him in playing with toys and with her 3-year-old son, and Dylan eventually calmed down and let his mother leave. However, this pattern continued for several weeks as Dylan adjusted to the new experience of being away from his mother each day in a relatively unfamiliar, albeit home, setting.

Several factors may explain why Dylan adapted to child care after a few weeks and his problems resolved. Importantly, both Dylan's mother and his caregiver were understanding and patient with him. Rather than become angry and annoyed at his noncompliance and clinginess, they both took his developmental level, level of understanding, and need to adapt to change into account. In addition, the caregiver was especially warm and skilled at redirecting him and involving him in interesting activities with her own son. Finally, Dylan and his mother had a warm relationship, and she made an effort to give him extra attention each evening before bed. These same behaviors, however, could potentially escalate into problems if the responsible adults were less patient and skilled and the child was less adaptable. Angry or neglectful responses on the part of adults might lead to increased tantrum behavior and separation anxiety, toilet-training difficulties, and other indicators of distress.

Three-year-old Timmy, in contrast, loved going to child care, but he came home some evenings in an angry mood, throwing frequent temper tantrums and lashing out at his younger sister, leading to frequent fights between his parents about how to handle his newly emerging defiance and aggression. Although Timmy had been much easier to handle as a toddler, he became more determined to do things his way soon after his third birthday, and he seemed to be constantly testing the limits of his parents' patience. Timmy's father was the disciplinarian and he had little patience for Timmy's defiance, especially after a day at work, preferring either to send Timmy to his room for time-out or even to spank him when he misbehaved. Timmy's mother thought that these acting-out behaviors were likely to be outgrown and that jealousy over the attention his younger sister was garnering, along with developmental changes indicative of a growing need for autonomy, largely explained his difficulties.

The outcome in this example will depend partly on how well the parents can work together to manage Timmy's difficult behavior by providing structure, firm limits, consistency, and appropriate attention to Timmy, while also meeting the needs of his younger sister. Continued and escalating family conflict over childrearing, inconsistency between his parents, and power-assertive disciplinary strategies might well lead to continued and even worsening behavior.

Three-and-a-half-year-old Sadie entered a new child care setting when her mother returned to work six months after the birth of her younger sister. Sadie tended to hover near the teacher and avoid contact with other children, refusing to play with others and joining group activities only reluctantly. Her mother was surprised to get these reports from the child care teachers because Sadie had been quite sociable in the past and had enjoyed attending child care at her old center. At home, she doted on her baby sister and was happy to help her mother whenever she was allowed to hold the baby or help give her a bath.

Both the stresses of sharing her mother with a new baby and the return to full-time child care in a new and unfamiliar setting appeared to trigger these reactions, which may resolve with sensitive and understanding reactions from adults or continue to be expressed as anxiety, shyness, and need for adult attention.

Five-year-old Jessie started kindergarten after several years attending a child care center. Although he had adjusted well to child care, he began acting out at school, getting into frequent fights with other children, pushing and shoving when it was time to line up for lunch or recess, and generally annoying other children, some of whom protested tearfully to the teacher.

Again, these reactions may be time-limited indications of Jessie's problems adapting to the demands of school, or they may reflect emerging problems that will ultimately predict more persistent difficulties with behavioral control, peer group relationships and friendships, and academic achievement. Outcomes will be partly a reflection of Jessie's earlier personality and ability to regulate negative emotions and impulses, and partly a reflection of how the school and his family deal with his initial difficulties.

The behaviors depicted in these vignettes are common and familiar to any adult who has been around young children on a regular basis.

These instances of separation anxiety, tantrums, defiance, aggression, or shyness often are typical behaviors evident during toddlerhood, the preschool period, and the school transition as children grapple with the challenges of regulating their behavior and emotions, establishing a sense of self, learning to cooperate with others in the peer group, and reaching out to form relationships with other adults in child care, preschool, or kindergarten settings. The degree to which children successfully meet these challenges will be determined by a complex mix of child characteristics, family relationships, and external supports. In the context of supportive relationships, these difficult behaviors are usually (but not always) time-limited, but when stress and family hardship are either serious and acute or more chronic and pervasive, children may have a more difficult time smoothly negotiating these developmental transitions and meeting adult expectations as they move from toddlerhood to preschool and kindergarten age. When problems do not easily resolve with development, parents and children alike may benefit from intervention services.

This chapter will discuss some of the major developmental advances evident from toddlerhood to kindergarten entry (roughly between ages 18 months and 5 years) and how normal transitions and life events may facilitate positive developmental changes or be associated with the onset of difficult behaviors. Family and social context effects will be discussed as well, with an emphasis on parenting and family relationships as contexts for either children's positive adaptation to life transitions and stresses or adjustment difficulties that may or may not be long-standing. Finally, this chapter will briefly discuss implications for prevention and early intervention.

DEVELOPMENTAL CHANGES, EXPECTATIONS, AND TRANSITIONS

In a recent volume, Brownell and Kopp (2007) discussed the profound "transitions and transformations" that occur from late infancy to toddlerhood, highlighting the major advances that typically characterize this phase of development. Between 18 and 36 months of age, children showing typical development achieve a set of interconnected competencies in social, communicative, cognitive, motor, and emotional domains that mark a major shift from infancy. These achievements are based on skills that develop by the end of the first year, including walking, using rudimentary language to communicate specific wants and needs, and using the parent as a secure base for exploring the wider social and object world. Expanding skills over the second year include a growing awareness of the self and others as distinct agents (Moore, 2007), marked advances in language acquisition and reciprocal conversation (Shatz, 2007), awareness of mental states in self and others (Hobson, 2007), the development of symbolic play (Lillard, 2007), the beginning of empathic concern for others (as distinct from emotion contagion) (Zahn-Waxler, Radke-Yarrow, Wagner, & Chapman, 1992), and the emerging ability to regulate emotion and behavior (Calkins, 2007; Kopp, 1989). There is also general agreement that these skills develop in a relatively integrated fashion across developmental systems (Brownell & Kopp, 2007) and that they build upon earlier social communicative skills and social-emotional experiences evident in infancy, such as joint attention and social referencing (Lillard, 2007; Shatz, 2007), with both earlier and later achievements strongly dependent on adult guidance, warmth, appropriate limit-setting, and support (Crockenberg & Litman, 1990; Kochanska, 2002; Thompson, 2006).

Between ages 3 and 5, children's language becomes increasingly complex; they also become better able to use language to control their own behavior and to talk about their own and other people's feelings and experiences (Shatz, 2007). At this developmental juncture, children's play also shows major shifts as parallel play gives way to much more nuanced social engagement with peers that includes turn-taking, role assignments, shared pretend play scenarios, and emerging friendships based on mutual liking as well as shared activities (Hughes & Dunn, 2007). Children also begin to express moral emotions such as guilt and concern for others, and they have an emerging sense of right and wrong as well as what is and is not acceptable behavior (Kochanska, 2002; Zahn-Waxler et al., 1992). These major developmental advances are partly a function of brain development, but they are also largely shaped by the quality of relationships with parents and other caregivers who are needed to support and scaffold children's social and emotional advances if they are to develop optimally (Brownell & Kopp, 2007; Campbell, 2002; Cummings, Davies, & Campbell, 2000; Sroufe & Fleeson, 1986). Furthermore, parents and other caregivers are potent role models for young children, and the nature of their relationships, not only with the child but with other children and adults, will have a profound influence on children's developmental trajectory.

In tandem with these remarkable developmental advances in children's social, emotional, cognitive, and linguistic skills, society places major demands upon young children. Most children today are in some form of out-of-home care by the time they are 24–36 months old (Shonkoff & Phillips, 2000), but the quality of care varies widely in terms of teacher-child ratios, teacher training, staff stability, and the ability of child care providers to anticipate, understand, and meet children's developmental and emotional needs. Child care quality also varies partly as a function of family resources (National Institute of Child Health and Human Development [NICHD] Early Child Care Research Network [ECCRN], 1996; 1997), with more affluent families able to afford higher-quality care and care for the working poor and for families in poverty more likely to vary widely in quality, as reflected in caregiver warmth, sensitivity, responsiveness, cognitive stimulation, and appropriate structure and limit-setting.

Around age 5, children are expected to make another major life transition from child care or preschool to elementary school as they enter kindergarten. The entry into kindergarten often involves other major changes as many children must adapt to a new school, a new set of mostly unfamiliar peers, and new teachers (Campbell & von Stauffenberg, 2007). Once children enter primary school, adults also have much higher expectations for their behavioral and emotional control that include conformity to classroom rules, cooperation with peers, and a focus on academic success. Children must possess a variety of regulatory strategies and social skills to cope successfully with these changing demands and expectations. For example, the transition to kindergarten requires a degree of independence and self-reliance that is not expected in child care or preschool, and often children must be able to function in a much larger group of peers with substantially less adult supervision. Children also must make new friends and learn to work cooperatively with other children in a more focused and goal-directed way than in preschool. They must follow teacher directions and inhibit impulses not to call out, push ahead in line, demand teacher attention, or be aggressive with peers. They must be able to follow a lesson and focus attention on challenging cognitive tasks. Many children also must cope with shyness and anxiety as they make the transition to school.

Although children gradually develop these social and regulatory skills in preschool and child care, the transition to kindergarten or first grade sometimes taxes young children's abilities in these areas. Moreover, children's entry into the school system is more often determined by age than by the acquisition of skills and competencies that indicate social and cognitive readiness for school. Thus, children enter school with widely different skills, and many are not quite ready for school (Campbell & von Stauffenberg, 2007; Rimm-Kaufmann, Pianta, & Cox, 2000). Poor school-readiness skills and lack of behavioral regulation are among the major concerns voiced by teachers, and they may set the stage for continuing difficulties in the classroom (Lin, Lawrence, & Gorrell, 2003; McClelland & Morrison, 2003; Rimm-Kaufmann et al., 2000), including escalating teacher-child conflict (Doumen et al., 2008).

Taken together, then, children make major developmental advances between the ages of 18 months and 5 years, with concomitant changes in societal expectations. Moreover, this is also a time when children may have to adapt to other normative life events such as the birth of a sibling, a family move, a parent's return to the workforce, entry into or a change in child care arrangements, or the death of a grandparent. Each of these life events may trigger negative reactions such as tantrums, defiance, the return to earlier forms of behavior (e.g., bedwetting or wanting a bottle), clinginess, and/or separation anxiety that may in turn be a short-lived and typical reaction to stress or may set the stage for more serious problems (Campbell, 2002, 2006). Given these normative developmental changes and life events, the many challenges facing young children are daunting, so it is hardly surprising that caregivers in child care settings and kindergarten teachers (Rimm-Kaufmann et al., 2000) often feel overwhelmed by the wide variability they see in the ability of the children in their classrooms to cooperate with adults and peers, follow directions, and adapt to classroom routines. These issues are exacerbated in the context of high levels of family stress and disruption, and in the absence of sensitive emotional support and structure across home and child care or school settings (NICHD ECCRN, 2002, 2003, 2004).

FAMILY AND SOCIAL CONTEXT: DEVELOPMENTAL MODELS AND CHILDREN'S ADJUSTMENT

It is obvious that children's development occurs in the context of the family and that the quality of the parent-child relationship is especially salient for children's adjustment. There is a large literature on infant-parent attachment that underscores the importance of sensitive, responsive early care that includes the ability to read infant signals appropriately, respond to infant distress, and anticipate needs such as hunger, fatigue, boredom, discomfort, and overstimulation. Sensitive responsiveness and attunement to infant communication undergirds early attachment security and a sense of basic trust (Ainsworth, Blehar, Waters, & Wall, 1978; Bowlby, 1969). A secure attachment and the quality of the parent-child relationship across early development are associated with the emerging sense of self in toddlerhood, expectations about early social relationships with others, and the willingness to seek out and form positive relationships with peers and other adults (Bretherton, 1985; Thompson, 2006), skills that are carried forward into other relationships across childhood (Sroufe & Fleeson, 1986).

Parents will be more able and more likely to provide their infant with sensitive responsive care when their own needs are met and when they themselves experienced adequate parenting as children (Serbin & Karp, 2004; Sroufe & Fleeson, 1986). Moreover, when confronting high levels of stress and hardship, parents may have a more difficult time responding to their infants' needs, for example, if they are overwhelmed with competing responsibilities due to financial problems, poverty, poor housing, job loss, and/or physical or mental illness (Ceballo & McLoyd, 2002; McLoyd, 1998).

Ecological (Bronfenbrenner, 1979), transactional (Sameroff, 1995), and family systems (Cox & Paley, 1997) models posit that children's development occurs in a complex web of reciprocal and changing social influences that begin with the child in the context of the parent-child relationship and move out to incorporate the influences of other relationships within the nuclear family system (e.g., the quality of the marital relationship, relationships with siblings, parent-sibling relationships) and relationships with extended family members (e.g., grandparents, aunts, and uncles). Other factors that influence children's development include community and social resources such as neighborhood safety; the availability and quality of child care, neighborhood schools, playgrounds, and libraries; and the availability of jobs, social services, adequate health care, and religious institutions (Bronfenbrenner, 1979).

These social and neighborhood resources have direct effects on children in their day-to-day interactions with others and indirect effects via their influences on parents' availability, sense of self-worth, and feelings of well-being. Furthermore, it is well established that children are both influenced by and have influences on parents and others in their social network (Sameroff, 1995), reflecting reciprocal processes that change from moment to moment during social interactions (for example, the give and take of a conversation or a play encounter with a peer) and that change over the course of development as a function of the history of relationships within the family (Cox & Paley, 1997;

Sroufe & Fleeson, 1986) and the nature of childrearing practices (e.g., a child's expectations, such as the anticipation of punishment or of a positive interaction, will vary with past experiences with a parent, and the parent's reaction to the child will vary based on the child's usual level of cooperation, language ability, etc.). In addition, the nature of parenting changes with children's development as needs for structure and direction change, for example from infancy to the "terrible twos," when children need more limit-setting and control, but when needs for autonomy must be recognized as well (see Campbell, 2002).

Thus, issues of child adjustment, parenting, and family interactions can be considered from multiple perspectives. Children living in relatively well-functioning families with adequate supports and generally positive parenting may react negatively to a difficult developmental transition, such as entry into preschool, or to a normative life event, like the birth of a sibling. In these situations, when parents are understanding and proactive, the overall parent-child relationship is positive and secure, and parents are able to consider the situation from the child's point of view, such adjustment reactions will most likely be time-limited and transient. Thus, basic parenting skills at times of developmental transitions and challenges can clearly support positive adjustment in young children (Campbell, 2002; Cummings et al., 2000; Shonkoff & Phillips, 2000). In contrast, if parents have a difficult time recognizing that their child's anger and aggression is likely to be age-related or reflects the child's anxiety, frustration, and need for reassurance in the face of change, they may become angry themselves, only adding to the child's anxiety and distress. In such instances, a battle of wills may ensue, only increasing the likelihood that the child's behavior may worsen, potentially developing into a more stable coping strategy that involves anger, aggression, non-compliance, and negative attention-seeking (Campbell, Shaw, & Gilliom, 2000).

In summary, children can show adjustment difficulties as they cope with typical, but challenging developmental transitions such as entry into child care; with typical life events such as a the birth of sibling, that force them to share their parents with another being and also alter their role in the family system; when they reach certain developmental milestones that include struggles over autonomy and limit-setting; and when parental expectations for more mature behavior (e.g., toilet training, modified bedtime rituals, better self-control, "big boy" table manners and trying new foods, getting along with siblings, playing cooperatively with peers) clash with children's habits and preferences.

The majority of families weather these transitory conflicts, which often become family lore, but for some children and families, these conflicts may be early signs of more entrenched and long-term difficulties. Furthermore, when developmental perturbations and early parent-child conflicts occur in families who are also dealing with more pervasive stresses or difficulties, problems may become exacerbated and require targeted interventions.

Child by Parenting Interactions

Decades of research in child development have highlighted the transactional nature of parent-child relationships as they relate to both positive adjustment and to adjustment difficulties (e.g., Belsky, 1984; Belsky, Hsieh, & Crnic, 1998; Sameroff, 1995, 2000; Thomas, Chess, & Birch, 1968). Thus, both child characteristics and parenting behaviors have been studied as predictors of adjustment outcomes. For example, children's early temperament or personality characteristics, such as high levels of irritability and fussiness and low levels of "soothability," are one precursor of early problems, but this is the case primarily when these child characteristics elicit less sensitive parenting in parents who are themselves more irritable and less attuned to their child's needs.

Several studies provide clear illustrations of this interaction between child characteristics and the nature of parenting behavior. For example, Bates, Pettit, Dodge, and Ridge (1998) reported that toddlers who were high in resistance to control showed better adjustment when their parents provided more structure and direction; in contrast, however, in the absence of positive, engaged, and structured parenting, toddlers who were noncompliant were more likely to demonstrate later externalizing problems as reported by teachers. In a classic study, Belsky et al. (1998) reported that infant irritability was exacerbated by harsh and intrusive parenting in toddlerhood, which in turn predicted externalizing problems at preschool age; whereas irritable infants who experienced more positive and sensitive parenting where not especially hard to manage in toddlerhood and the preschool period. These findings were also replicated by van Zeijl and colleagues (2007), who found that toddlers exhibiting difficult behaviors showed higher levels of externalizing problems when their mothers used negative disciplinary techniques, but lower levels of behavior problems and aggression when mothers were positive and proactive. On the other hand, children with more easygoing temperaments who were less irritable and demanding showed less variability in behavioral outcomes regardless of their mothers' disciplinary strategies.

Taken together, these and other studies (e.g., Holden, 1983; Kochanska, Philibert, & Barry, 2009; Leve et al., 2009) demonstrate the importance of parental involvement that includes a mix of sensitivity to the child's point of view, warmth, structure, and proactive control. For example, in toddlerhood and the preschool period, proactive parenting includes the ability to anticipate situations that may lead children to become overwhelmed or noncompliant, and then to have strategies to redirect them as a way of avoiding conflicts or outbursts. In contrast, when parents are harsh, negative, power assertive, use physical restraint or punishment as means of control, or fail to consider the child's perspective, children often respond with angry reactions, defiance, and escalating difficulties at home and child care or school (Campbell et al., 2000). In addition, these patterns of interaction and responsiveness to parental control attempts, both positive and negative, seem to be more evident in children who show particular personality styles that include greater emotional reactivity and less ability to regulate negative emotions including sadness and anger.

These studies illustrate what Belsky, Bakermans-Kranenberg, and van IJzendoorn (2007) call "differential susceptibility to rearing influences" and a growing number of studies have now documented this effect across contexts, including child care. Pluess and Belsky (2009) used data from the NICHD Study of Early Child Care to examine the interaction of infant temperament and child care quality in predicting adjustment and social competence. Consistent with the differential susceptibility hypothesis, infants who were fussier and more difficult to calm down when upset and who also attended lower-quality child care were later rated as showing more externalizing problems and lower social competence than were fussy infants attending higher-quality child care and infants who were generally more easygoing regardless of child-care quality. Thus, problems in children exhibiting difficult behavior will be more likely to be exacerbated by harsh treatment but will be more clearly ameliorated in the context of responsive, positive caregiving. Furthermore, these effects are apparent across family and child care settings. Overall, temperamental difficulties are less likely to be stable when parents are responsive and sensitive and firmly, but gently, enforce age-appropriate limits. In addition, some young children who tend to be more positive and adaptable may be less affected by less engaged and responsive parenting than children who show more irritability and noncompliant behavior. Excessively structured, intrusive, and harsh parenting, however, may elicit resistance even in children at lower temperamental or genetic risk (Leve et al., 2009).

These recent findings reflecting gene by environment interaction have important implications for intervention, because they make it evident that some children who exhibit difficult behavior and some high-risk families will be especially receptive to early intervention. This will be discussed in more detail in the section on implications for intervention.

Family Risk Factors Associated with Adjustment Difficulties

Children with special needs, be they cognitive, social, physical, or some combination of these, often grow up in families grappling with many stresses that challenge their ability to provide consistent, sensitive, and responsive care for their young children. The fragmentary nature of service delivery systems and the lack of easy access for some families, especially in rural areas, to pediatric, social, and educational services that treat the child in the context of the family, school, and community may further exacerbate problems (Atkins, Hoagwood, Kutash, & Seidman, 2010; Melton, 2010; Stiffman et al., 2010).

The need for comprehensive, family-based services is highlighted by a voluminous research literature identifying a range of risk factors that are associated with adjustment difficulties in children, including poverty, teen parenting, single parenting, family separation and disruption, parental mental illness, parental unemployment, family violence, substance use/abuse, and low social support. These difficulties often co-occur, placing children at especially high risk for behavioral, emotional, and learning problems that spill over to affect the child's functioning in child care, preschool, and kindergarten settings. Children living in families experiencing this range of adversities show a myriad of adjustment difficulties including aggression, noncompliance, attention problems, disruptive behavior, social withdrawal, and delays in acquiring age-appropriate cognitive and school readiness skills. These difficulties often tax the resources of preschool and kindergarten teachers, making referrals to external services necessary.

Ecological and transactional models of development and accruing research on risk and resilience indicate that children who experience this range of adversities at home enter group settings with few role models for positive social behavior with peers, poor ability to regulate anger and impulses, and poor social skills like sharing, turn-taking, and negotiating to solve disputes. Language delays may exacerbate these difficulties by making children less responsive to adult requests, and because these children are less able to use language in their social interactions with peers, they may resort to aggression such as hitting, fighting, or grabbing toys when they cannot make their needs or wants understood (Tremblay, 2000).

Studies that have examined the development of children in the context of family adversity have tended to focus on specific problems that include maternal depression (Goodman, 2007), single parenting (Jones, Forehand, Brody, & Armistead, 2002), family violence and abuse (Cicchetti & Toth, 1995; Yates, Dodds, Sroufe, & Egeland, 2003), and poverty (Aber, Jones, & Cohen, 2000; McLoyd, 1990, 1998), although it is well known that these tend to co-occur (Appleyard, Egeland, van Dulmen, & Sroufe, 2005; Deater-Deckard, Dodge, Bates, & Pettit, 1998; Jones et al., 2002). In trying to understand the processes linking adverse family experiences, both direct and indirect effects have been examined. Direct effects impinge directly on the child and include factors like poor nutrition and lack of health care that may result from poverty, or fearfulness in the face of family violence. Indirect or mediated effects emphasize the impact of family adversity on the quality of parenting, which in turn affects the child's development. Maternal depression serves as one good example of mediated effects in the context of co-occurring risk factors for adjustment problems. In other words, maternal depression is associated with parenting difficulties, which generally explain the links between maternal depression and child outcomes. In addition, maternal depression tends to co-occur with other psychosocial stresses that may cause the depression, be effects of the depression, or merely correlate with depressive symptoms.

A wealth of research on maternal depression indicates that when mothers are depressed, they are also less positive, warm, and engaged with their children across infancy and early childhood (Campbell, Matestic, von Stauffenberg, Mohan, & Kirchner, 2007; NICHD ECCRN, 1999), more likely to become irritable and angry (Eamon & Zuehl, 2001; Lyons-Ruth, Easterbrooks, & Cibelli, 1997), less likely to use proactive controls to prevent misbehavior (Kochanska, Kuczynski, Radke-Yarrow, & Welsh, 1987), and less likely to talk to and stimulate their children's cognitive development (see Goodman [2007] for a thorough review). Their children in turn may show less advanced cognitive and linguistic development (Lyons-Ruth et al., 1997; NICHD ECCRN, 1999), less cooperation and higher levels of externalizing problems (Lyons-Ruth et al., 1997; NICHD ECCRN, 1999), and elevated rates of insecure attachment, especially disorganized attachment (Campbell et al., 2004). It is widely accepted that the links between maternal depression and child adjustment are partly explained or mediated by parenting behavior (Goodman, 2007; NICHD ECCRN, 1999) because depressed mothers' less engaged and stimulating parenting styles and their difficulty setting limits are less likely to foster cognitive advances and emotion regulation. In addition, the persistence over time of maternal depressive symptoms and their associations with other indicators of family adversity predict adjustment difficulties in young children.

For example, using data from the NICHD Study of Early Child Care, Campbell and colleagues (2007) reported that high levels of both chronic and concurrent depressive symptoms in mothers predicted more adjustment difficulties during the transition to first grade as reflected in both mother and teacher reports and cognitive test scores. Moreover, because maternal depression may be associated with marital distress (Cummings et al., 2000), parenting by a single adolescent mother (Leadbeater, Bishop, & Raver, 1996), and poverty (McLoyd, 1990, 1998), elevated depressive symptoms may be a proxy for multiple risk factors that tend to co-occur. Indeed, the NICHD Study (NICHD ECCRN, 1999), found an interaction between the chronicity of maternal depressive symptoms and financial stress such that mothers who were depressed and had limited resources were significantly less sensitive with their infants and toddlers, and this was especially marked at 24 months, when children were likely to test limits and seek autonomy. Children's adjustment to first grade was also partly explained by more general family adversity, including low income and family disruption, as teacher reports of problems in children whose mothers were depressed were no longer significant once other measures of family adversity were controlled statistically (Campbell et al., 2007). Other research suggests that the combination of maternal depression and other stresses, especially marital dissatisfaction and dissolution (see review by Cummings et al. [2000]), bodes poorly for young children's early adjustment and development, consistent with a multiple risk model.

As already noted, over and above maternal depression, other indicators of family stress, including low educational level, poverty, and limited social support for parents, seem to have similar effects on parenting behavior. These stresses are also reflected in less patient, sensitive, engaged, and proactive parenting; parents who are under high levels of stress and adversity are more likely to use physical punishment, demand immediate compliance rather than explain, and engage in negative and angry interactions with their children. Their children, in turn, are more likely to respond with noncompliance or outright defiance, throw temper tantrums, and model their parents' aggressive behavior by fighting with peers and destroying toys. Consistent with a transactional model, this escalating pattern of coercive exchanges can permeate the family system, as negative parent-child interactions may be mirrored in negative marital and sibling relationships as well. Furthermore, expectations of negative interactions will prime family members to be argumentative and belligerent in future encounters. Thus, negative, punitive, and harsh childrearing practices are one mechanism that links family risk to children's adjustment difficulties.

A large body of research also indicates that negative, punitive, and harsh parenting tends to co-occur with other risks that include poverty, mental illness, marital dysfunction or single parenting, and other stressful life events (Appleyard et al., 2005; Ceballo & McLoyd, 2002; Deater-Deckard et al., 1998; McMahon, Grant, Compas, Thurm, & Ey, 2003; NICHD ECCRN, 2004, 2005; Sameroff, 2000). In general, findings indicate that risks tend to be nonspecific in predicting negative outcomes (McMahon et al., 2003) and that cumulative risk—that is, the increasing number of co-occurring risks—is more likely to be associated with adjustment problems than one specific risk. Some studies report a threshold effect such that two or more risks predict more serious adjustment problems (Jones et al., 2002), whereas other studies suggest a linear relationship between the number of risks and children's outcomes (Appleyard et al., 2005). In general, however, as risk factors accumulate, children not surprisingly have more adjustment difficulties that are reflected in some combination of aggression, noncompliance, peer problems, anxiety and sadness, and academic and learning problems.

The timing of risk matters as well. Appleyard et al. (2005) found that cumulative risk in early childhood predicted later problems even after later risk was controlled statistically. The NICHD Study of Early Child Care (NICHD ECCRN, 2005) found that poverty in infancy and early childhood predicted more social and academic problems in elementary school than did concurrent poverty, but chronic poverty that lasted across the child's life was associated with the most academic and behavior problems. Furthermore, cumulative risk tended to be reasonably stable in a small subsample of children who also showed the highest levels of aggression from toddlerhood to elementary school (NICHD ECCRN, 2004). Taken together, these studies underscore the importance of family context and parenting for children's adjustment, including the number, timing, and long-term stability of family stresses.

Despite these challenges to parents and young children, children's adjustment outcomes will be partly determined by the balance of risk and protective factors (Luthar & Cicchetti, 2000; Masten, 2007). Protective factors are generally conceptualized as child characteristics and environmental supports that can counteract risks for children facing family adversity. Child characteristics, such as an easygoing personality and high intelligence, are often identified as protective (Masten, 2007) because children who are more easygoing and positive may be less upset or blame themselves less often for negative events or because their personality and intelligence help them to develop coping strategies and enlist the support of others. Maternal involvement and stimulation, despite elevated risk, is one potent protective factor (e.g., Jaffee, 2007). In considering protective factors, most emphasis has been placed on the role of caring adults who may take over from a stressed, depressed, or otherwise emotionally unavailable or harsh parent. In single-parent families, an involved noncustodial father (Coley & Hernandez, 2006; Masten, 2007) and/or a caring grandparent may serve an important protective role for young children. Similarly, when a mother is depressed, paternal and grandparental involvement may be crucial for young children's adaptation and developmental progress. Other recent work underscores the general importance of father involvement for young children's development and adjustment to school (Tamas-Lamonda, Shannon, Cebrera, & Lamb, 2004; NICHD ECCRN, 2004). Studies also point to the importance of a caring teacher, child care provider, or other adult who can at least temporarily help a young child cope with developmental challenges (Pianta, Steinberg, & Rollins, 1995; Shonkoff & Phillips, 2000). High-quality child care and preschool programs are often developed primarily with the goal of protecting young children from risk, and the need to work with the family and even the broader community is increasingly recognized (Brooks-Gunn, 2003; Shonkoff & Phillips, 2000).

EARLY PREVENTION AND INTERVENTION PROGRAMS AND CHILDREN'S FUNCTIONING

There are numerous prevention programs meant to help children and families living in adverse circumstances before problems develop or escalate (Dishion et al., 2008), and early intervention programs are meant to provide help to young children and their families before problems worsen (Gardner, Hutchings, Bywater, & Whitaker, 2010). Most programs emphasize work with the parents and focus on both relationship building and childrearing. Thus, programs include teaching parents how to play with their child by tuning into their child's communications and letting the child take the lead in play. They also emphasize parenting practices by teaching parents to use positive, proactive, and anticipatory methods of limit-setting; establish child-rearing goals and priorities; ignore some inappropriate behavior; and avoid the use of physical punishment (Eyberg, Nelson, & Boggs, 2008; Gardner, Burton, & Klimes, 2006; Webster-Stratton, 1998). In general, studies suggest that these methods can be effective in the short term as both prevention and intervention strategies. In a recent meta-analysis of 77 studies, Kaminski, Valle, Filene, and Boyd (2008) concluded that programs that included relationship building and also coached parents in the use of time-out and the importance of consistency tended to be more effective than programs that did not include these components. Other studies suggest that home visiting can lead to positive change (Olds, 2006) and effectively prevent child abuse in families experiencing risk in poor and dangerous neighborhoods. Still other studies emphasize the importance of moving beyond the parent-child dyad to promote parent well-being and to enhance the marital and co-parenting relationship (Trivette, Dunst, & Hamby, 2010).

Because intervention effects may be nonspecific, studies evaluating the impact of prevention and intervention programs have moved beyond asking whether a particular intervention is effective to asking *why* the program works (i.e., what processes are changed and, therefore, explain or mediate treatment effects) and *for whom* (i.e., are some children and families more likely to improve than others or what moderates treatment effects). Although a thorough review of this voluminous literature is beyond the scope of this chapter, the conclusions emerging from these studies are consistent with the transactional, ecological, and family systems models that inform our understanding of normative development and the development of problems. For example, some studies suggest that changes in parenting styles and strategies are the "active ingredient" that ultimately leads to de-escalating parent-child conflict and to better adjustment across settings (Eyberg et al., 2008).

For example in a large, multisite randomized controlled trial of a prevention program for parents and toddlers at high risk for externalizing behavior problems because of poverty and other indicators of family risk, Dishion et al. (2008) reported that improvements in parents' positive behavior and support for the toddler at age 2 accounted for improvements in child behavior at ages 3 and 4. Similar findings have been reported in other studies that specifically examine whether positive changes in parenting behavior account for treatment effects (e.g., Forgatch & DeGarmo, 1999; Gardner et al., 2010). Dishion and colleagues have also found that decreases in maternal depression (Shaw, Connell, Dishion, Wilson, & Gardner, 2009) and improvements in couple satisfaction (Linville et al., 2010) partially explain treatment effects as well. That is, as mothers' depressive symptoms declined and couple satisfaction increased, children's behavior problems improved. These results are consistent with a family systems perspective in suggesting not only the importance of positive parenting, but also that improved maternal mental health and more marital harmony have direct effects on children via improvements in family climate and indirect effects via more skillful childrearing.

Attempts to identify moderators of prevention and intervention effects have been less consistent (Eyberg et al., 2008), although there is growing evidence that families with multiple risk factors, including poverty, low education, and single parenting, respond to parenting interventions, and there is suggestive evidence that catching problems early, especially in boys, may be beneficial (Gardner et al., 2010). Gardner et al. (2010) also found that young children whose mothers reported more depressive symptoms showed a decline in problem behaviors after their mothers participated in a 12-week group-based parenting intervention, whereas children in the control condition showed a marked increase in problem behavior when their mothers also reported elevated depression. This may reflect the fact that mothers experiencing depression who attended the intervention group received social support from other parents and also learned better child-management skills, both of which may have alleviated their depressive symptoms. In another study, using the same sample as Dishion et al. discussed above, Gardner et al. (2009) reported that two-parent families were more responsive to the parenting intervention than were single-parent families, possibly because of the social support derived from co-parenting.

There is clearly a need for further studies that examine the acceptability and feasibility of parent training and supportive interventions for various cultural and ethnic groups with different values and belief systems as well as families coping with different types of stressful life events and conditions (Alegria, Atkins, Farmer, Slaton, & Stelk, 2010). Recent studies and several reviews and meta-analyses, however, suggest that children living in a range of family situations do benefit from structured interventions that support more positive parenting, while also providing broad support for families and increasing feelings of self-confidence and efficacy in parents (Eyberg et al., 2008; Kaminski et al., 2008; Trivette et al., 2010). Given the wealth of data linking family context and childrearing practices to young children's social adjustment and academic success, the need for comprehensive but didactic and structured programs remains a priority. In addition, child care workers and teachers need support and strategies to deal with children showing adjustment and other difficulties during the transition to out-of-home settings with an emphasis on bringing parents and teachers together to help young children cope (Atkins et al., 2010).

Other considerations include better preparation of new parents for their role as caregivers, better preparation of child care providers for handling problem behaviors, and continued efforts to improve the quality of child care. More comprehensive, available, and equitable family-leave policies and flexible work schedules that support family transitions are also needed (Campbell, 2002; Shonkoff & Phillips, 2000).

SUMMARY AND CONCLUDING COMMENTS

An ecological, transactional, and family systems framework for understanding children's early development and adjustment in the family and community underscores the complex mix of child, parenting, and family factors that are associated with young children's adjustment across toddlerhood and the preschool years. This is an especially challenging time for young children as they go through fundamental shifts in their cognitive and social development that will set them on a pathway toward good adjustment or emerging problems. The importance of the parent-child relationship and childrearing practices cannot be overestimated, but family climate, extended family support, and community resources also play a central role in young children's development. In particular, the availability and affordability of high-quality child care, preschool, and kindergarten programs will have implications for children's social and academic success. Further, policies that support families more broadly by facilitating warm, involved, and responsive parenting and that also provide child caregivers and primary school teachers with the tools and supports to optimize young children's adjustment to school and to the peer group are also a priority. Research indicates that structured prevention and early intervention programs focused on childrearing and the parent-child relationship can be effective in improving children's behavior and alleviating other aspects of family conflict. We know a good deal about the needs of children and families. The goal now is to translate this knowledge into practice.

References

Aber, J. L., Jones, S., & Cohen, J. (2000). The impact of poverty on mental health and development of very young children. In C. H. Zeanah (Ed.), *Handbook of Infant Mental Health* (2nd ed., pp. 113–128). New York: Guilford Press.

Ainsworth, M., Blehar, M., Waters, E., & Wall, S. (1978). *Patterns of attachment: A psychological study of the strange situation*. Hillsdale, NJ: Erlbaum.

Alegria, M., Atkins, M., Farmer, E., Slaton, E., & Stelk, W. (2010). One size does not fit all: Taking diversity, culture, and context seriously. *Administration and Policy in Mental Health and Mental Health Services Research, 37*, 48–60.

Appleyard, K., Egeland, B., van Dulmen, M., & Sroufe, L. A. (2005). When more is not better: The role of cumulative risk in child behavior outcomes. *Journal of Child Psychology and Psychiatry, 46*, 235–245.

Atkins, M. S., Hoagwood, K. E., Kutash, K., & Seidman, E. (2010). Toward the integration of education and mental health in the schools. *Administration and Policy in Mental Health and Mental Health Services Research, 37*, 40–47.

Bates, J. E., Pettit, G. S., Dodge, K. A., & Ridge, B. (1998). Interaction of temperamental resistance to control and restrictive parenting in the development of externalizing behavior. *Developmental Psychology, 34*, 982–995.

Belsky, J. (1984). The determinants of parenting: A process model. *Child Development, 55*, 83–96.

Belsky, J., Bakermans-Kranenberg, M., & van IJzendoorn, M. (2007). For better *and* for worse: Differential susceptibility to rearing influences. *Current Directions in Psychological Science, 16*, 300–304.

Belsky, J., Hsieh, K., & Crnic, K. (1998). Mothering, fathering, and infant negativity as antecedents of boys' externalizing problems: Differential susceptibility to rearing experiences? *Development and Psychopathology, 10*, 301–319.

Bowlby, J. S. (1969). *Attachment*. New York: Basic Books.

Bretherton, I. (1985). Attachment theory: Retrospect and prospect. In I. Bretheton & E. Waters (Eds.), *Growing points in attachment theory and research. Monographs of the Society for Research in Child Development, 50* (Serial no. 209), 3–35.

Bronfenbrenner, U. (1979). *The ecology of human development*. Cambridge, MA: Harvard University Press.

Brooks-Gunn, J. (2003). Do you believe in magic? What we can expect from early childhood intervention programs. *SRCD Social Policy Report, 17*(3), 1–14.

Brownell, C. A., & Kopp, C. B. (2007). Transitions in toddler socioemotional development: Behavior, understanding, and relationships. In C. A. Brownell & C. B. Kopp (Eds.), *Socioemotional development in the toddler years: Transitions and transformations* (pp. 1–40). New York: Guilford Press.

Calkins, S. D. (2007). The emergence of self-regulation: Biological and behavioral control mechanisms supporting toddler competencies. In C. A. Brownell & C. B. Kopp (Eds.), *Socioemotional development in the toddler years: Transitions and transformations* (pp. 261–284). New York: Guilford Press.

Campbell, S. B. (2002). *Behavior problems in preschool children: Clinical and developmental issues* (2nd ed.). New York: Guilford Press.

Campbell, S. B. (2006). Maladjustment in preschool children: A developmental psychopathology perspective. In K. McCartney & D. Phillips (Eds.), *The Blackwell Handbook of Early Childhood Development* (pp. 358–378). London: Blackwell.

Campbell, S. B., Brownell, C. A., Hungerford, A., Spieker, S., Mohan, R., & Blessing, J. (2004). The course of maternal depressive symptoms and maternal sensitivity as predictors of attachment security at 36 months. *Development and Psychopathology, 16*, 231–252.

Campbell, S. B., Matestic, P., von Stauffenberg, C., Mohan, R., & Kirchner, T. (2007). Trajectories of maternal depressive symptoms, maternal sensitivity, and children's functioning at school entry. *Developmental Psychology, 43*, 1202–1215.

Campbell, S. B., Shaw, D. S., & Gilliom, M. (2000). Early externalizing behavior problems: Toddlers and preschoolers at risk for later maladjustment. *Development and Psychopathology, 12*, 467–488.

Campbell, S. B., & von Stauffenberg, C. (2007). Child characteristics and family processes that predict behavioral readiness for school. In A. Booth and A. C. Crouter (Eds.), *Early disparities in school readiness: How do families contribute to successful and unsuccessful transitions into school?* (pp. 225–258). Mahwah, NJ: Erlbaum.

Ceballo, R., & McLoyd, V. C. (2002). Social support and parenting in poor and dangerous neighborhoods. *Child Development, 73*, 1310–1321.

Cicchetti, D., & Toth, S. L. (1995). A developmental psychopathology perspective on child abuse and neglect. *Journal of the American Academy of Child and Adolescent Psychiatry, 34*, 541–565.

Coley, R. L., & Hernandez, D. (2006). Predictors of paternal involvement for resident and non-resident low-income fathers. *Developmental Psychology, 42*, 1041–1056.

Cox, M. J., & Paley, B. (1997). Families as systems. *Annual Review of Psychology, 48*, 243–267.

Crockenberg, S., & Litman, C. (1990). Autonomy as competence in 2-year-olds: Maternal correlates of child defiance, compliance, and self-assertion. *Developmental Psychology, 26*, 961–971.

Cummings, E. M., Davies, P., & Campbell, S. B. (2000). *Developmental psychopathology and family process: Research, theory, and clinical implications*. New York: Guilford Press.

Deater-Deckard, K., Dodge, K. A., Bates, J. E., & Pettit, G. S. (1998). Multiple risk factors in the development of externalizing behavior problems: Group and individual differences. *Development and Psychopathology, 10,* 469–493.

Dishion, T., Shaw, D. S., Connell, A., Gardner, F., Weaver, C., & Wilson, M. (2008). The Family Check-Up with high-risk indigent families: Preventing problem behavior by increasing parents' positive behavior support in early childhood. *Child Development, 79,* 1395–1414.

Doumen, S., Verscherueren, K., Buyse, E., Germeijs, V., Luyckx, K., & Soenens, B. (2008). Reciprocal relations between teacher-child conflict and aggressive behavior in kindergarten: A three-wave longitudinal study. *Journal of Clinical Child and Adolescent Psychology, 37,* 588–599.

Eamon, M. K., & Zuehl, R. M. (2001). Maternal depression and physical punishment as mediators of the effect of poverty on socio-emotional problems of children in single-mother families. *American Journal of Orthopsychiatry, 71,* 218–226.

Eyberg, S., Nelson, M. M., & Boggs, S. R. (2008). Evidence-based psychosocial treatments for children and adolescents with disruptive behavior. *Journal of Abnormal Child Psychology, 37,* 215–237.

Forgatch, M. S., & DeGarmo, D. S. (1999). Parenting through change: An effective prevention program for single mothers. *Journal of Consulting and Clinical Psychology, 67,* 711–724.

Gardner, F., Burton, J., & Klimes, I. (2006). Randomized controlled trial of a parenting intervention in the voluntary sector for reducing child conduct problems: Outcomes and mechanisms of change. *Journal of Child Psychology and Psychiatry, 47,* 1123–1132.

Gardner, F., Connell, A., Trentacosta, C., Shaw, D. S., Dishion, T., & Wilson, M. N. (2009). Moderators of outcome in brief family-centered intervention for preventing early problem behavior. *Journal of Consulting and Clinical Psychology, 77,* 543–553.

Gardner, F., Hutchings, J., Bywater, T., & Whitaker, C. (2010). Who benefits and how does it work? Moderators and mediators of outcome in an effectiveness trial of a parenting intervention. *Journal of Clinical Child and Adolescent Psychology, 39,* 568–580.

Gardner, F., Sonuga-Barke, E., & Sayal, K. (1999). Parents anticipating misbehavior: An observational study of strategies parents use to prevent conflict with behavior problem children. *Journal of Child Psychology and Psychiatry, 40,* 1185–1196.

Goodman, S. (2007). Depression in mothers. *Annual Review of Clinical Psychology, 3,* 107–135.

Hobson, R. P. (2007). Social relations, self-awareness, and symbolizing: A perspective from autism. In C. A. Brownell & C. B. Kopp (Eds.), *Socioemotional development in the toddler years: Transitions and transformations* (pp. 423–450). New York: Guilford Press.

Holden, G. W. (1983). Avoiding conflict: Mothers as tacticians in the supermarket. *Child Development, 54,* 233–240.

Hughes, C., & Dunn, J. (2007). Children's relationships with other children. In C. A. Brownell & C. B. Kopp (Eds.), *Socioemotional development in the toddler years: Transitions and transformations* (pp. 177–200). New York: Guilford Press.

Jaffee, S. R. (2007). Sensitive, stimulating caregiving predicts cognitive and behavioral resilience in neurodevelopmentally at-risk infants. *Development and Psychopathology, 19*, 631–648.

Jones, D. J., Forehand, R., Brody, G., & Armistead, L. (2002). Psychosocial adjustment of African-American children in single mother families: A test of three risk models. *Journal of Marriage and the Family, 64*, 105–115.

Kaminski, J. W., Valle, L. A., Filene, J. H., & Boyle, C. L. (2008). A meta-analytic review of components associated with parent training program effectiveness. *Journal of Abnormal Child Psychology, 36*, 567–589.

Kochanska, G. (2002). Mutually responsive orientation between mothers and their young children: A context for the early development of conscience. *Current Directions in Psychological Science, 11*, 191–195.

Kochanska, G., Kuczynski, L., Radke-Yarrow, M., & Welsh, J. D. (1987). Resolution of control episodes between well and affectively ill mothers and their young child. *Journal of Abnormal Child Psychology, 15*, 441–456.

Kochanska, G., Philibert, R., & Barry, R. A. (2009). Interplay of genes and early mother-child relationship in the development of self-regulation from toddler to preschool age. *Journal of Child Psychology and Psychiatry, 50*, 1331–1338.

Kopp, C. B. (1989). Regulation of distress and negative emotions: A developmental view. *Developmental Psychology, 25*, 343–354.

Leadbeater, B., Bishop, S., & Raver, C. (1996). Quality of mother-toddler interaction, maternal depressive symptoms, and behavior problems in preschoolers of adolescent mothers. *Developmental Psychology, 32*, 280–288.

Leve, L. D., Gordon, G. T., Ge, X., Neiderheiser, J. M., Shaw, D., Scaramella, L. V., & Reiss, D. (2009). Structured parenting of toddlers at high versus low genetic risk: Two pathways to child problems. *Journal of the American Academy of Child and Adolescent Psychiatry, 48*, 1102–1109.

Lillard, A. (2007). Pretend play in toddlers. In C. A. Brownell & C. B. Kopp (Eds.), *Socioemotional development in the toddler years: Transitions and transformations* (pp. 149–176). New York: Guilford Press.

Lin, H. L., Lawrence, F. R., & Gorrell, J. (2003). Kindergarten teachers' views of school readiness. *Early Childhood Research Quarterly, 18*, 225–237.

Linville, D., Chronister, K., Dishion, T., Todahl, J., Miller, J., Shaw, D., et al. (2010). A longitudinal analysis of parenting practices, couple satisfaction, and child behavior problems. *Journal of Marital and Family Therapy, 36*, 244–255.

Luthar, S. S., & Cicchetti, D. (2000). The construct of resilience: Implications for intervention and social policies. *Development and Psychopathology, 12*, 857–885.

Lyons-Ruth, C., Easterbrooks, M. A., & Cibelli, C. D. (1997). Infant attachment strategies, infant mental lag, and maternal depressive symptoms: Predictors of internalizing and externalizing problems at age 7. *Developmental Psychology, 33*, 681–692.

Masten, A. S. (2007). Resilience in developing systems: Progress and promise as the fourth wave rises. *Development and Psychopathology, 19*, 921–930.

McMahon, S. D., Grant, K. E., Compas, B. E., Thurm, A. E., & Ey, S. (2003). Stress and psychopathology in children and adolescents: is there evidence of specificity? *Journal of Child Psychology and Psychiatry, 44*, 107–133.

McClelland, M., & Morrison, F. J. (2003). The emergence of learning-related social skills in preschool children. *Early Childhood Research Quarterly, 18*, 206–224.

McLoyd, V. C. (1990). The impact of economic hardship on Black families and children: Psychological distress, parenting and socioemotional development. *Child Development, 61,* 311–346.

McLoyd, V. C. (1998). Socieconomic disadvantage and child development. *American Psychologist, 53,* 185–204.

Melton, G. (2010). Putting the "community" back into "mental health": The challenge of a great crisis in the health and well-being of children and families. *Administration and Policy in Mental Health and Mental Health Services Research, 37,* 173–176.

Moore, C. (2007). Understanding self and other in the second year. In C. A. Brownell & C. B. Kopp (Eds.), *Socioemotional development in the toddler years: Transitions and transformations* (pp. 43–65). New York: Guilford Press.

NICHD Early Child Care Research Network. (1996). Poverty and patterns of child care. In J. Brooks-Gunn and G. Duncan (Eds.), *Consequences of growing up poor* (pp. 100–131). New York: Russell Sage Foundation.

NICHD Early Child Care Research Network. (1997). Familial factors associated with characteristics of nonmaternal care for infants. *Journal of Marriage and the Family, 59,* 389–408.

NICHD Early Child Care Research Network. (1999). Chronicity of maternal depressive symptoms, maternal sensitivity, and child functioning at 36 months. *Developmental Psychology, 35,* 1399–1413.

NICHD Early Child Care Research Network. (2002). Structure>Process>Outcome: Direct and indirect effects of caregiving quality on young children's development. *Psychological Science, 13,* 199–206.

NICHD Early Child Care Research Network. (2003). Social functioning in first grade: Associations with earlier home and child care predictors and with concurrent classroom experiences. *Child Development, 74,* 1639–1662.

NICHD Early Child Care Research Network. (2004). Trajectories of aggression from toddlerhood to middle childhood: Predictors, correlates, and outcomes. *Monographs of the Society for Research in Child Development, 69,* whole no. 4.

NICHD Early Child Care Research Network. (2005). Duration and developmental timing of poverty and children's cognitive and social development from birth through third grade. *Child Development, 76,* 795–810.

Olds, D. L. (2006). The Nurse-Family Partnership: An evidence-based preventive intervention. *Infant Mental Health Journal, 27,* 5–25.

Pianta, R. C., Steinberg, M. S., & Rollins, K. B. (1995). The first two years of school: Teacher-child relationships and deflections in children's classroom adjustment. *Development and Psychopathology, 7,* 295–312.

Pluess, M., & Belsky, J. (2009). Differential susceptibility to rearing experience: the case of childcare. *Journal of Child Psychology and Psychiatry, 50,* 396–404.

Rimm-Kaufmann, S. E., Pianta, R. C., & Cox, M. J. (2000). Teacher's judgments of problems in the transition to kindergarten. *Early Childhood Research Quarterly, 15,* 147–166.

Sameroff, A. J. (1995). General systems theories and developmental psychopathology. In D. Cicchetti & D. Cohen (Eds.), *Developmental Psychopathology, Vol. I: Theory and methods* (pp. 659–695). New York: Wiley.

Sameroff, A. J. (2000). Developmental systems and psychopathology. *Development and Psychopathology, 12,* 297–312.

Serbin, L., & Karp, J. (2004). Intergenerational transfer of psychosocial risk: Mediators of vulnerability and resilience. *Annual Review of Psychology, 55*, 333–363.

Shatz, M. (2007). Revisiting *A Toddler's Life* for the toddler years: Conversational participation as a tool for learning across knowledge domains. In C. A. Brownell & C. B. Kopp (Eds.), *Socioemotional development in the toddler years: Transitions and transformations* (pp. 241–260). New York: Guilford Press.

Shaw, D. S., Connell, A., Dishion, T. J., Wilson, M. N., & Gardner, F. (2009). Improvement in maternal depression as a mediator of intervention effects on early childhood problem behavior. *Development and Psychopathology, 21*, 417–440.

Shonkoff, J., & Phillips, D. (2000). *From neurons to neighborhoods.* Washington, DC: National Academy Press.

Sroufe, L. A., & Fleeson, J. (1986). Attachment and the construction of relationships. In W. Hartup & Z. Rubin (Eds.). *The nature and development of relationships* (pp. 51–71). Hillsdale, NJ: Erlbaum.

Stiffman, A. R., Stelk, W., Horwitz, S. M., Evans, M. E., Outlaw, F. H., & Atkins, M. (2010). A public health approach to children's mental health services: possible solutions to current service inadequacies. *Administration and Policy in Mental Health and Mental Health Services Research, 37*, 120–124.

Tamas-LaMonda, C., Shannon, J., Cabrera, N., & Lamb, M. (2004). Fathers and mothers at play with their 2- and 3-year-olds: Contributions to language and cognitive development. *Child Development, 75*, 1806–1820.

Thomas, A., Chess, S., & Birch, H. (1968). *Temperament and behavior problems in children.* New York: New York University Press.

Thompson, R. (2006). The development of the person: Social understanding, relationships, self, and conscience. In W. Damon and R. M. Lerner (Eds.), N. Eisenberg (Vol. Ed.), *Handbook of Child Psychology: Vol. 3. Social, emotional, and personality development* (6th ed., pp. 24–98). New York: Wiley.

Tremblay, R. E. (2000). The development of aggressive behavior during childhood: What have we learned in the past century? *International Journal of Behavioral Development, 24*, 129–141.

Trivette, C. M., Dunst, C. J., & Hamby, D. W. (2010). Influences of family systems intervention practices on parent-child interactions and child development. *Topics in Early Childhood Special Education, 30*, 3–19.

Van Zeijl, J., Mesman, J., Stolk, M. N., Alink, L. R., van IJzendoorn, M. H., et al. (2007). Differential susceptibility to discipline: The moderating effect of child temperament on the association between maternal discipline and early childhood externalizing problems. *Journal of Family Psychology, 21*, 626–636.

Webster-Stratton, C. (1998). Preventing conduct problems in Head Start children: Strengthening parenting competencies. *Journal of Consulting and Clinical Psychology, 66*, 715–730.

Yates, T. M., Dodds, M. F., Sroufe, L. A., & Egeland, B. (2003). Exposure to partner violence and child behavior problems: A prospective study controlling for child-directed abuse and neglect, child cognitive ability, socioeconomic status, and life stress. *Development and Psychopathology, 15*, 199–218.

Zahn-Waxler, C., Radke-Yarrow, M., Wagner, E., & Chapman, M. (1992). The development of concern for others. *Developmental Psychology, 28*, 126–136.

Chapter 8

Supporting Young Children with Social and Behavioral Challenges

Sharon Doubet and Rob Corso

A growing body of research shows that promoting the emotional wellness of young children and fostering secure, warm relationships between children, their parents and other caregivers are keys to healthy development and later school success (Denno, Phillips, Harte, & Momaw, 2004; Hyson, 2004; Knitzer, 2000; NICHD, 2003; Raver, 2002; Zigler, 2004; Zins, Bloodworth, Weissberg, & Walberg, 2004). Educators, researchers, and policy makers are becoming increasingly aware that many young children are beginning school without the requisite emotional, social, and behavioral skills that increase the likelihood of success. Although specific estimates of prevalence rates vary depending on the sample and criteria used, the significant rates at which emotional and behavior problems occur in young children are now well documented. For example, data from the Early Childhood Longitudinal Study revealed that 10 percent of kindergarteners arrive at school with problematic behavior (West, Denton, & Germino-Hausken, 2000). Furthermore, children from low-income families are even more likely to develop behavior problems, with prevalence rates that approach 30 percent (Qi & Kaiser, 2003). The significance of the early display of externalizing-type problems (e.g., aggression and property destruction) for later behavior has been well established; therefore, intervening as early as possible is critical (Kaiser & Rasminsky, 2007; Stormont, Lewis, Beckner, & Johnson, 2008). The longer a child uses challenging behaviors to get his or her needs met, the more difficult it is to change these patterns of interaction (Webster-Stratton, 1997). Not surprising, a growing body of research points to the correlation between social competence and school success (Raver, 2002).

Because more young children enter school displaying severe problem behaviors, there is an increased interest in providing early intervention to children during the preschool years (Shonkoff & Phillips, 2000). The primary settings in which these efforts are likely to occur are early childhood programs. Unfortunately, many early childhood programs are not prepared to meet the needs of children who are emotionally delayed or have problem behavior (Kaufmann & Wischmann, 1999). Often, children with complex and intensive social and emotional needs are removed or are at risk for being removed from inclusive settings as a result of their challenging behaviors (Gilliam, 2005; Raver & Knitzer, 2002). In a national study, Gilliam found that on average, 6.67 preschool-age children in state-subsidized prekindergarten classrooms were expelled per 1,000 enrolled, a rate 3.2 times higher than for students in K–12 classrooms.

Because of the intensive, ongoing needs of children with more problematic behaviors, simply placing these children in Head Start programs, preschools, child care centers, and other early childhood environments is not enough. Typically, teachers have applied generic strategies (e.g., time-out) and rules to complex problem behaviors, which in turn often cause problem behaviors to accelerate rather than diminish (Sprague et al., 2001). Rather, children with high levels of challenging behaviors need to have access to ongoing positive relationships and environments that support their social and emotional development. At the same time, these children also need individual support so that they can learn appropriate ways to express what they want or need, rather than using challenging behaviors. In sum, these children need more systematic behavioral approaches that go beyond typical intervention strategies (Sandall & Schwartz, 2002).

In response to the need for systematic behavioral approaches, the content of this chapter will focus on the current state of support for young children with social and behavioral challenges. In support of this topic, the experiences of the players (i.e., children and families, teachers, administrators), their roles, and current support strategies will be described. The next section of the chapter focuses on current service delivery systems, including professional development and a framework for a pyramid model using a tiered system of support. Stories of successful implementation of the pyramid model in diverse settings are included in the third section of the chapter. The final section includes discussion of Response to Intervention and mental health consultation, both current support approaches in the field.

THE PLAYERS AND THE SUPPORTS

Children and Families

The demographic description of young children with social and behavioral challenges is inconsistent. The children may or may not have Individual Family Service Plans (IFSPs) or Individual Education Plans (IEPs); likewise, they may be typically developing or have atypical development. Family demographics are also very diverse as there does not appear to be a consistent descriptor of families with children exhibiting social or behavioral challenges.

The Impact of Challenging Behaviors on Children and Families

Challenging behaviors has a substantial impact on all members of a family system (Fox, Vaughn, Dunlap, & Bucy, 1997). Family stress and family isolation are reoccurring topics in studies focusing on the impact of parenting a child exhibiting challenging behaviors (Guralnick, 2000; Hoppe, 2005). For example, as previously noted, young children may be expelled from a child care program because of their behavior (Gilliam, 2005), adding stress to a family system. For many parents, one of the most difficult issues they confront surrounds their child's behavior (Boulware, Swartz, & McBride, 1999).

Doubet, Ostrosky, and Hemmeter (2007) conducted an interview study with seven parents of children ages 3–5 in child care settings in a Midwestern county. Each child was at risk for expulsion or had been expelled from one or more child care programs due to their challenging behaviors. Parents reported instances when either the whole family did not attend public events, or other plans were made so that the child with challenging behavior stayed home with one of the parents while the rest of the family attended the event. Such choices impact families' abilities to go places as a unit. One parent spoke of staying home due to her son's unpredictable behavior, "We don't go to that many places, 'cause he'll fall apart. Wherever we're at, he does it." This influence extends to sibling relationships. Parents who discussed the effect on older siblings reflected on missed activities and attempts to help their other children understand absences from their extracurricular activities. The need to plan ahead to avoid problem situations was tiresome, and the stress on intra-family relationships was evident.

In addition, parent confidence in their parenting skills is affected when community and family members express concern about the role of the parent in the behaviors of the child. Parents report hearing negative comments from community members expressing blame toward the parents for the child's behavioral problems (Hutton & Caron, 2005). Parents in the Doubet, Ostrosky, and Hemmeter (2007) study also described how they began to doubt their parenting skills and abilities. When asked about the impact of a child exhibiting challenging behaviors on her family, one mother replied, "Stressful, embarrassing. Like 'Oh, she can't control her kids.' And really—I can't."

In response to the impact of challenging behaviors on families, positive behavior support (PBS) stresses the importance of a family-centered approach when providing support and services. Fox, Dunlap, and Cushing (2002) describe the family as "the overwhelmingly dominant influence on a child's behavioral development and functioning" (p. 151). Family-centered support emerged as a focus for service providers in the last 20 years and is reflected in the service delivery systems in place today. The early childhood field has defined "family-centered" as practices that value family strengths, needs, priorities, input, and privacy (Boone & Crais, 2002).

This attitude toward the parent-professional relationship is echoed in national policy. Under IDEA, early intervention programs are required to use a family-centered approach, which guides the development and implementation of intervention strategies (Hoppe, 2005). Outcomes of any child support plan are not independent of family functioning. For example, Fox, Vaughn, et al. (1997) found children's progress was inextricably tied to the functioning of the family as a whole. Family-centered positive behavior support has the potential to result in lifestyle improvements for the child and other family members (Lucyshyn, Dunlap, & Albin, 2002).

Effective early education programs include a parent-training component. Parent instruction focuses on behavior management skills, increasing positive interactions, increasing children's prosocial behavior, and child guidance procedures (Strain & Timm, 2001; Webster-Stratton, Reid, & Hammond, 2001). In light of the research supporting a family-centered approach (Hoppe, 2005; Trivette & Dunst, 2005), early childhood programs continue to investigate ways to increase their parent support and educational opportunities on the topic of young children's social and emotional development.

Teachers: The Workforce That Supports the Development of Young Children

Over the last two decades, there has been growing acceptance among policy makers that early childhood professionals (e.g., teachers, assistants, care providers, directors) are in a position to design programs that foster children's social and emotional development as well as their cognitive skills. Many early research studies have reported that the early years of children's lives form the social-emotional foundation for later learning and school success (Thompson, 1994; Zero to Three, 1992). However, due to inconsistency in the quality of care, it is unrealistic to expect that every child in a child care setting will be provided with the supports and opportunities they need for healthy social and emotional development.

For example, the early care and education workforce is often underpaid and undervalued, receives little professional development training, and works in difficult physical and emotional environments. Additionally, child care staff often feel overwhelmed with the responsibilities of caring for multiple children in group care. More than in most professions, child care providers must collaborate, share space, be flexible, and coordinate almost every aspect of their day—a challenge for any group of workers with varied histories, experiences, cultures, and beliefs about children (Johnston & Brinamen, 2006). Furthermore, early childhood teachers find that working with a child exhibiting challenging behaviors adds much stress to an already difficult situation. Unfortunately, teacher stress and burnout, as well as high levels of teacher turnover, may negatively impact the social and emotional development of students.

Job Satisfaction

Teachers report that working with children exhibiting challenging behaviors affects their overall job satisfaction (Joseph, Strain, & Skinner, 2004). Many early childhood staff members feel ill prepared to meet the needs of children who are emotionally delayed or who exhibit social and emotional problems. Early childhood teachers report that (1) challenging behaviors is one of their greatest challenges,

(2) there seems to be an increasing number of children who have challenging behaviors, (3) they do not feel competent in handling children exhibiting challenging behaviors, and (4) all of this negatively affects job satisfaction and leads to stress and burnout (Hemmeter, Corso, & Cheatham, 2006).

Low job satisfaction may lead to high levels of staff turnover. Low wages and poor working conditions in the child care profession have created conditions in which many teachers have minimal education and training, and more than a third of the teachers in child care leave their positions each year (Hyson, 2004). In fact, the child care staff turnover rate hovers around 30 percent each year (U.S. Bureau of Labor Statistics, 1998), which, according to Shonkoff and Phillips (2000), is among the highest of any profession tracked by the Department of Labor. Staff turnover rates negatively affect the social and emotional development of children. According to the National Research Council and Institute of Medicine (2000b), there is a strong correlation between high-quality programs, highly qualified staff, very minimal teacher turnover, and positive developmental outcomes for young children.

Personnel Development of the Workforce

Teachers note an increasing number of children exhibiting disruptive behaviors and cite these behaviors as one of the greatest challenges they face in providing a quality program (Arnold, McWilliams, & Arnold, 1998). Unfortunately, there exists a critical shortage of service providers available to work with young children with social-emotional delays, challenging behaviors, and disabilities (Klein & Gilkerson, 2000). Furthermore, there is a lack of personnel who have relevant training in social-emotional development and intervention to assist with evaluation, IFSP or IEP development, and service provision at these key points of entry (Kopel, 2004). Similar numbers are evidenced for teachers working with young children exhibiting challenging behaviors (U.S. Department of Education [USDOE], 2007). At the same time, teachers qualified to work with children with emotional disturbance represent the area in which the least amount of progress has been made. In a national survey, Bruder (2004) found that fewer than 50 percent of state administrators surveyed believed that special educators and social workers in their state were adequately prepared for their roles in early intervention. In part, shortages of service providers adequately prepared to address the social-emotional needs of children result from the fact that many early childhood staff members are not well trained before entering the field, nor are they adequately supervised (Johnston & Brinamen, 2006).

Accordingly, early care and education providers often report that addressing challenging behaviors is one of their most significant training needs (Child Care Resource Services [CCRS], 2003; Joseph et al., 2004). For example, the results of a survey study of 88 child care and at-risk pre-kindergarten teachers revealed that 65 percent chose "learning how to support children exhibiting challenging behaviors" as their highest in-service training priority (Doubet, Ostrosky, & Corso, 2007). In a larger survey study of 400 child care providers, 73 percent selected the issue of "controlling children's problem behaviors" as a primary in-service training need (Dinnebeil, McInerney, Fox, & Juchartz-Pendry, 1998). Clearly, early childhood educators have voiced their need for training in the area of working with young children exhibiting challenging behaviors.

Teachers' Responses to Challenging Behaviors

Many teachers do not feel confident in their abilities to address challenging behaviors, and this perception impacts their overall view of how effective they are as a teacher. Nungesser and Watkins (2005) surveyed 45 preschool teachers in Head Start, at-risk prekindergarten, and private preschool classrooms to learn how early education teachers perceived and reacted to challenging behaviors. The strategies and interventions that teachers reported using most frequently when responding to challenging behaviors were reactive and punitive types of intervention approaches (e.g., time-out, restraint, loss of privileges) versus proactive or preventative approaches (e.g., functional analysis, choices, use of emotion words).

Doubet and Ostrosky (2009) reported similar results in a descriptive study where participants were 11 early childhood teachers. Seventy-three percent of the teachers who were interviewed used punitive strategies in response to challenging behaviors. The most cited reactive and punitive responses were sending the child to sit in the administrator's office, expulsion, and time-out. Only 33 percent of the teachers in this study reported using proactive and prevention strategies (i.e., teach rules and schedules, problem solving, how to ask for help, emotion words, calming strategies).

When reviewing teachers' responses to challenging behaviors, another point to consider is the theory that teachers' reactions and responses to children's challenging behaviors may be a combination of their own life experiences and training. For example, staff members have their own life history and social circumstances that inform their practices and classroom choices. Often the style of parenting a teacher experienced as a child will exert more power over his or her teaching style than years of training (Johnston & Brinamen, 2006).

Support for Teachers

Given the multiple levels and complexity involved with implementing promotion, prevention, and intervention strategies, an equally multi-faceted training and support system for teachers must be employed (Sandall & Schwartz, 2002). More intensive training programs are needed with follow-up support to help teachers and child care providers feel more competent when working with children exhibiting challenging behaviors (Winton, McCollum, & Catlett, 1997). In turn, children are more likely to feel comfortable and safe, and teachers will be able to use time that was previously spent addressing challenging behaviors on teaching academic, social, and emotional skills.

Teachers of young children exhibiting challenging behaviors may experience difficulties finding support services for their students or helping families access community resources, resulting in few children with early signs of problem behaviors receiving support (Kazdin & Kendall, 1998). Given that more favorable outcomes for young children exhibiting challenging behaviors are realized when intervention begins at a young age (Strain & Timm, 2001), delays in accessing services and support for teachers is a concern.

Administrators

High-quality early education environments are related to positive outcomes in children's social and emotional development and reduced challenging behaviors. Providing a high-quality environment is an essential foundation for the implementation of promotion and intervention practices (Burchinal, Peisner-Feinberg, Bryant, & Clifford, 2000; NICHD, 1999). Strong administrative knowledge and skills must be in place to provide high-quality environments, training, and support for early care and education professionals.

Specific policies and procedures regarding training, support, and collaboration must be developed to sustain a system of this magnitude. These program policies and procedures should include processes for teaching social-emotional skills; screening, assessing, and monitoring young children's social-emotional development; involving families in supporting their child's social-emotional development; addressing challenging behaviors and supporting children with persistent challenging behaviors; and providing training, technical assistance, and ongoing support to staff addressing young children's social emotional competence and challenging behaviors (Fox & Hemmeter, 2009).

Implementing recommended practices in support of young children and their families requires a review of current policies, procedures, and systems change (Sandall, Hemmeter, Smith, & McLean, 2005).The success in implementing these changes will be improved when administrators (1) are knowledgeable in recommended practice in early childhood, (2) share resources with other community programs, and (3) engage in systems change (Smith, 2000). Without strong policies and procedures in place to support social and emotional development of young children, punitive and reactive responses that minimally influence challenging behaviors are more evident. In a study conducted by Doubet and Ostrosky (2009), early childhood teachers reported that they often send a child exhibiting challenging behaviors to the office to "spend time" with the director or administrator. According to one teacher, sending children exhibiting challenging behaviors to the office "affects them [director] so they can't do their jobs. They can't do what they're supposed to be doing because they're dealing with this child." Another teacher noted: "I think it affects everyone, the whole system. I think it affects the other children in the room. And then, in turn, I'm so stressed that I affect the directors."

The Doubet and Ostrosky (2009) study also found that several teachers felt unsupported by the administrators when they were working with children exhibiting challenging behaviors. In fact, these teachers believed that the administrators lacked the necessary skills to support them. In addition to a desire for administrator time and skills, teachers expressed a desire for program policies addressing challenging behaviors. Examples of administrative support teachers discussed included help with problem solving, communicating with parents, and investigating options for assistance from outside agencies.

SERVICE DELIVERY SYSTEMS

Even though the increased rate of young children exhibiting challenging behaviors has been recognized, adequate service delivery is lacking.

For young children who show early signs of problem behaviors, it has been estimated that fewer than 10 percent receive support services for these difficulties, and parents who seek supportive services for their children may encounter difficulties in accessing appropriate services and supports (Kazdin & Kendall, 1998). As a result, 50 percent of preschool children with externalized challenging behaviors continue to demonstrate problems during their school years, leading to long-term, serious difficulties (Stormont, Lewis, & Beckner, 2005).

Fox, Dunlap, and Cushing (2002) wrote about the lack of a system focused on young children with behavior problems. According to Fox and colleagues, there are 39 different governmental sources of funding for early childhood mental health services, each with differing policies, procedures, and eligibility standards. As a result of the lack of coordination, services do not reach all children who qualify. Furthermore, the early childhood mental health system is fragmented and difficult for families to navigate. The point of entry into a community support system of mental health services is often unclear. Families with young children may already be overburdened, and difficulty accessing a system of support may be one reason why some families do not pursue community services.

In a literature review conducted by Smith and Fox (2003a), much support was found for a system of service delivery for young children at risk of or who have challenging behaviors. Smith and Fox reviewed approximately 90 articles of relevant literature from 1982 to 2002, leading to conclusions in support of family-oriented systems. They recommend that families should (1) help design systems of care, (2) be in the center of decisions related to supports, and (3) have their individual family needs and strengths taken into consideration when designing a plan for support.

A challenge to the field is to blend the multiple existing services into a cohesive, collaborative system (Smith & Fox, 2003b). According to Fox et al., (2002), this type of interconnected system of care has been effective with older children and adults in serving their behavioral needs: "It is reasonable to conclude that the knowledge and technology for achieving behavior change for young children exhibiting challenging behaviors is known; the challenge that remains is the delivery of the support in ways that reach the most vulnerable families" (p. 217). This challenge extends to teachers who must have the knowledge and resources to help families access supports and services for young children with persistent challenging behaviors. Early intervention systems need to address the barriers to service delivery and develop family-friendly outreach practices that meet the unique needs of families who may already be facing difficulties (Knitzer, 2000).

Office of Special Education Child Outcomes

In 2005, the Office of Special Education Programs (OSEP) began requiring State Early Intervention and Preschool Special Education programs to report on child outcomes. Two out of the three required outcomes for states related to children's social and emotional development and behavior. Specifically, states are required to report on the percentage of infants and toddlers with IFSPs or preschool children with IEPs who demonstrate improved positive social-emotional skills (including social relationships), acquisition and use of knowledge and skills (including early language/communication [and early literacy]), and use of appropriate behaviors to meet their needs. A great deal of effort has gone into this initiative, including funding of the national Early Childhood Outcomes (ECO) Center. Since its inception in 2003, the ECO Center has provided technical assistance and conducted research to support states in the development of outcome measurement systems that provide valid and reliable data for federal reporting and program improvement.

Systems for Professional Development

Many early childhood professionals lack specific training that prepares them to work with children with behavioral disabilities (Dinnebeil et al., 1998). Addressing the need for highly qualified staff, Knitzer (2000) called for states to strengthen systems of training for early care providers to include a focus on children at risk of atypical social and emotional development.

Community or system-wide change is required for sustainable improvements to the current responses that many early childhood programs use when young children have challenging behaviors (i.e., punitive reactions to behavior, expulsion). Recommendations from Smith and Fox (2003b) list ways to support social and emotional development and address challenging behaviors through evidence-based practices. This list includes a systems focus on (1) providing a range of services from promotion to prevention to intervention, (2) offering comprehensive and family-centered services and supports, and (3) supporting personnel with the resources to provide evidence-based services.

CURRENT STATE: EARLY CHILDHOOD POSITIVE
BEHAVIOR SUPPORT

One model that has been demonstrated to be effective in providing the various levels of support and intervention needed to address the often complex behavioral needs of children while providing support and training to teachers is school-wide positive behavior support (PBS) (Sugai, Sprague, Horner, & Walker, 2000). PBS utilizes a focused, team-based, comprehensive approach to support all children, including those exhibiting challenging behaviors. The focus of PBS is on teaching children social skills and promoting appropriate behavior while preventing problem behaviors (Lewis & Sugai, 1999; Sugai et al., 2000). It emphasizes the adoption of evidence-based intervention practices and the use of data to understand issues related to problem behaviors. School-wide PBS not only supports the needs of children exhibiting challenging behaviors, but it is also designed to support their teachers and providers in efforts to implement effective teaching practices. Some key elements of support for teachers include professional development plans, teacher training, and school-wide processes for responding to problem behaviors. Such efforts may result in teachers feeling adequately supported and competent in addressing the needs of all children, including those with persistent challenging behaviors.

Although school-wide PBS has proven effective with school-age (K–12) populations, less is known about the effectiveness of this model with children under the age of 6. However, some of the critical components of PBS are applicable to young children, including (1) staff and administrative buy-in when developing and implementing school-wide and individual plans, (2) clear goals and expectations for all children, (3) using prevention strategies and teaching social skills, and (4) individualized interventions for children with more intensive needs. Yet, other components, such as rewards and tracking systems for behaviors, were seemingly in need of revision or modification to align more closely with developmentally appropriate early childhood practices. Additionally, some components that are not typically a part of PBS systems in primary or secondary school settings that would be critical in early childhood settings include (1) parental/family involvement, (2) teaming with professionals (e.g., therapists, behavior specialists, etc.), (3) assessing current program policies and procedures related to behavior, and (4) providing and maintaining support and training for staff (Fox & Hemmeter, 2009; Quesenberry & Hemmeter, 2005).

Unfortunately, many early childhood programs do not have all of these essential elements in place, thus teachers do not feel well supported in their efforts to include children exhibiting challenging behaviors in their classrooms. A first step for many programs is to develop program policies and procedures that outline key issues that often arise in early childhood programs. After developing comprehensive policies and procedures, programs must ensure that stakeholders (e.g., administrators, teachers, support staff, parents) are aware of the content of the policies and procedures and their role in implementing them.

Conceptual Framework: The Pyramid Model for Supporting the Social and Emotional Competence of Infants and Young Children

The Pyramid Model has been proposed for promoting the social and emotional development and addressing challenging behaviors of young children (Fox, Dunlap, Hemmeter, Joseph, & Strain, 2003). Shown in Figure 8.1, this multitiered model describes the levels of prevention, promotion, and intervention that must be in place to address the needs of young children within early childhood programs.

Prevention, Promotion, and Intervention: A Comprehensive System of Support

Early education and care environments should be structured to provide universal (prevention), secondary (promotion), and individual intervention practices. There are promising data indicating that the adoption of this model as a program-wide approach results in positive outcomes for children, families, and the programs that support them (Dunlap, Fox, & Hemmeter, 2004). Given the relationship between children's social and emotional competencies and academic success (Hyson, 2004; Zigler, 2004), prevention, promotion, and intervention is necessary to address young children's social and emotional challenges.

Details and descriptions of these tiers of the Pyramid Model will be discussed in the following three sections of this chapter. Readers may wish to refer to the Center on the Social and Emotional Foundations for Early Learning (CSEFEL) Web site at http://www.vanderbilt.edu/csefel for in-depth information in these areas.

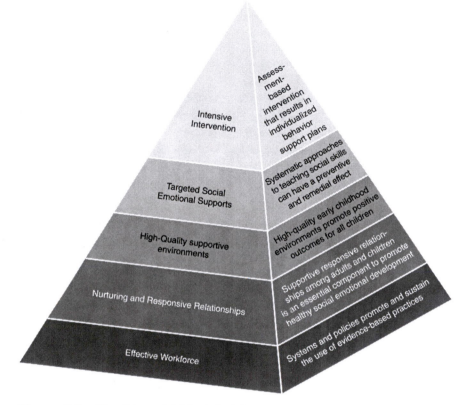

Figure 8.1   The Pyramid Model of Strategies for supporting positive relationships with children, families, and co-workers.

Universal Level: Prevention—Relationships

The Pyramid Model details the provision of universal strategies to support building positive relationships with children, families, and coworkers and creating high-quality supportive environments. With regard to the process of *building positive relationships*, Hyson (2004) explains that developing such relationships provides a secure foundation for all areas of development, including emotional development. There is a strong link between the quality of children's relationships with adults and their emotional development (Denno et al., 2004; Hamre & Pianta, 2001). Research about the brain and resiliency reveals that consistent, nurturing relationships are a child's best protection against risk—including the risk of challenging behaviors. These positive, relationship-based experiences typically lead to less challenging and aggressive behavior (Peisner-Feinberg et al., 2001).

A close relationship with a teacher brings a child "strong and persistent" benefits (Hamre & Pianta, 2001). In their book *A Matter of Trust: Connecting Teachers and Learners in Early Childhood Classrooms*, Howes and Ritchie state, "The quality of children's early relationships with their teachers is an important predictor of these children's future social relations with peers, their behavior problems, and school satisfaction and achievement" (2002, p. 6). Research has documented that teachers with warm, responsive, affective interaction styles are more likely to engage children for longer periods of time and at higher levels, thus leading to more opportunities to develop positive relationships (Denno et al., 2004).

The relationships that we build with children, families, and colleagues are at the foundation of everything that we do. Children learn and develop in the context of relationships that are responsive, consistent, and nurturing. The adults who interact with young children have many opportunities throughout the day to build and sustain a strong relationship with the children and families in their care. Warmly greeting a child and their parent as they enter a child care center in the morning builds a sense of trust between all involved. Spending time playing alongside a child, having a conversation with a child, recognizing family events (e.g., new baby), and inviting parents to spend time in the classroom are a few ways that teachers can build and sustain relationships. It is these experiences that children with the most challenging behaviors need, yet their behaviors often prevent them from benefiting from those relationships.

Universal Level: Prevention—Environment

At the next level, *classroom preventative practices* or *creating supportive environments*, adults ensure that the physical and social environments are supportive of fostering social emotional competence among children. All early childhood educators should design environments to include predictable schedules with minimal transitions, visual reminders of rules/expectations, time and attention for appropriate behavior, positive reinforcement to promote appropriate behavior, choices where appropriate, and maximum child engagement to minimize problem behaviors (Strain & Hemmeter, 1999). Additional environmental supports may include assigning class jobs or developing books to tell the "story of our day." For a child who is awake during naptime, a special "naptime backpack" could be filled with quiet items and favorite books. The child could access his special backpack as an alternative choice.

When designing supportive environments, early childhood professionals should review the following components: physical environment; schedules, routines, and transitions; large- and small-group activities; directions; rules; positive attention; and descriptive feedback and encouragement. Across each of these elements, early care providers need to consider each area and ask themselves if each child can be successful in this environment and consider what adaptations or enhancements could be made to ensure success for all children.

A helpful tool to use when assessing the classroom environment (and the other pyramid levels) is the Inventory of Practices (Center on the Social and Emotional Foundations for Early Learning [CSEFEL], 2006). This instrument can be found at http://www.vanderbilt .edu/csefel/modules/module1/handout4.pdf and used by individuals or teams in a reflective manner to identify areas of training and support. There are skills and indicators listed that reflect practices to promote social-emotional competence in young children. The users can determine at which level this skill is demonstrated in their classroom and use the Action Plan to determine their next steps.

Secondary Level: Promotion—Social-Emotional Teaching Strategies

At the secondary level, *social-emotional teaching strategies* can be used to develop skills that children may be lacking (e.g., language, social, emotional). Research indicates that systematic efforts to promote children's social competence can have both preventive and remedial effects (Webster-Stratton & Reid, 2004). Proactive teaching would include topics such as friendship skills, rules and classroom schedules, how to ask for help, emotion words, problem solving, and calming strategies. It is important to remember that children need to have opportunities to learn social and emotional skills, to practice the skills, and to be acknowledged for using the skills.

Teachers in the Doubet and Ostrosky study (2009) discussed their frustration with students who won't talk when they get angry. One teacher explained:

John will clam up a lot. He will get angry, and he just won't say anything, and if he does say anything, it's screaming at you. So I am just trying to get him to say, "I am angry," and trying to get him to understand what that feeling is, and how we can deal with that feeling.

In response to instances such as the one described above, teachers have used calming strategies such as offering a soft space (e.g., refrigerator box with pillows and books) where children can go to cool off, calm down, and relax. The turtle technique, or Tucker Turtle, is a strategy that was originally developed to teach adults anger management, then successfully adapted for school-age children (Schneider, 1974), and since then adapted for young children (Webster-Stratton, 1990). With this approach, once the child recognizes that they are angry, they stop, go inside their "shell," take three deep breaths, and think calm thoughts. When they are calm, the child is encouraged to think of solutions to the problem. This technique helps children learn to replace aggressive, reactive responses with more effective and efficient behavioral alternatives. Young children have responded well to using techniques such as Tucker Turtle to help them think about their emotions and to act on them in a healthy way.

Tertiary Level: Individual Interventions

Even when these two levels of prevention promotion strategies are in place, some children will still exhibit persistent challenging behaviors. For these children at the tertiary level, *intensive individualized interventions* are needed to address their challenging behaviors (Dunlap & Fox, 1999; Sugai et al., 2000). When addressing the needs of these children, a functional assessment should be conducted to determine the function or the *why* of the behavior. Functional assessment conducted through observations, document analysis, and interviews helps to determine what triggers and maintains a problem behavior. Once adequate information is gathered, a behavior hypothesis is written synthesizing all of the data collected about the child's behavior. After the behavior hypothesis is written, a behavior support plan is developed for the child by a team of individuals who know the child best (Lucyshyn et al., 2002). This plan includes prevention strategies, replacement skills, and new responses by the adults and peers to both the problem behaviors and to the appropriate behaviors or replacement skills that are being taught.

The effectiveness of this intervention depends on consistent implementation across natural environments such as home, child care, and community settings (Dunlap & Fox, 1996). It requires that staff and administrators collaborate with families and community partners to access and coordinate needed resources and supports (National Research Council and Institute of Medicine, 2000a).

Guidance for implementing assessment-based interventions at the tertiary (or intervention) level can be found in the Division for Early Childhood concept paper *Identification of and Intervention with Challenging Behavior* (2007). In this paper, five areas of focus are described:

1) Appropriate screening and assessment (variety of settings, comprehensive, reliable and valid measure and observation, involve parents and caregivers, consideration of culture, link assessment information and intervention strategies, use a team-based process).
2) Ensuring effective partnerships between families, service providers, and caregivers.
3) Utilizing individualized interventions that are based on understanding the behavior in the context in which it occurs.
4) Using an FBA to identify the triggers and maintaining consequences and functions of the behavior.
5) Developing an intervention plan that is tailored to fit the unique circumstances of the child, their family, and any programs they are involved in. The plan must be designed for the family and caregivers to implement and should include strategies to teach the child new skills, and prevention strategies.

Systems Level

The pyramid approach also applies to the community or system level. On the bottom of the pyramid, at the universal level, all children and families in a community benefit from nurturing relationships, health care, parent education, screening, quality early care, etc. Moving into the prevention and promotion levels of the pyramid, communities, children, and families who are at risk will benefit from programs and activities such as parenting support and education, health care, home visiting, quality early care, family supports and services, screening and assessment, service coordination and case management, and mental health consultation. At the top of the pyramid, the tertiary level, systems can provide children with persistent challenging behaviors and their families with family-centered interventions focused on targeted outcomes.

SUCCESS STORIES

In many communities across the nation, early childhood programs have responded to the need to support young children's social and emotional development by implementing a system of support referred to as program-wide PBS, or a system of support. Parents, teachers, administrators, and community members have come together to develop plans for supporting young children's social and emotional development. The focus of the following section is to share some of their experiences with the intention of encouraging others to work collaboratively in this effort.

A large National Association for the Education of Young Children (NAEYC)–accredited Head Start program, SEK-CAP in southeast Kansas, has been involved in PBS since 2001 (Fox, Jack, & Broyles, 2005). A complete description of their implementation process and experiences can be found online at http://www.challengingbehavior.org/do/resources/documents/sek_cap_booklet.pdf. Their stated purpose for starting PBS was to increase the amount of time spent teaching by decreasing the amount of time they spent dealing with children's challenging behaviors. A staff member commented, "[PBS] was difficult at first, but the more you use it, the better it is, and it is life changing" (p. 12). With PBS in place, staff members and administrators have noticed improvements in individual child development, environments, relationships with parents, and staff well-being. A staff member commented, "Everyone has been a part of the culture change from classroom staff to secretaries" (p. 7).

While the story of SEK-CAP describes the experiences of a large rural program covering a wide geographical area, similar PBS implementation experiences were shared from a smaller program housed at one location in a Midwest urban community. Valeska Hinton Early Childhood Education Center (VHECEC) is a facility serving 400 children through a variety of funding sources (e.g., public school, Special Education, Head Start, Early Head Start, state-funded prekindergarten, Title I). At approximately the same time SEK-CAP was developing their PBS project, VHECEC was also in the implementation stages of their PBS project (Hemmeter, Fox, & Doubet, 2006).

The development of center-wide PBS for this NAEYC-accredited program gave staff members many opportunities to have in-depth discussions about the programs' philosophy, policies, and procedures. An important lesson learned through this process was the need to establish expectations, not just for children's behavior, but also for adults' behavior. Thus, the expectations developed by the VHECEC Leadership Team, including being respectful, safe, and a team player (p. 8) reflect a commitment to holding staff accountable for demonstrating these same behaviors in their interactions with children, colleagues, and families. Outcomes of the VHECEC PBS approach have included program-wide agreement and focus on positive behavior support, an increased feeling of unity among staff members, shared language surrounding children's behaviors, and a reduction in children being "sent (taken) to the office."

The experiences of SEK-CAP and VHECEC give readers insight into publicly funded programs. The final success story shared is a review of the PBS process for a group of family-owned child care centers in the Midwest. Rogy's Learning Place operates 19 centers, which serve a total of 2,300 children. They are accredited by the National Association of Child Care Professionals. In 2007, the owners decided to improve their support of young children's social and emotional development and piloted PBS at a center serving 230 children and their families.

The administrators in the center wanted to implement center-wide PBS because although they were a high-quality program, they felt unsure about supporting young children with persistent challenging behaviors. Following the steps included in PBS Benchmarks of Quality (Center on the Social and Emotional Foundations for Early Learning, 2006), the administrators started the process by explaining PBS at a monthly staff meeting and then asking for teachers from each age level (i.e., birth through school age), a variety of staff (e.g., kitchen staff, secretarial, bus driver), and parents to consider joining the Leadership Team to develop the PBS implementation plans. This team committed to meeting monthly for at least the first year of planning and implementing the pyramid model in their center. During this time, professional development was conducted for all staff members, and they received coaching and support to implement strategies. Two members of the child care center team chose to receive more in-depth training and coaching to support children needing individualized behavior support plans.

Team members decided to start each Leadership Team meeting with success stories. Teachers shared encouraging stories and continued to become more enthused with their new role as PBS leaders. One teacher talked about how she and the classroom assistant implemented what they learned about transitions and schedules.

We don't rush into naptime anymore. We realized how much stress our lunch and transition to nap was causing for the children and for us. We changed our schedule so that lunch is a little earlier, and now we are both in the room while we clean up from lunch and get ready for nap. Such a simple thing has made a big difference!

The child care staff also grew in their relationships with parents. A teacher of 4-year-old children explained:

In our room, we have gotten better at talking to parents about their children. Before PBS, we mostly wrote behavior information on the Daily Notes. Now we talk personally to a parent and we try to start out by talking about good things and then about the problems we are having. We use the Oreo cookie approach. We always start with the positive, then talk about the challenges, and finish up with another positive comment.

Staff members from this center had the opportunity to explain the pyramid model of support and describe their PBS experiences to directors and assistant directors from the other Rogy's child care centers. The center director described her experiences:

Before PBS, it seemed that teachers thought the only response to challenging behaviors was to send a child down to the office to sit until he or she was calm enough to go back to the classroom. We didn't really have a plan. We weren't teaching the child anything. We've changed that. Now teachers seem more confident in their skills to work with a child with difficult behavior. They know we are a team, and we support each other, the child, and the parents.

As a result, directors from other Rogy's locations expressed interest in adopting the Pyramid Model, and the owners decided to begin the PBS process in all of their centers. Staff members involved in piloting the original PBS effort are now guiding the other centers as they go through the PBS process. Training is conducted both at centers and through satellite education. Support and coaching is scheduled each week and also as needed. As their organization continues down the path toward full implementation, an owner shared that she feels the majority of the staff members are now experiencing less stress, feel more supported, and have more confidence in their role in the growth and develop of the young children in their care.

These success stories are only a few of many examples in communities where early childhood professionals, families, and community members are collaborating to support young children's social-emotional development and address challenging behaviors. As the early childhood field continues to move toward a model of prevention, promotion, and intervention, more success stories for programs, parents, and children will be told.

TIERED MODEL AS REFLECTED IN OTHER CURRENT APPROACHES

Using a Response-to-Intervention Framework to Promote Young Children's Social Development

Over the past few years, Response to Intervention (RtI) has provided another tiered model to instruction that uses a systematic problem-solving approach focusing on students' responses to interventions as a basis for determining instructional needs and intensity. RtI has multiple levels or tiers of instructional support available so children can be matched with the appropriate level of support. Similar to PBS, RtI uses a progress-monitoring approach to make sure an intervention is working. Fox, Carta, Strain, Dunlap, and Hemmeter (2009) note that a pyramid is often used to illustrate the three tiers of RtI.

Tier 1: Evidence-based core curricula and instructional practices provided to *all* children.

Tier 2: More *intensified* instruction for children not demonstrating adequate growth in Tier 1. Increased opportunities to practice skills from Tier 1 curriculum.

Tier 3: More *focused* intervention for children not showing adequate growth in Tier 2 or for children well below Tier 1 benchmark.

Importantly, similar to the Pyramid Model, RtI focuses on learning or behavioral problems. RtI does not replace existing systems for evaluating or determining eligibility for special education services and procedural safeguards. Children with disabilities can be found at all tiers. Fox, Carta, et al. (2009) also describe the necessary infrastructure features that support the implementation of RtI and the Pyramid, including (1) the development of clear procedures for screening, progress monitoring, and the delivery of more intensive tiers of intervention to children; (2) the development of strategies and systems for family involvement within each tier; (3) professional development and ongoing support to teachers for implementation fidelity; (4) access to expertise in the design and implementation of tier 2 and tier 3 interventions; and (5) procedures for efficient and meaningful data collection and data-based decision making.

Early Childhood Mental Health Consultation

All young children need to form strong, loving relationships with their caregivers to achieve social and emotional well-being. These relationships and supportive experiences foster resiliency and set children on a trajectory for future school readiness and positive relationships. Currently, mental health consultants focus much energy on screening and identifying children with behavior problems, with less emphasis on increasing promotion and prevention activities, and limited attention to the mental wellness of families and staff (Perry, Kaufmann, & Knitzer, 2007). Furthermore, special prevention techniques are needed to support children at risk for behavioral problems because of stressful experiences (e.g., witnessing domestic violence) that may disrupt their brain development and impair their ability to cope with stress and regulate emotions (National Scientific Council on the Developing Child, 2003). To truly promote mental wellness, it is important to meet the social and emotional needs of all children, regardless of whether they are currently manifesting mental health problems or not.

To this end, there is a movement to redefine early childhood mental health consultation as a "problem-solving and capacity-building intervention implemented within a collaborative relationship between a professional consultant with mental health expertise and, typically, child care staff" (Cohen & Kaufmann, 2000, p. 4). According to Cohen and Kaufmann, there are two subtypes of consultation: child- or family-centered, and programmatic consultation. The former and more traditional type of consultation aims to address the needs of an individual child (or family) exhibiting challenging behaviors. In contrast, programmatic consultation takes a more preventive and systemic approach, focusing on "improving the overall quality of the program and/or assisting the program to solve a specific issue that affects more than one child, staff member and/or family" (p. 8). To optimize children's social and emotional outcomes and truly embed evidence-based mental health practices, consultants must attend to both levels and adopt a capacity-building approach to consultation. Within this approach, consultants do not provide direct therapeutic services but instead model techniques and provide coaching to families and staff so that they can effectively implement evidence-based practices and interventions for individual or groups of young children.

The emphasis on capacity building (as opposed to direct service provision) within early childhood mental health consultation underscores one of the primary challenges facing consultants—confusion over the consultant role and, subsequently, the skills and competencies needed to perform this role effectively (Allen, 2008). Mental health consultation is a fundamentally different approach than the one-on-one therapeutic mental health services for which mental health practitioners are typically trained. It is a relationship-based, capacity-building, indirect service provided to those caring for young children and, as such, requires a unique set of skills. In support of the redefinition of mental health consultation, Perry et al. (2007) advocate the use of the pyramid approach and underscore the need for a continuum of services and supports that span promotion, prevention, and intervention.

CONCLUSION

In summary, this is a critical period in the early childhood care and education field. As we continue to increase the number of children who are served in group care settings, we are also seeing a rise in the number of children who exhibit challenging behaviors. These issues intensify the need for a comprehensive approach to providing support for young children's healthy social and emotional development. There is promise in the pyramid, or tiered-framework, model, which addresses prevention, promotion, and individual levels of support. Encouraging research points toward a high level of success when the promotion of emotional wellness begins with young children.

REFERENCES

Allen, M. D. (2008). Attributes of effective Head Start mental health consultants: A mixed methods study. Portland State University.

Arnold, D. H., McWilliams, L., & Arnold, E. H. (1998). Teacher discipline and child misbehavior in preschool: Untangling causality with correlational data. *Developmental Psychology, 34,* 276–287.

Boone, H. A., & Crais, E. (2002). Strategies for achieving family-driven assessment and intervention planning. *Young Exceptional Children Monograph Series #4.*

Boulware, G., Schwartz, I., & McBride, B. (1999). Addressing challenging behaviors at home: Working with families to find solutions. *Young Exceptional Children, 3,* 21–27.

Bruder, M. (2004). Credentialing early intervention providers. Presented at OSEP Joint Personnel Preparation/State Improvement/CSPD Conference, Washington, DC.

Burchinal, M. R., Peisner-Feinberg, E. S., Bryant, D. M., & Clifford, R. M. (2000). Children's social and cognitive development and child care quality: Testing for differential associations related to poverty, gender, or ethnicity. *Applied Developmental Science, 4,* 149–165.

Center on the Social and Emotional Foundations for Early Learning (CSEFEL). (2006, August). *Module 4: Leadership Strategies.* Retrieved from http://www.vanderbilt.edu/csefel/modules/module1/handout4.pdf

Child Care Resource Services (CCRS). (2003). *FY03 Needs assessment summary.* University of Illinois at Urbana-Champaign.

Cohen, E., & Kaufmann, R. (2000). *Early childhood mental health consultation.* Washington, DC: Center for Mental Health Services, SAMHSA, U.S. Department of Health and Human Services.

Denno, D., Phillips., L., Harte, H., & Moomaw, S. (2004). Creating a supportive classroom environment. In S. H. Bell, V. Carr, D. Denno, & L. Johnson (Eds.), *Challenging behaviors in early childhood settings* (pp. 62–83). Baltimore: Paul H. Brookes.

Dinnebeil, L. A., McInerney, W., Fox, C., & Juchartz-Pendry, K. (1998). An analysis of the perceptions and characteristics of child care personnel regarding inclusion of young children with special needs in community-based programs. *Topics in Early Childhood Education, 18*(2), 118–136.

Division for Early Childhood. (2007). *Identification of and intervention with challenging behavior.* Concept Paper. Retrieved from http://www.dec-sped.org/uploads/docs/about_dec/position_concept_papers/ConceptPaper_Chal_Behav_updated_jan2009.pdf

Doubet, S., & Ostrosky, M. M. (2009, October). *Childcare teachers' experiences as they support young children with challenging behavior.* Poster presented at the meeting of the Division for Early Childhood of the Council for Exceptional Children, Albuquerque, NM.

Doubet, S., Ostrosky, M. M., & Corso, R. (2007). *Survey of early educators.* Manuscript in preparation.

Doubet, S., Ostrosky, M. M., & Hemmeter, M. L. (2007, October). *Mapping parents' journeys: Support for young children with challenging behavior.* Paper presented at the meeting of the Division for Early Childhood of the Council for Exceptional Children, Niagara Falls, Ontario, Canada.

Dunlap, G., & Fox, L. (1996). Early intervention and serious problem behaviors. In L. K. Koegel, R. L. Koegel, & G. Dunlap (Eds.), *Positive behavioral support: Including people with difficult behavior in the community* (pp. 31–50). Baltimore: Paul H. Brookes.

Dunlap, G., & Fox, L. (1999). A demonstration of behavioral support for young children with autism. *Journal of Positive Behavior Interventions, 2,* 77–87.

Dunlap, G., Fox, L., & Hemmeter, M. L. (2004, April). *Program-wide approaches for addressing children's challenging behavior.* Symposium conducted at the meeting of the National Training Institute on Effective Practices: Supporting Young Children's Social/Emotional Development, Clearwater Beach, FL.

Fox, L., Carta, J., Strain, P., Dunlap, G., & Hemmeter, M. L. (2009). *Response to intervention and the pyramid model.* Tampa, FL: University of South Florida, Technical Assistance Center on Social Emotional Intervention for Young Children.

Fox, L., Dunlap, G., & Cushing, L. (2002). Early intervention, positive behavior support, and transition to school. *Journal of Emotional and Behavioral Disorders, 10*(3), 149–157.

Fox, L., Dunlap, G., Hemmeter, M. L., Joseph, G. E., & Strain, P. S. (2003, July). The teaching pyramid. *Young Children, 58*(4), 48–52.

Fox, L., & Hemmeter, M. L. (2009). A program-wide model for supporting social emotional development and addressing challenging behavior in early childhood settings. In W. Sailor, G. Dunlap, G. Sugai, & R. Horner (Eds.), *Handbook of positive behavior support* (pp. 177–202). New York: Springer.

Fox, L., Jack, S., & Broyles, L. (2005). *Program-wide positive behavior support: Supporting young children's social-emotional development and addressing challenging behavior.* Tampa, FL: University of South Florida, Louis de la Parte Florida Mental Health Institute.

Fox, L., Vaughn, B., Dunlap, G., & Bucy, M. (1997). Parent-professional partnership in behavioral support: A qualitative analysis of one family's experience. *Journal of the Association for Persons with Severe Handicaps, 22,* 198–207.

Gilliam, W. S. (2005). *Pre-kindergarteners left behind: Expulsion rates in state prekindergarten systems.* Yale University Child Study Center. Retrieved from: http://info.med.yale.edu/chldstdy

Guralnick, M. J. (2000). Early childhood intervention: Evolution of a system. In M. L. Wehmeyer & J. R. Patton (Eds.), *Mental retardation in the 21st century* (pp. 37–58). Austin, TX: PRO-ED.

Hamre, B. K., & Pianta, R. C. (2001). Early teacher-child relationships and the trajectory of children's school outcomes through eighth grade. *Child Development, 72,* 625–638.

Hemmeter, M. L., Corso, R., & Cheatham, G. (2006, February). *Issues in addressing challenging behaviors in young children: A national survey of early childhood educators.* Paper presented at the Conference on Research Innovations in Early Intervention, San Diego, CA.

Hemmeter, M. L., Fox, L., & Doubet, S. (2006). Together we can! A program-wide approach to addressing challenging behavior. *Young Exceptional Children Monograph Series No. 8,* 1–13.

Hoppe, S. (2005). Parent perceptions: Communication, interaction, and behavior in autism. *Teaching Exceptional Children Plus, 1*(4), Article 5. Retrieved from http://escholarship.bc.edu/cgi/viewcontent.cgi?article=1109&context=education/tecplus

Howes, C., & Ritchie, S. (2002). *A matter of trust: Connecting teachers and learners in the early childhood classroom.* New York: Teachers College Press.

Hutton, A. M., & Caron, S. L. (2005). Experiences of families with children with autism in rural New England. *Focus on Autism and Other Developmental Disabilities, 20*(3), 180–189.

Hyson, M. (2004). *The emotional development of young children: Building an emotion-centered curriculum.* New York: Teachers College Press.

Johnston, K., & Brinamen, C. (2006). *Mental health consultation in child care: Transforming relationships among directors, staff, and families.* Washington, DC: Zero to Three.

Joseph, G., Strain, P., & Skinner, B. (2004). *Survey of children's challenging behavior in early care and education setting.* Unpublished manuscript. University of Colorado at Denver.

Kaiser, B., & Rasminsky, J. (2007). *Challenging behavior: Understanding, preventing, and responding effectively.* (2nd ed.) Boston: Pearson Education.

Kaufmann, R., & Wischmann, A. L. (1999). Communities supporting the mental health of young children and their families. In R. N. Roberts & R. R. Magrab (Eds.), *Where children live: Solutions for serving young children and their families* (pp. 175–210). Stamford, CT: Ablex.

Kazdin, A., & Kendall, K. (1998). Adolescent mental health: Prevention and treatment programs. *American Psychologist, 48,* 127–141.

Klein, R., & Gilkerson, L. (2000). Prenatal development and the brain. In L. Gilkerson (Ed.), *Teaching and learning about the brain and early development.* Manuscript in preparation, Erikson Institute.

Knitzer, J. (2000). Early childhood mental health services: Policy and systems development perspective. In J. P. Shonkoff & S. M. Meisels (Eds.), *Handbook of early childhood intervention* (2nd ed., pp. 416–438). New York: Cambridge University Press.

Kopel, C. C. (2004). Early intervention social emotional component expands statewide. *Social Work Networker, 63,* 7–11.

Lewis, T., & Sugai, G. (1999). Effective behavior support: A systems approach to proactive schoolwide management. *Focus on Exceptional Children, 31*(6), 1–24.

Lucyshyn, J. M., Dunlap, G., & Albin, R. W. (2002). *Families and positive behavior support.* Baltimore: Paul H. Brookes.

National Institute of Child Health and Human Development (NICHD). (1999). Chronicity of maternal depressive symptoms, maternal sensitivity, and child functioning at 36 months. *Developmental Psychology, 35,* 1297–1310.

National Institute of Child Health and Human Development (NICHD), Early Child Care Research Network. (2003). Does amount of time spent in child care predict socio-emotional adjustment during the transition to kindergarten? *Child Development, 74,* 976–1005.

National Research Council and Institute of Medicine. (2000a). *Early childhood intervention: Views from the field* (J. P. Shonkoff, D. A. Phillips, & B. Keilty, Eds.). Washington, DC: National Academy Press.

National Research Council and Institute of Medicine. (2000b). *From neurons to neighborhoods: The science of early child development.* Committee on Integrating the Science of Early Childhood Development (J. P. Shonkoff & D. A. Phillips, Eds.). Board on Children, Youth, and Families, Commission on Behavioral and Social Sciences and Education. Washington, DC: National Academy Press.

National Scientific Council on the Developing Child. (2003). Excessive stress disrupts the architecture of the developing brain. Cambridge: Center for the Developing Child.

Nungesser, N. R., & Watkins, R. V. (2005). Preschool teachers' perceptions and reactions to challenging classroom behavior: Implications for speech-language pathologists. *Language, Speech, and Hearing Services in Schools, 36,* 139–151.

Peisner-Feinberg, E. S., Burchinal, M. R., Clifford, R. M., Culkin, M. L., Howes, C., Kagan, S. L., et al. (2001). *The children of the cost, quality, and outcomes study go to school: Technical report.* Chapel Hill: Frank Porter Graham Child Development Center, University of North Carolina.

Perry, D. F., Kaufman, R. K., & Knitzer, J. (2007). *Social and emotional health in early childhood: Building bridges between services and systems.* (pp. 121–146). Baltimore: Paul H. Brookes.

Qi, C., & Kaiser, A. (2003). Behavior problems of preschool children from low-income families: Review of the literature. *Topics in Early Childhood Special Education, 23,* 188–216.

Quesenberry, A., & Hemmeter, M. L. (2005, October). *Implementing a program wide model of positive behavior supports in early childhood settings.* Paper presented at the Annual DEC International Early Childhood Conference on Children with Special Needs, Portland, OR.

Raver, C. (2002). Emotions matter: Making the case for the role of young children's emotional development for early school readiness. *Social Policy Report/Society for Research in Child Development, 16*(3). Retrieved from http://www.srcd.org/spr.html

Raver, C., & Knitzer, J. (2002). *Ready to enter: What research tells policymakers about strategies to promote social and emotional school readiness among three- and four-year-old children.* New York: National Center for Children in Poverty, Columbia University Mailman School of Public Health. Retrieved from http://cpmcnet.columbia.edu/dept/nccp/ProEmoPP3.html

Sandall, S., Hemmeter, M. L., Smith, B. J., & McLean, M. E. (2005). *DEC recommended practices: A comprehensive guide for practical application.* Longmont, CO: Sopris West.

Sandall, S. R., & Schwartz, I. S. (2002). *Building blocks for teaching preschoolers with special needs.* Baltimore: Paul H. Brookes.

Schneider, M. (1974). Turtle technique in the classroom. *Teaching Exceptional Children, 7,* 21–24.

Shonkoff, J., & Phillips, D. (Eds.). (2000). Nurturing relationships. In J. Shonkoff & D. Phillips (Eds.), *From neurons to neighborhoods: The science of early development* (pp. 225–266). Washington, DC: National Academy Press.

Smith, B. J. (2000). The federal role in early childhood special education policy in the next century: The responsibility of the individual. *Topics in Early Childhood Special Education, 20*(1), 7–13.

Smith, B. J., & Fox, L. (2003a). *Synthesis of evidence related to systems of services, Center for Evidence-Based Practice: Young Children with Challenging Behavior.* Retrieved from http://www.challengingbehavior.org

Smith, B. J., & Fox, L. (2003b). *Systems of service delivery: A synthesis of evidence relevant to young children at risk of or who have challenging behavior.* Tampa, FL: University of South Florida, Center for Evidence-Based Practice: Young Children with Challenging Behavior.

Sprague, J., Walker, H., Golly, A., White, K., Myers, D., & Shannon, T. (2001). Translating research into effective practice: The effects of a universal staff and student intervention on indicators of discipline and school safety. *Education and Treatment of Children, 24,* 495–511.

Stormont, M., Lewis, T., & Beckner, R. (2005). Positive behavior support systems: Applying key features in preschool settings. *Teaching Exceptional Children, 37* (6), 42–49.

Stormont, M., Lewis, T. J., Beckner, R., & Johnson, N. W. (2008). *Implementing positive behavior support systems in early childhood and elementary settings.* Thousand Oaks, CA: Corwin Press.

Strain, P., & Hemmeter, M. L. (1999). Keys to being successful. In S. Sandall & M. Ostrosky (Eds.), *Young exceptional children: Practical ideas for addressing challenging behaviors* (pp. 17–28). Longmont, CO: Sopris West; and Denver, CO: DEC.

Strain, P. S., & Timm, M. A. (2001). Remediation and prevention of aggression: An evaluation of the RIP Program over a quarter century. *Behavioral Disorders, 26,* 297–313.

Sugai, G., Sprague, J. R., Horner, R. H., & Walker, H. M. (2000). Preventing school violence: The use of office discipline referrals to assess and monitor schoolwide discipline interventions (Electronic version). *Journal of Emotional and Behavioral Disorders, 8,* 94–101.

Thompson, R. A. (1994). Emotion regulation: A theme in search of a definition. *Monographs of the Society for Research in Child Development, 59*(2–3, Serial No. 240), 25–52.

Trivette, C. M., & Dunst, C. J. (2005). DEC recommended practices: Family-based practices. In S. Sandall, M. L. Hemmeter, B. J. Smith, & M. McLean (Eds.), *DEC Recommended Practices* (pp. 107–120). Longmont, CO: Sopris West.

U.S. Bureau of Labor Statistics. (1998). *Occupational projections and training data.* Washington, DC: U.S. Department of Labor.

U.S. Department of Education (USDOE). (2007). *Teacher Shortage Areas Nationwide Listing: 1990–91 thru 2006–07.* U.S. Department of Education Office of Postsecondary Education Policy & Budget Development Staff.

Vaughn, B., Dunlap, G., Fox, L., Clarke, S., & Bucy, M. (1997). Parent professional partnership in behavioral support: A case study of community-based intervention. *Journal of the Association for Persons with Severe Handicaps, 22,* 186–197.

Webster-Stratton, C. (1990). Long-term follow-up of families with young conduct problem children: From preschool to grade school. *Journal of Clinical Child Psychology, 19,* 144–149.

Webster-Stratton, C. (1997). Early intervention for families of preschool children with conduct problems. In M. J. Guralnick (Ed.), *The effectiveness of early intervention: Second generation research* (pp. 429–454). Baltimore: Paul H. Brookes.

Webster-Stratton, C., & Reid, J. M. (2004). Strengthening social and emotional competence in young children—The foundation for early school readiness and success. Incredible Years Classroom Social Skills and Problem-Solving Curriculum. *Infants and Young Children 17,* 96–113.

Webster-Stratton, C., Reid, J., & Hammond, M. (2001). Preventing conduct problems, promoting social competence: A parent and teacher training partnership in Head Start. *Journal of Clinical Child Psychology 30,* 283–302.

West, J., Denton, K., & Germino-Hausken, E. (2000). *America's kindergartener: Findings from the early childhood longitudinal study, kindergarten class of 1998–99, fall*

1008. Washington DC: U.S. Department of Education, National Center for Educational Statistics.

Winton, P. J., McCollum, J. A., & Catlett, C. (Eds.). (1997). *Reforming personnel preparation in early intervention: Issues, models, and practical strategies* (pp. 409–664). Baltimore: Paul H. Brookes.

Zero to Three: National Center for Clinical Infant Programs. (1992). *Head Start: The emotional foundations of school readiness*. Arlington, VA: Author.

Zigler, E. (2004). Foreword. In M. Hyson (Ed.), *The emotional development of young children* (pp. vii–viii). New York: Teachers College Press.

Zins, J. E., Bloodworth, M. R., Weissberg, R. P., & Walberg, H. J. (2004). The scientific base linking social and emotional learning to school success. In J. E. Zins, M. R. Weissberg, M. C. Wang, & H. J. Walberg (Eds.), *Building academic success on social and emotional learning: What does the research say?* (pp. 3–22). New York: Teachers College Press.

Chapter 9

Specific Issues on Developmental Disability: Autism (Including New Strategies in Testing, Diagnosis, and Treatment)

Juliann Woods and Rachel Whittington Saffo

E nter an early care and education program, Head Start, toddler dance class, or Sunday school and observe the children at play. You will see boys and girls, some with smiling faces who will pause to look at you, and others who will stay engrossed in activity. Some will be in groups, and others alone; some will be talking, while others are quiet. Can you identify the child with Autism Spectrum Disorder (ASD) in this observation? It is not likely. Children with ASD are not identified by their physical features, motor skills, or through a brief interaction. This disorder is not always obvious in young children. However, with the prevalence rate at one occurrence for every 110 children (Centers for Disease Control, 2009), one or more of the children you observe could have ASD, a group of developmental disabilities with symptoms typically present before the age of 3. Current estimates are that in the United States alone, one out of 70 boys is diagnosed with autism. Let us meet three children with a diagnosis of ASD and their families. The unique characteristics of each child will help us define and describe ASD in young children.

Amir. Amir is an only child and 18 months of age, and has been cared for primarily by his mother on maternity leave from her law firm. At his last checkup, his pediatrician recommended that his parents consider enrolling him into a group setting so he could talk and play with other children his age. He noticed some communication and social delays compared to other children.

Ms. Myra, the director of Kids Incorporated, a private community early care and education program, welcomes Amir and his parents on a sunny spring day. His dad, a successful accountant, carries Amir into the classroom and continues to hold him throughout the tour of the facilities. Amir does not look around or ask to join the other children as they eat breakfast or play in their centers. He doesn't seem to notice the sand and water tables or elaborate outdoor playground equipment. He is quiet and content in his dad's arms. He does not respond to Ms. Myra or the other children's invitations to join in the fun. When asked about concerns, Amir's parents shared that other people don't understand what he says, he prefers to play alone, and he is a picky eater. They estimate that he has at least 50 words, but he doesn't use them very often. They describe him as affectionate but not interested in others. Both parents acknowledge that they have been protective of their firstborn son, but also comment they are sure he is just fine and only needs some socialization opportunities. Amir's dad believes that he is showing an emerging independence from his parents by being self-sufficient in his play, preferring to be left alone with his blocks and DVDs.

Katie. Katie, 30 months, and her little brother, Ben, 15 months, are taking a bath before getting ready for bed. Ben is dumping and pouring water, splashing and squealing. Katie is squealing, too, but not joyfully. It is her own special version of a high-pitched hum that no one else can quite imitate. It is clear however, that she wants out of the tub and away from Ben's activities, but her mom wants to shampoo her hair. Her mom calls her name, offers her a cloth to cover her eyes from the water, and tries to gain her attention with some special tub toys. Katie continues to squeal and increases the tension and flexion in her hands by clenching and unclenching her fists. She senses the bath routine is going to change, and she begins to rock back and forth. Mom knows from experience that washing her hair is not going to be easy. Ben continues to enjoy the playtime and shows Katie the bubbles on his hair. Without a sideways glance to Ben or Mom, Katie climbs out and refuses to return to the water. As Katie's rocking and squealing increases, Mom worries she will hurt herself or Ben. She scoops her up into her lap to quiet her and washes her hair quickly with a cloth.

Mom wishes that bath time could be as much fun with Katie as it is with Ben. If Katie would just tell her when she needed help or when she had enough, she could avoid the tantrums that make any routine or activity a major challenge. Katie just seems to hate interacting with her environment and others more every day.

Dante. Dante just turned 4 and is fascinated with the stickers he collects. He looks at his sticker books, talks about his stickers, and requests more stickers wherever he goes. At school, his teacher finds the stickers get in his way of participating in the activities planned throughout the day and often interfere with his social interactions with his classmates. Other children ride bikes, swing, and play in the sand while outside, but Dante prefers to sit alone with his sticker books. He carries them with him to center and table activities in the classroom, and he has no interest in sharing the stickers with his classmates.

His mom and dad add to his supply of stickers and sticker books as a strategy for getting him to do his chores around the house, to keep him busy during car travel, and to teach him advanced math and reading concepts. They work well for Dante's parents and his older siblings. The family is very proud of his advanced vocabulary, math, and reading skills and is encouraging him to expand his knowledge with computer games and learning tools.

DEFINING AUTISM SPECTRUM DISORDER (ASD)

Amir, Katie, and Dante have a diagnosis of ASD. They have different clusters of behavioral characteristics and are affected by the characteristics differently. ASD ranges in the number and types of symptoms and is described as a spectrum ranging on the continuum from mild to severe. To receive a diagnosis of ASD, impairments of social interaction and communication as well as restricted, repetitive, and stereotyped patterns of behavior, interests, or play must be evidenced within the first three years of life (APA, 2000). For example, Dante is highly verbal, interested in numbers and letters, and carries on adult-like conversations, while Katie has limited vocalizations and uses challenging behaviors instead of words to make simple requests and protests. Amir is quiet, communicates primarily with his parents, and even then, infrequently. None of the children actively engaged in play or socialized with their peers. Dante and Amir demonstrate restricted interests, with Dante preferring stickers over play with other children, while Amir is gaining interest in blocks and DVDs and becoming more object-focused. Katie illustrates rocking, squealing, and clenching as repetitive behaviors. The saying, "If you've met one child with autism, you've met one child with autism," is used frequently because autism is not a clear-cut, easy-to-identify disability—it is a spectrum disorder, with no two children displaying the same pattern of characteristics. Research also shows that the symptoms may change over time (Mitchell et al., 2006; Wetherby et al., 2004), as evidenced by Amir's growing interest in object play with specific toys.

Autism is a complex neurodevelopmental disorder. It is described as a lifelong condition with no known cure (American Academy of Pediatrics, Council on Children with Disabilities [AAP-CCD], 2006.) Outcomes for children with ASD span a broad continuum, with a small percentage achieving independence and full employment as adults (Howlin, Goode, Hutton, & Rutter, 2004). However, it is important to note that some children improve from early interventions to the degree that they no longer meet the eligibility criteria for the disorder (Dawson et al., 2010). Milder symptoms may persist, but can be managed. The true impact of early intervention will be seen in the next generation of adults.

No one knows the exact cause of ASD, and many believe there are multiple causal factors. Scientists have shown that genetics plays a role, but while many different chromosomal and genetic abnormalities have been identified, no single one is present for all children (AAP-CCD, 2006). Twin and family studies strongly suggest that some people have a genetic predisposition to autism. If a family has a child identified with ASD, then it is more likely a sibling will also be identified (Bishop, Maybery, Wong, Maley, & Hallmayer, 2006). Mundy and Burnette (2005) suggest that an initial neurological deficit in infants with autism may lead to an early impairment in social orienting and joint attention, which contributes to subsequent neurodevelopmental pathology by an attenuation of social input. ASDs may co-occur with medical conditions such as Fragile X syndrome and tuberous sclerosis (CDC, 2009). This disorder can also co-occur with many other developmental disabilities and learning problems. Research is underway in many areas to further knowledge of the causes of autism.

ASDs occur in all racial, ethnic, and socioeconomic groups, but are four times more likely to occur in boys than in girls. More young children than ever before are being diagnosed with ASD. It is unclear how much of this increase is due to a broader definition of ASD and better efforts in diagnosis (CDC, 2009). Public awareness of and attention to early identification of ASD has increased markedly in the past few years. The result of greater attention is a growth in general knowledge in the disorder and its spectrum. Children with milder symptoms are being identified and served. However, a true increase in the number of people with an ASD cannot be ruled out. The most reasonable answer for the increase in ASD diagnosis is a combination of these factors (CDC, 2009).

Core Deficits of ASD and Outcomes

Children with ASD are likely to have delays and disorders in both expressive and receptive communication and language. Delays or differences in communication are often the first concerns noted by parents. Parents often wonder if their children have hearing loss, because they do not turn to look when their names are called and do not follow simple directions or identify common objects—all symptoms of hearing loss (AAP-CCD, 2006). Joint attention, another deficit noted early for many children with ASD, involves sharing and shifting gaze between a communication partner and an object or activity. This dyadic and triadic interaction is a sophisticated way in which the child and partner can share an object or activity. Words need not accompany this interaction; it can be completely nonverbal.

Children with ASD also experience difficulty socializing with others and later understanding others' points of view. Dante plays alone with his stickers without concern for the interest of the other children in his preschool. Children with ASD may exhibit unconventional or odd behaviors in social situations that an outsider might deem rude, unacceptable, or offensive. Lack of awareness and understanding of these behaviors further estrange them from children with typical development, even society as a whole. Excessive focus on objects rather than people, restricted interests in play, repetition of specific behaviors, and ritual actions are frequently observed in young children with ASD. Children, such as Amir, may be able to play independently but do not generate new or more complex interactions with the objects and have limited play schemas; they simply repeat the behaviors, Other children with ASD may exhibit repetitive motor mannerisms (e.g., flapping hands, spinning body), repetitive movements with objects, preoccupations with restricted interests or parts of objects, excessive adherence to routines, and marked distress over change. The impact children's behaviors have on families and caregivers also varies (Sperry, Whaley, Shaw, & Brame, 1999). Amir's parents value his independence, while Dante's parents encourage his pre-academic interests. Katie's mom compares her to her younger brother and worries about her future.

Communicative competence may be the primary factor determining the extent to which individuals with ASD can develop relationships with others and participate in daily activities and routines at school, home, and in the community. In this area, results of research are hopeful. A number of longitudinal studies provide evidence of a relationship between early social communication skills and language outcomes. Mundy, Sigman, and Kasari (1990) found that responding to and initiating gestural joint attention at a mean age of 3 years, 9 months were significant predictors of language development 13 months later for children with ASD, while none of the other nonverbal measures, initial language scores, mental age, chronological age, or IQ were significant predictors. These findings were further substantiated in a long-term follow-up study demonstrating that initial joint attention skills of 51 children with autism at a mean age of 3 years, 11 months predicted gains in expressive language at a mean age of 12 years, 10 months (Sigman & Ruskin, 1999).

The level of communicative competence achieved by persons with ASD is closely related to the development of social behavior and functional outcomes (Wetherby & Woods, 2008). Charman et al. (2003) found that measures of joint attention late in the second year predicted language at 3 years of age. Wetherby, Watt, Morgan, and Shumway (2007) examined a larger set of predictive measures and found that many measures including joint attention predicted language outcome at age 3, but that understanding of language in the second year was the strongest predictor. The presence of fluent speech before the age of 5 continues to be a good prognostic indicator of intelligence or IQ, language measures, adaptive skills, and academic achievement in adolescence (Dawson et al., 2010). Moreover, improvements in receptive and expressive communication, especially in the youngest children, have been found to prevent problem behaviors and maintain reductions of these behaviors (Powell, Dunlap, & Fox, 2006).

The severity of the symptoms of ASD reflects the interaction of the two core diagnostic domains. A student who has deficits in social communication, and who has intense preoccupations with narrow interests or ritualized patterns of behavior and excessive resistance to change, is at great risk for challenging behavior. Difficulties with emotional expression, interpretation of nonverbal social cues, and mood regulation are widely noted in the ASD literature (Klin & Volkmar, 2003). For children with ASD, there is often a mismatch between a child's ability to remain actively engaged, adapt to novel stimuli, and inhibit impulsive reactions and the expectations for that child regarding appropriate and socially conventional behavior in a given context (Laurent & Rubin, 2004; Miller, Robinson, & Moulton, 2004). The combination of deficits in social communication and the presence of unusual behaviors can have a significant impact on a child's access to educational and social opportunities (Bishop, Richler, & Lord, 2006; Wetherby et al., 2007).

EARLY IDENTIFICATION

Why Diagnose Earlier?

The past decade of research has introduced new behaviors that contribute to an earlier diagnosis of ASD. A diagnosis of autism at age 2 is reliable, valid, and stable (Lord et al., 2006). Presently, the mean age for diagnosis of ASD in the United States is over 4 years of age (Centers for Disease Control and Prevention Department of Health and Human Services [CDC-HHS], 2007; Yeargin-Allsopp et al., 2003). In socioeconomically disadvantaged groups, the age of diagnosis might be even older (Mandell, Listerud, Levy, & Pinto-Martin, 2002). Most children identified as having ASD demonstrate symptoms within the first two years of life. and their families generally express concern to their pediatrician by the time their child is 18 months old (Wimpory, Hobson, Williams, & Nash, 2000). Observational studies of social communication skills in children under 2 years of age with ASD are emerging from two different sources of information, retrospective analyses of home videotapes and prospective longitudinal designs. The largest cohort of retrospective analyses is based on home videotapes from first birthday parties of children later diagnosed with ASD. Osterling and colleagues (Osterling & Dawson, 1994; Osterling, Dawson, & Munson, 2002) found that children with ASD could be distinguished at their first birthday party with four features—lack of pointing, showing, looking at faces, and orienting to name—however, children with general developmental disabilities also showed the first two features. The time between first concern and diagnosis can impact the early specialized services and supports that a child may receive and ultimately, his prognosis for future outcomes.

There are several reasons why early identification is delayed. Lack of professional training on the early signs of autism by early care and education or medical professionals, as well as limited health-care plan coverage contribute to the postponement of identification (Woods & Wetherby, 2003). Multiple efforts are underway to increase earlier identification of autism. The CDC and national partners launched a campaign encouraging public awareness of the early signs of autism. The "Learn the Signs. Act Early." Web site (http://www.cdc.gov/ncbddd/actearly) provides developmental checklists in both interactive and printable formats for easy access. The AAP-CCD recommends that pediatricians screen all 18- to 24-month-olds for autism (AAP, 2006; Johnson & Myers, 2007). They, and other national organizations such as the American Academy of Neurology, have published clinical guidelines regarding early screening and diagnosis of ASD (Filipek et al., 2000). *Autism Speaks* (http://www.autismspeaks.org), an international organization devoted to public awareness for autism, has a high media profile, including a presence on the Internet and television, with multiple resources for improving early identification, including a video library that illustrates the early red flags of autism for professionals and families.

The Beginning: Who and How?

Parents or caregivers, including early care and education professionals, generally are the first to notice differences or changes in the child's development. Familiarization with the developmental milestones of young children is important for families and caregivers. Not only does it educate them about their child's development, it provides them with information to share with their child's pediatrician during well-baby checkups. Informed parents are able to express their concerns about their child's development in relation to these developmental milestones. Several organizations post charts of developmental milestones for families. A friendly Web site is First Signs (http://www.firstsigns .org/about/earlyid.htm), an organization developed by a parent of a child with autism, to educate parents and professionals about the early signs of autism and similar disorders. Another site with resources for families is First Words (http://www.firstsigns.org/concerns/parent _doc.htm), which includes a developmental checklist for families and physicians (see Table 9.1).

Table 9.1   Early Signs of Autism

The traits below distinguish children with autism from children with developmental delays and typical development.

Atypical development in or lack of:

- Social Communication
  - Decreased presence of showing
  - Decreased presence of coordinated nonverbal communication
  - Decreased presence of response to name
  - Decreased presence of shared/joint attention and eye gaze
  - Decreased presence of ability to shift gaze and respond to joint attention (i.e., gaze point follow)
  - Less positive affect and social, back-and-forth smiling
  - Decreased presence of social concern/awareness or mutual enjoyment (sans physical cues/touch, such as tickling)
  - Decreased presence of gestures
  - Decreased rate of pointing
- Play
  - Decreased rate of symbolic play

(Continued)

Table 9.1 (Continued)

- • Decreased rate of imitating actions with objects
- • Repetitive actions with toys (e.g., spinning, wobbling, rolling)
- • Language and Cognition
  - • Decreased rate of communication
  - • Atypical prosody (inflection of voice)
  - • Loss of words or social-emotional reciprocity
  - • Lack of social, reciprocal babbling by 12 months
  - • No single words by 16 months
- • Repetitive and Stereotyped Behaviors or Interests
  - • Repetitive movements with body or body posturing
  - • Atypical visual examination of objects
- • Atypical regulatory functions
  - • Gastrointestinal
  - • Feeding (e.g., picky eater, PICA)
  - • Sleep attention

Source: Adapted from Filipek et al. (2000); Wetherby et al. (2007); Wetherby et al. (2004).

Pediatricians should be knowledgeable about young children's developmental milestones, for they often are the first person to whom a concerned parent speaks. Very young children change rapidly (day to day, month to month) across many domains and benefit from routine surveillance for developmental markers. A typical developmental screening instrument concentrates on five key areas of development: gross motor, fine motor, adaptive, social-communication (including speech-language), and cognition. Generally, autism affects a child's social-communication, cognitive, and motor (including sensory) abilities. During well-baby checks, medical personnel screen for developmental disabilities. A secondary screener specific to the signs of ASD is also in order if any questions about red flags occur. This allows for a focus on children for autism and related disorders by observing a child's behaviors and asking the parent(s) questions about the child's development (e.g., words a child might say; if child responds to her name). Table 9.2 details common autism-specific screeners. If red flags for autism on an autism-specific screener are identified, the doctor should refer the child for a specific autism diagnostic evaluation.

The red flags for the three children in our chapter vary significantly. Amir's pediatrician noted potential delays in social interaction and communication and recommended an immediate intervention to increase opportunities to participate with others and engage in developmentally appropriate play. As first-time parents with professional careers, his parents may have limited social reference for their son's development. They readily acknowledge their attention and admiration of "everything Amir." They have not participated previously in community parent-child groups or any consistent child care programs and will be looking to his professional team for information and resources. His provider's interest in Amir's communication and play

Table 9.2   Developmental/Broadband Screeners and Autism-Specific Screeners

The *CSBS DP Infant-Toddler Checklist* (ITC; Wetherby & Prizant, 2002) is a social-communication screener that a caregiver completes when their child is 6–24 months of age. This tool identifies children with delays in communication who are in need of further evaluation. The ITC is not an autism-specific screener, although it contains many red flags for autism. http://firstwords .fsu.edu/pdf/checklist.pdf

The *Modified-Checklist for Autism in Toddlers* (M-CHAT; Robins, Fein, Barton, & Green, 2001) helps doctors and other professionals identify early signs of autism in children 16–30 months of age. Although this tool does not provide a diagnosis of autism, it indicates "risk for" autism and the need for further assessment. This 23-item checklist can be administered during a child's well-baby visits.

>   http://www.firstsigns.org/downloads/m-chat.pdf

>   http://www2.gsu.edu/~psydlr/Diana_L._Robins,_Ph.D._files/ Robins_JADD01.pdf

The *Screening Tool for Autism in Two-Year-Olds* (STAT; Stone et al., 2000, 2004) is an interactive measure of 12 activities that take approximately 20 minutes to complete. This play-based, autism-specific screener initially was developed for children 24–36 months of age. However, recent work has suggested the STAT's effectiveness in detecting autism in children younger than 2 years of age (Stone, McHahon, & Henderson, 2008). Although prior training is necessary, a variety of professionals, including SLPs, pediatricians, preschool teachers, and early interventionists can administer this measure. http:// kc.vanderbilt.edu/triad/training/page.aspx?id=821

The *Social Communication Questionnaire* (SCQ; Rutter, Bailey, & Lord, 2003) is a parent questionnaire that evaluates the child's social-communication skills to determine whether further diagnostic testing for autism or autism spectrum disorder is warranted. Formally known as the *Autism Screening Questionnaire*, this 10-minute instrument can be used with children 4 years and older, with a mental age of 2 years or older. This brief measure has been validated in the literature (e.g., Charman et al., 2004). Clinician and educators may give this measure to screen for autism spectrum disorder.

skills helps her begin to gather information about his overall development as well as potential areas of concern.

Eighteen-month-olds would be expected to be communicating frequently through gestures and vocalizations to make requests, to protest, and to draw attention to self, even if they were not using many words. Word usage should be on the increase, with words added to the child's vocabulary every week. Most toddlers his age would also have a variety of play interests that included people as well as objects. Seeking out others to share enjoyment, surprises, and sadness is common, even if they are less likely to want to share or give up the preferred object of their attention! Repetitive behaviors for Amir related to his limited range of play interests, foods he will eat, and his intense interest in activities, watching DVDs, or building with blocks, that are difficult to interrupt. Amir smiles and notices others in his environment, but does not maintain attention or communicate his interests to others.

Katie, at 30 months, is showing more of the symptoms that have been traditionally associated with ASD. She has obvious verbal and nonverbal communication delays, squeals and uses challenging behaviors when frustrated instead of words, has aversions such as with water and shampooing, and displays repetitive behaviors with the clenching and rocking. She does not respond when her mother calls her name. Her diagnosis of ASD occurred around her second birthday, when her family sought an evaluation from their local early intervention program supported by the Individuals with Disabilities Education Act (IDEA). ASD impacts Katie and her family. Katie does not have functional communication, and her younger brother Ben is surpassing her with gestures and words. Like most daily routines with Katie, bath time is not fun; it is a chore, and one that is exhausting for her caregiver. She does not play with her toys; displays many sensory issues such as sensitivity to noise, temperature, and textures; and gets frustrated with any change that occurs. These behaviors affect her willingness to explore her environments and to learn from them.

Dante is at the other end of the spectrum. His language skills could be described as advanced in understanding and use of vocabulary, grammar and syntax, and complexity of structures. He talks like an adult and actually prefers talking to them rather than his peers. However, his social use of communication and his restricted topics and interests challenge those around him. Dante is missing the social or pragmatic components of his communication skills and talks at people rather than with them. He is more interested in what he has to say than what others around him are saying to him. His restricted interests in stickers and computer games allow him to continue his one-way interactions. His advanced language and academic skills lead his family to question that there is anything "wrong" with Dante and wonder why the early childhood providers at his program want to make a referral for evaluation.

Early childhood professionals should routinely include observations of the children's play, social, and communication strengths and concerns with an eye for red flags of ASD. Some red flags may be seen as early as six months, while others evolve throughout the second year of life, or become more obvious around 24 months. As a consistent caregiver in the child's life, early childhood professionals should know the red flags for autism and be able to collaborate with the family to refer the child for an autism-specific screener or evaluation, when concerns arise. While early care and education professionals are not likely to have the training or experience to administer autism-specific screening or diagnostic tools, they are a first-line informant that should be both knowledgeable about red flags and comfortable asking for help in validating their concerns with other professionals. Early interventionists—e.g., psychologists, speech-language pathologists (SLPs), occupational therapists, developmental specialists, educators, and others specifically trained in autism—can recognize early signs of ASD. Information about referring to an ASD-specific screener or for an evaluation should be provided through each state's Child Find initiatives.

What: The Screening Tools

Currently no biological markers for ASD or autism exist, so diagnosis must be derived from behavioral features (APA, 2000). As previously discussed, autism is defined by atypical development in the key areas of social interaction, communication, and repetitive and stereotyped behaviors or interests, and many behaviors comprise each of the domains. There are a number of developmental screening tools that highlight early signs of autism. Pediatricians or professionals can use these tools as a first step to identifying if further testing is warranted. Note: These tools *screen for and/or indicate the possible existence of* developmental delays and autism; they *do not* diagnose these conditions.

When

The earlier, the better! Identifying children with autism and beginning intervention within the first three years of life will have greater impact on a child's and family's outcomes than waiting until the child is school-aged. Studies have begun to document the effectiveness of early intervention in young children with ASD (Dawson et al., 2010). Recent focused studies in young children by Kasari, Freeman, and Paparella (2006) and Yoder and Stone (2006) have also shown effects of brief interventions on social communication. Bono, Daley, and Sigman (2004) found that the relation between amount of intervention and gain in language for children with ASD depended upon their ability to respond to joint attention as well as initial language skills. Landa, Holman, and Garrett-Mayer (2007) noted changes in children with autism's joint attention abilities from age 14 months to 24 months. Kasari and colleagues' intervention studies revealed increases in joint attention correlated with increases in expressive language in children with autism (Kasari, Freeman, & Paparella, 2006; Kasari, Paparella, Freeman, & Jahromi, 2008). These findings illustrate the impact of early social and communication interventions.

DIAGNOSIS

Who Is on the Team?

After a child has tested positive on an autism screener, the next step is to conduct an evaluation for autism spectrum disorder. Filipek et al. (2000) recommends a multidisciplinary team in the diagnosis of autism. The child's current team will help expand (if need be) to include a team of specialists to evaluate the presence of ASD. The type and number of members vary, depending upon each child's individual needs. Team members may include the child and family, a speech-language pathologist, developmental psychologist, pediatrician, neurologist, teacher(s)/educators, and other developmental therapists. Members of the team play different roles at different times, yet at the heart of this team are the child and the family.

What Is the Role of the Family and Caregivers?

Parents/caregivers are the experts on their child. They know and understand their child the best. Therefore, the parents' role is vital in the diagnosis of autism. They make the decision to participate in this process, provide a family and child medical history, and support their child throughout the evaluation process. Caregivers also provide rich and abundant information about their child's development and current behaviors when offered opportunities to participate through methods that support their cultural and linguistic diversity (Westby, 2009). Other team members need this information to make an accurate and differential diagnosis (i.e., ruling out other possible, competing diagnoses). Parents perform multiple roles as informants, guides, and validators for the evaluators, but more importantly, they are the child's parent: nurturer, teacher, advocate, and friend for life. A diagnosis of autism brings many changes to the family's life. Any diagnosis of delay or disability evokes many and different emotions for a family; ASD is certainly no different. The range of child outcomes that are possible and the challenges at making early predictions for future quality of life increases the fear and anxiety for many families. The more the family is involved in the diagnostic process, and the more opportunities they have to learn about the disorder, to ask and answer questions, and to be a part of the assessment and intervention process, the more prepared for the future the family will be (Johnson & Myers, 2007; Sperry et al., 1999).

What Does the Team Do?

Typically, the family and the current team will seek out professionals who diagnose autism—for example, pediatric neurologists, developmental psychologists, and speech-language pathologists with specialization in autism. These professionals may employ a variety of tools to achieve an accurate behavioral assessment of the child, such as observations of the child in her natural environment and curriculum-based measures; natural language and play samples; and standardized measures. It is important to understand, at this time, there is no medical procedure, neurological examination, or psychometrically irrefutable measure that can determine if a child has autism. Behavioral measures administered by a team of experts with specialized knowledge of autism spectrum disorders are the tools used for diagnosis. Diagnosis should always be multidisciplinary, include multiple measures, and be completed over more than one time and setting. The good news is that there is a growing body of research that indicates that diagnosis by age 2 is both accurate and stable when completed by an experienced team (Bishop, Gahagan, & Lord, 2007).

Observation and Informal Measures

It is important to observe a child with autism in a variety of environments because each setting may elicit different behaviors/red flags for autism. Parent-teacher questionnaires and observations of the child in his natural environments can help to bridge this gap and offer more insight into a child's social-communication abilities, or lack thereof. The *Autism Diagnostic Instrument—Revised* (ADI-R; LeCouteur, Lord, & Rutter, 2003) is the caregiver companion piece to the *Autism Diagnostic Observation Schedule* (ADOS; Lord, Rutter, DiLavore, & Risi, 1999), discussed subsequently. Here, a diagnostician interviews the parent about their child and his abilities. Parent report is an important and reliable source of information about the child's development. Another parent interview is the *Vineland Adaptive Behavior Scales, Second Edition* (VABS-II; Sparrow, Cicchetti, & Balla, 1984), which explores a child's daily functioning/adaptive abilities by asking parents questions about their child's personal and social skills. These assessments accentuate the features of autism to determine if further diagnostic testing for autism is warranted.

Natural Language and Play Samples

Natural language and play samples offer rich information about the child's independent, cognitive, and symbolic abilities. Because children with autism evidence delays in social-communication skills, it is essential to assess their *independent* language and play skills. Team members— e.g., caregivers, speech-language pathologists—collect natural language samples of a child during her daily interactions to evaluate expressive language. These samples might encompass various settings (e.g., home and school) and comprise a variety of routines (e.g., free play, outdoor play, center time, dinner time). Multiple samples will help the team to gather and decode the child's complete repertoire of expressive and symbolic actions and offer insight into cognitive processes.

Direct Assessment and Standardized Measures

Speech-language evaluations assess a child's receptive (comprehension) and expressive language. Decreased receptive language skills or lack of talking by 15 months of age indicate a need for further evaluation. A measure of language is important because of the relationship of language delays to ASD, and also because most behavioral assessments use language—e.g., directions to the child, symbols—to complete the assessments. Depending upon the child's age, the designated team members will administer various communication and developmental assessments, such as the *Communication Symbolic Behavior Scales Developmental Profile* (CSBS DP; Wetherby & Prizant, 2002), Preschool Language Scale, fourth edition (PLS-4; Zimmerman, Steiner, & Pond, 2002), *Early Social Communication Scales* (ESCS; Mundy, Delgado, & Block, 2003), *Mullen Scales of Early Learning* (MSEL; Mullen, 1995), or the *Bayley Scales of Infant-Toddler Development, Third Edition* (Bayley, 2005). These assessments are comprehensive and highlight many features of autism, such as gaze shifts, play, repetitive and stereotyped behaviors or interests, and communication. They also may test for social concepts, problem solving, or cognitive abilities. Incorporating developmental and language testing is required to interpret the child's behavior in the context of his overall developmental strengths and needs. In addition to speech-language evaluations, hearing evaluations are very important to rule out the possibility of a hearing loss that could cause a child to have decreased receptive or expressive language. These evaluations are necessary before any diagnosis of autism would be given. It is important to note, however, that autism can co-occur with other diagnoses, such as hearing loss, anxiety, intellectual impairment, Fragile X, seizures, and attention deficit hyperactivity disorder (ADHD; Filipek et al., 2000; Johnson & Myers, 2007).

A further step in the process is to administer an autism-specific measure. One such assessment is the Autism Diagnostic Observation Scales (ADOS) developed by Lord and colleagues (1999). There are four versions of this assessment: for toddlers (under field testing), preschoolers, children, and teens/adults. The ADOS measures a child's communicative, social interactive, and play/imaginative abilities to determine if he qualifies for a diagnosis of autism. While other measures are available, the ADOS has the strongest psychometric ratings for young children. Again, sound diagnoses can now be made at age 2. The diagnosis is important to ensure that appropriate and adequate interventions are initiated early.

INTERVENTION

As noted previously, there is mounting evidence demonstrating the effectiveness of intensive early intervention using a range of behavioral, developmental, and blended approaches with a substantial proportion of young children with ASD (e.g., Dawson et al., 2010; Kasari, Freeman, & Paparella, 2006; Whalen & Schreibman, 2003). For children with ASD, research indicates that intervention provided before age 3½ has a much greater impact than intervention provided after age 5; this finding is consistent with early intervention research with other populations (Lord & Paul, 1997). More recent studies are showing that the benefits of interventions initiated prior to the child's second birthday have even greater results. However, the most widely used outcome measures in intervention research for children with ASD have been changes in IQ and proportion of children placed in a regular classroom after intervention (NRC, 2001). Such outcome measures are problematic because they may reflect increased compliance or parent preference in placement, rather than meaningful changes. Furthermore, these measures are not applicable with infants and toddlers.

It is widely believed that there is no single best intervention/treatment package for all children with ASD. Decisions about the best intervention, or combination of interventions, should be made by the parents with the assistance of their team based upon the unique needs of the child and family and scientific knowledge about the intervention (NRC, 2001). The NRC conducted a systematic review of research on educational interventions for children with ASD from birth through 8 years of age (NRC, 2001). They concluded that a large body of research has demonstrated significant progress in response to intervention with a substantial proportion of children with ASD using a range of techniques. However, few well-controlled studies with random assignment are available, and therefore, it is not yet known whether particular intervention approaches are more effective than others. Furthermore, children's outcomes are variable, with some making substantial progress and others showing slow gains. The committee concluded that there is a convergence of evidence that the following characteristics are essential active ingredients of effective interventions for young children with ASD:

1) Entry into intervention programs as soon as ASD is suspected.
2) Active engagement in intensive instruction for a minimum of five hours per day, five days a week.
3) Use of repeated planned teaching opportunities that are structured over brief periods of time.
4) Sufficient individualized adult attention on a daily basis.

5) Inclusion of a family component, including parent training.

6) Mechanisms for ongoing assessment with corresponding adjustments in programming.

7) Priority for instruction on: (1) functional, spontaneous communication, (2) social instruction across settings; (3) play skills with a focus on peer interaction; (4) new skill maintenance and generalization in natural contexts; and (5) functional assessment and positive behavior support to address problem behaviors.

Due to the nature of autism, young children with ASD are at risk for impoverished social interactions. Recent studies have shown that parent-implemented interventions, beginning in the second year of life, can affect joint attention and social communication and, consequently, developmental outcomes (Schertz & Odom, 2007; Wetherby & Woods, 2006). Early intervention provides young children with opportunities and support to interact with their caregivers in functional daily routines and activities. Studies further support the benefits of inclusive preschool programs on language, cognitive, and social outcomes (Boulware, Schwartz, Sandall, & McBride, 2006; Rogers & Vismara, 2008; Yoder & Stone, 2006). Thus an urgent need exists for young children to be identified earlier so that they might receive intervention as soon as possible.

Principles for Supporting Young Children with ASD and Their Families

The amount of information, resources, and intervention strategies available and meaningful to support young children with ASD and their families is overwhelming and far beyond a single chapter. Just search on any Internet browser and watch for the multimillions of hits for ASD. A dozen basic principles related to the NRC's components with resources for more information are offered.

1) *Children with ASD are first and foremost children; they are members of families, and they live in a community* (Wolery & Garfinkle, 2002). Always remember, children with ASD have much in common with other children. They have physical attributes, personalities, interests, and unique ways to get your attention, to share information, and to challenge your knowledge/skills as a caregiver just like all children. If you focus only on the differences or the symptoms of ASD, you could easily lose sight of who the child is: a blue-eyed, blonde ball of energy

fascinated with books, music, and his pet dog who enjoys going to the park with his dad and brother. As caregivers of children with ASD, it is important to see the child, not the disorder, and to support the child within the family as they live, learn, and play in their community.

2) *Start now . . . move forward . . . measure success.* If you observe red flags for ASD, you do not have to wait for a diagnosis to begin providing supports and instruction. Engage the child in developmentally appropriate social, communication, and play activities systematically, increasing the amount of active engagement for the child and expanding interests and interactions with others. Caregivers may be able to compensate for a child's deficits in joint attention by ensuring a common focus of attention when modeling language. Join the child in their play, music, or books and provide words, gestures, and enjoyment. Engaging the child frequently and with increasing expectations is important to decrease the potential for restricted interests and repetitive behaviors. Amir's family followed the pediatrician's advice to enroll him in a community program. However, it is important that they not stop with the addition of focused intervention. *A diagnosis is important.* Caregivers and team members need to support the family in the referral process and share observations, developmental information, and encouragement. A diagnosis the first step in the development of an individualized plan that is carefully and consistently reviewed for progress. The child's plan, developed by the family, caregivers, and team of professionals, must be monitored consistently for progress. Children change rapidly, and every minute counts with early intervention for ASD. Consistent progress monitoring ensures that the team maintains their coordinated efforts to focus on the children's most essential learning priorities, that adequate intensity of active engagement occurs, and that new outcomes or program revisions support the children's maximum success. Because we know there are many effective interventions available, it is important to monitor the effectiveness of those identified and to communicate as a team. Each intervention should not be seen as separate, but rather as a coordinated and collaborative plan.

3) *Partnerships with families are essential.* Families are maximally involved in the services and supports for young children with ASD by the simple fact of the child's age and reliance on parents for nurturance. The diagnosis of ASD, as well as the ongoing intervention program, immerses the family into a cycle of information gathering, giving, and decision making. Partnerships promote family participation when team members respect their priorities, concerns, and interests (Woods &

Wetherby, 2003). The team has significant knowledge and expertise to share with the family to support informed decision making. The family knows what will be compatible with their values and beliefs, their resources, and their expectations for their children. Dante's family values his academic skills and encourages his focus on books and computer games rather than social play with peers. Additional information on social skills development and their importance for future academic outcomes, strategies to support his interactions with others that build on his strengths, and encouragement to his family to identify opportunities for social interactions with Dante can establish the family's role as important contributors.

Providers must recognize that time spent by parents working with their child can enhance their confidence and competence to interact with their child, increase the child's independence in family activities, and improve the quality of the family's life (Sperry et al., 1999). While the amount and type of participation by parents in the intervention process varies significantly from the role of primary teacher to an observer and informant, two results are clear. First, evidence of effectiveness of parent-implemented intervention in children with varying types of developmental delays and specifically for children with ASD has been consistently documented across a wide range of adaptive, behavioral, social, and communication child outcomes (Meadan, Ostrosky, Zaghlawan, & Yu, 2009). Second, caregivers are able to learn a variety of broad and specific intervention strategies to teach their children functional and meaningful outcomes. Teaching caregivers to implement intervention strategies during everyday activities is a logical method to achieve the intensity of active engagement needed for young children with ASD.

4) *Children with ASD need a comprehensive curriculum* to include developmentally appropriate content across learning areas. Comprehensive treatment models (CTM) are broad in scope in that they "address core deficits in autism including language, social, cognition, and play" (Rogers & Vismara, 2008, p. 9). CTMs are generally intended to be long term, have a broad scope of skills and behaviors for development, promote sufficiency and intensity of intervention to maximize learning, have specialized or highly qualified personnel for the intervention, and may include components that have an established evidence base. CTMs are comprehensive in nature and address the range of developmental and behavioral needs of children (Boulware et al., 2006). However, CTMs are not "one size fits all." They vary by the theoretical perspective they are based on, the specialized personnel identified as

team members, the role of the family, and the outcomes to be achieved. As CTMs designed for young children become more widely available, research will be needed to study the relationship between child characteristics, specific treatment procedures, and specific outcomes. Such research findings will help families and team members prioritize intervention goals and select specific intervention strategies appropriate to the CTM and those that are comfortable and meaningful to family members implementing them. Caregivers and team members must carefully examine the unique strengths of each child and family and match for key variables when choosing a CTM (Strain, McGee, & Kohler, 2001). Examples of some comprehensive curricular approaches for young children with ASD are briefly reviewed in Table 9.3.

Table 9.3   Selected Comprehensive Treatment Models

DIR (Developmental, Individual-Difference, Relationship-Based) and Floortime

Brief Description

DIR (Developmental, Individual-Difference, Relationship-Based) and Floortime approach focuses on helping children master the building blocks of relating, communicating, and thinking (Greenspan & Weider, 2006). Based on a developmental theoretical perspective, DIR/Floortime views social relationships and play as critical to a child's development.

Key Features

- Developmental: Understanding where the child is developmentally is critical to planning a treatment program. Ongoing assessment of the child occurs to monitor healthy emotional and intellectual growth.
- Individual-Difference: Each child is recognized as a unique learner; individual sensory and motor challenges that may be interfering with the child's ability to grow and learn, e.g. understanding and responding to the environment (sights, sounds, etc.) is examined.
- Relationship-Based: Building relationships between children and their primary caregivers is essential to promote the children's development. Floortime, the centerpiece of the DIR approach, teaches parents and others important in the children's life to interact and communicate in developmentally enhancing exchanges that helps them learn.

Source: Greenspan, S., & Weider, S. (2006). *Engaging autism: Using the floortime approach to help children relate, communicate, and think.* Cambridge, MA: DiCopa Press.

(Continued)

Table 9.3   (Continued)

SCERTS Model

Brief Description

The SCERTS model is derived from a developmental theoretical perspective as well as a research-based foundation on communication and social-emotional development in children with and without special needs. Developed by Barry Prizant, PhD, and Amy Wetherby, PhD, the comprehensive assessment and curriculum model uses everyday activities and routines as the primary contexts in which children learn, and in which progress is measured. The model prioritizes Social Communication, Emotional Regulation, and Transactional Support as the core challenges that must be addressed in a program for children with Autism Spectrum Disorder.

Key Features

- SC (Social Communication)
- ER (Emotional Regulation)
- TS (Transactional Support)

The SCERTS Model focuses on children's development of spontaneous, functional communication and secure, trusting relationships with children and adults, and the ability to maintain a well-regulated emotional state for learning and interacting. The model supports children, their families, and professionals to maximize positive social experiences across home, school and community settings.

References

Prizant, B., Wetherby, A., Rubin, E., & Laurent, A. (2007). The SCERTS model manual: Enhancing communication and socioemotional abilities of young children with ASD. Baltimore: Paul. H. Brookes.

Prizant, B., Wetherby, A., Rubin, E., Laurent, A., & Rydell, P. (2007). *The SCERTS Model: A comprehensive educational approach for children with Autism Spectrum Disorders, Volume II-Intervention.* Baltimore: Paul. H. Brookes.

TEACCH

Brief Description

The TEACCH model was developed by Eric Schopler, PhD, and is based on understanding the needs of the individual with autism, adopting appropriate adaptations, and creating a broadly-based intervention strategy that builds on existing skills and interests.

Key Features

- Structured teaching through organizing the physical environment, developing schedules and adaptive materials, making expectations clear and explicit, and using visual materials.

(Continued)

Table 9.3   (Continued)

- Focus on developing communication skills, and pursuing social and leisure interests.
- Cultivating strengths and interests, rather than drilling solely on deficits is priority in TEACCH. Capitalizing on children's relative strengths in visual skills, recognizing details, and memory, among other areas, these skills are the basis of instructional strategies. TEACCH also capitalizes on children's individual interests to increase their motivation and an understanding of what they are doing.

Reference: http://www.teacch.com

LEAP

Brief Description

Learning Experiences: Alternative Programs for Preschoolers and Parents (LEAP) was established by Phil Strain and colleagues in 1981 as a model demonstration site. It uses a blend of applied behavioral analysis with naturalistic teaching methods within inclusive community preschool programs. The belief is that preschool classrooms with children with ASD and typically developing peers (peer-mediated intervention) provide the most developmentally appropriate context for learning.

Key Features

- Maintains that early intervention is key, with a classroom environment that mirrors typical early childhood settings.
- Co-teaching approach between early childhood educators. All special therapies occur within the classroom context.
- Strong ABA background, use of incidental teaching and other naturalistic communication strategies through embedded individualized instruction in natural routines and activities.
- Peer-mediated instruction (typically developing children teach those with ASD) with an emphasis on social skill strategies and practice in real-world situations.
- All parents required to spend 12 hours per week in training at the onset of the intervention. Opportunities for systematic parent training continue throughout program.

Reference: http://www.ttoolbox.com/teacher_training.htm

5) *Build predictable, functional daily routines.* Daily caregiving and play routines identified by family members and caregivers are the primary contexts for embedded intervention with young children with ASD because of their repetition, frequency, systematic implementation, functionality, cultural appropriateness, and brevity (Woods &

Wetherby, 2003). While the types and level of independence in care-giving, play, and academic routines and activities evolve as the child grows, they are constant in children's lives. The documentation supporting the use of daily routines and activities as an organizational structure to enhance participation includes many studies conducted with preschool children with ASD (NRC, 2001). The development of routines with individuals with ASD is a long-standing intervention strategy (Kashinath, Woods, & Goldstein, 2006; Woods, Kashinath, & Goldstein, 2004) and is particularly useful with young children who spend large amounts of time engaged in daily living and play routines with caregivers. Many routines result in positive outcomes for the child, such as a drink, music, a piece of fruit, or a story and snuggle time with dad, and are motivating and reinforcing to the child, increasing the likelihood that engagement and participation will occur.

The routine sequence and its frequent repetition provide familiarity, predictability, and security for the child, thereby developing a framework for the child to anticipate and produce an appropriate response. While important for all children, predictability has been identified as critical for both learning new skills and decreasing challenging behaviors for children with ASD (Powell, Dunlap, & Fox, 2006; NRC, 2001). With the routine framework to support the child, new information or experiences can be added to increase the child's ability and lead to increased independence. Routines also support interaction between the child and the caregiver by providing clear roles and responsibilities that can be learned to increase engagement, communication, and social interaction, the core deficits associated with ASD. For younger children and caregiver-implemented interventions, the procedures are embedded into the preferred routines identified by the family. For example, getting a drink can become a framework for Katie's mother to embed meaningful targets such as requesting help with vocalizations and gestures, making choices between milk or juice, showing an empty cup to request more, smiling and looking toward the communication partner as a social exchange, and placing the empty cup on the kitchen counter to indicate satisfaction. The roles provide systematic patterns of interactions for reciprocity and turn taking, further enhancing the quality of the intervention. Katie's mother responds to her signal that initiates the routine and may imitate Katie's request or model a more sophisticated communication target and then signal to Katie to respond. As Katie responds, her gaze is directed to her mother's face. The adult may also use exaggerated facial expressions, or comments to share enjoyment with the child's response. The child is following the adult's actions that are integral to the routine—not establishing eye contact to the verbal prompt, "look at me" (McGee, Morrier, & Daly, 1999). The sequence of the routine and familiarity with the materials provide a scaffold of support to the family implementing the intervention. They can predict when the next opportunity for communication or social interaction will occur in the routine and be prepared to support their child's response positively. These everyday experiences also make intervention more meaningful and consistent with their family and intervention priorities.

6) *Many, if not most teaching or intervention strategies used for children with ASD are also effective with other children* in your class or program (Boulware et al., 2006; Strain et al., 2001.) While teaching children with ASD has the best outcomes when it is systematic and intentional, the evidence-based strategies promoted for children with ASD are good teaching for all children (Carnahan, Musti-Rao, & Bailey, 2009). Following the child's lead, expanding communication, encouraging initiation of social interaction, embedding intervention into daily routines, using visual supports, and including peers as mentors are developmentally appropriate teaching strategies and easily incorporated in most small group settings and classrooms. The amount and level of support needed for the child with ASD will vary based on the child's needs. Amir benefits from systematic support during snack time by providing food and drink choices for him to request, waiting for a response, helping him work with a peer to clean up after snack, and providing him with a choice board to transition to his next activity. Amir joins in story time by responding with his peers. During block play, his favorite activity, he takes the lead, with the adult imitating his motor and communication bids. She expands on his single words by commenting on the objects (e.g., "Mickey book") describing them (e.g., "car go"), or making requests (e.g., "more blocks"). The caregiver gently interrupts when needed to get his attention, makes him work too, and expands his play repertoire by bringing in some cars and trucks to the block center to build roads and houses. Throughout the day, Amir has multiple different routines where his priority outcomes are embedded to ensure adequate practice. Katie works with her mom at home throughout the day on multiple outcomes to increase her use of pictures to make requests and protests. Katie's mom uses very systematic prompts and visual supports to help Katie make choices and learn that communication is powerful. She will soon be attending an early childhood special education program within her community school, where she will benefit from a

comprehensive curriculum and specialized team members, including an occupational therapist and a speech-language pathologist. Specialized instruction coordinated across the team benefits the child and family the most (Woods & Wetherby, 2003).

7) *Environment matters—set the stage for learning.* Caregivers can design the environment to encourage the initiation of communication, social interaction, and play; however, it has to be meaningful and predictable for children with ASD. "Engineering," or arranging the environment to provide opportunities and reasons for children to initiate, is important to prevent a more passive or responder role. The contemporary behavioral literature has described specific strategies to occasion language use, such as to delay at critical moments in natural routines and to interrupt chains of behavior by removing an object needed to complete the activity (Boulware et al., 2006). By making the initiation of communication a priority, natural opportunities for communicating can be capitalized upon in all settings.

Caregivers must also maintain appropriate physical proximity to be available for interaction with children and to support their active engagement. Planning for individual attention, pairs, small groups, and larger, less structured times necessitates careful examination of who will be where, when, and prepared to support the children's learning objectives. Strategies as simple as providing children with a place for their materials can support organization and clear expectations. A place for everything and everything in its space has significance for children with ASD. Classroom or family rules provide concrete guidance for the children, and many children with ASD are proficient at following rules, just as they do routines. Children with ASD often have visual strengths. The use of visual supports provides concrete representation and memory supports that are not available in auditory directions. Early preliteracy programs can help children to capitalize on their memory and visual strengths to build school-readiness skills. Providers may label their classrooms areas and toys with text and real pictures. The use of daily schedule boards (again with pictures and text) to help a child transition between activities has been shown to be useful (Massey & Wheeler, 2000). It is also important to examine the environment—e.g., home, classroom, and materials—for their sensory qualities. Observe children's responses to stimulation—e.g., lights, heat, noise—to ascertain if modifications or adaptations would benefit the children's engagement and learning (Miller et al., 2004).

8) *Focus attention of intervention on priority outcomes.* The emphasis on successful interactions is one of the most critical components of education programs for children with ASD found in current literature from both behavioral and developmental perspectives (Paul, Chawarska, Cicchetti, & Volkmar, 2008). While the methods or teaching strategies may vary across theoretical perspectives, the focus does not; social communication and play are essential. Caregivers must not ignore the core deficit of limited or restricted play repertoires in young children with ASD. What this means is that you may need to teach the child to play, and not just use play as a context to teach other skills. A formal assessment of play skills provides important developmental detail that may be lacking in comprehensive developmental curriculum based assessments. Building on the child's play strengths and needs will produce growth in play skills that will also foster growth in communication and social skills. Thus, play is an important feature of a young child's development, particularly symbolic play. Symbolic play parallels a child's language development, and both may be delayed when either one or the other does not develop. Play is a developmentally appropriate way to help very young children learn how to interact with others, socialize, problem solve, and build literacy skills (Kasari et al., 2008). This is a winning combination for all children and one that is essential for children like Dante.

9) *Without a doubt, behavior communicates.* Learn how each child communicates with you and respond consistently. When a child with ASD can only get attention by squealing, pinching, or kicking, then she will engage in inappropriate behavior because it is successful. Inappropriate behaviors are not about children being bad. They are about children not having acceptable ways to communicate that are as effective as the unacceptable ones. Katie did not have words, pictures, gestures, or easy-to-read signals to communicate with her mother and used what she knew would work—screaming and throwing herself on the floor. If you respond to children's early communication behaviors such as taking your hand, standing close to the desired object, or looking at it, then you can model a more appropriate communication and prevent a challenging one

"Challenging behaviors" is a simple term for an extensive topic. It may include: biting, hitting, kicking, pinching (self or others), head banging, screaming, running away, defecating, ingesting feces, throwing, or slapping, to name a few. It may also include repetitive or stereotyped behaviors, such as flapping of arms or limbs, finger flicking, body rocking, rubbing body, or rubbing body against an object (Fox, Dunlap, & Cushing, 2002). Most people are not trained in autism and view these behaviors negatively, perhaps as a threat, so they try to stop them by inhibiting the action. Unfortunately, their intervention often fails, and the child's behavior increases or becomes disruptive to others. Careful investigation into these behaviors reveal their purpose and meaning and often reveals a resolution to change or shape them.

Observation and interview strategies can uncover the meaning behind the behaviors and facilitate the development of communication skills to replace them. For example, a functional assessment of challenging behaviors requires observing a child with autism in various environments (home, school, grocery store) on several occasions and organizing the challenging behaviors that were observed into patterns that describe the reason(s) for the behavior (Powell, Dunlap, & Fox, 2006). A variety of prevention and intervention strategies have empirical support for reducing the challenging behaviors but, more importantly, developing communication skills that promote socially appropriate interaction, including the use of Augmentative, Alternative Communication (AAC; Yoder & Stone, 2006). For more information about challenging behaviors or about Positive Behavior Support, see http://www.challengingbehavior.org.

10) *Teach social skills deliberately.* Although social skills deficits are a central feature of ASD, few children receive adequate social skills programming (Hume, Bellini, & Pratt, 2005). Communication and play skills may set the stage for the development of social skills, but there is a need to start early and provide systematic instruction to ensure the social skills are meaningful and fun. There are a variety of strategies to support social skills, including the use of modifications to the physical and social environment that promote social interactions between children with ASD and their peers. When interesting or engaging materials are systematically shared or exchanged, opportunities are available for social skill teaching. Peer opportunities must be supported to be successful. Dante will benefit from adult-supported engagement with his peers. Specific instruction on initiating and responding to social interactions may be included with related skills, such as play, language, problem solving, or during lunch or cleanup time. Peer-mediated interventions involving training typically developing peers to direct and respond to the social behaviors of children with ASD during activities have a strong database for support (Strain et al., 2001).

Social stories are a developmentally appropriate way to help a child with some early or emerging language skills understand the rules of certain social situations—for example, how to greet a friend and request to play. Rather than approaching a peer and demanding that he play with him, a social story could be developed for Dante showing him how to tap the child on the shoulder to gain his attention, smile, ask him politely if he would like to play, and to offer the friend an opportunity to identify what he would like to play. Social stories are written at the child's linguistic level, using pictures or drawings to illustrate appropriate actions, and follows a scripted format to increase the child's comprehension of what to do as well as what not to do and why. Team members can develop social stories to address a specific social concern with a child. While each story addresses only a single social concern, the story interventions have also been shown to build language and literacy skills (Fox, Dunlap, & Cushing, 2002).

11) *The team, with the family as guide, provides group intelligence.* The team coordinates goals, methods, and plans for the child. As recommended previously, children with ASD benefit from a team approach guided by the family's priorities and concerns. The team's input will result in a meaningful plan and their consistent communication will ensure the good ideas generated by the team will support child's learning. Meeting with the team regularly keeps the team up to date on the child's progress and facilitates program change when needed. The team approach also facilitates transition from one program or service to another. Children are less likely to engage in challenging behaviors when the team plans ahead and prepares the children for change. Children with ASD usually prefer routine and sameness and may have difficulty with transitions. Before rearranging the room, changing teachers, taking a field trip, or even transitioning to a different activity, prepare the child. You may want to take photos of the new setting, write a story for the child about what he will do at the post office, and slowly introduce him to the new teacher by meeting with her briefly for several days before joining the group, or provide a visual schedule of the day's activities. Time spent in preparation will be saved later in helping the child adjust.

12) *Believe in all children and value their contributions to a diverse and evolving society.* We end the basic principles as we began—with the child. Capitalize on the child's strengths and interests. Incorporate the special skills the child has with blocks or puzzles, naming letters or drawing lines into activities with other children. This allows you

to encourage the child's competence and comment on his work and contributions to the group. Make a portfolio of his work. Share the pictures or papers with his parents, take a photo of him helping his classmates, or include him in a story for the group. Embrace his uniqueness and share it with others.

FUTURE IMPLICATIONS

While there is still much to learn about young children with ASD, more is known now than ever, and more is learned every day. Research and advocacy groups continue to search for accurate diagnostic evaluation methods and comprehensive treatments as well as developing effective specific interventions to address the wide range of needs for individuals with ASD (AAP-CCD, 2006). Everyone can play an important role in helping to address the needs of young children with ASD and their families. We can continue to search for the cause, seek early identification, and most importantly, help support the growth and development of all young children with ASD. Identified early, the prognosis for improvement is excellent. The future is ripe for discovery and change. The next decade will bring great growth in knowledge of autism spectrum disorder.

ANNOTATED WEB RESOURCES

Autism Speaks (http://autismspeaks.org). This interactive Web site includes up-to-date information on early identification and intervention for ASD across the age span. Of particular interest is the video library that illustrates early red flags helpful to early identification.

First Signs (http://www.firstsigns.org): First Signs is dedicated to educating parents and professionals about autism and related disorders. Developed and maintained by a parent of a child with autism to support early identification, the site helps parents to share their concerns with their pediatrician. Its focus on early identification includes a review of various methods and measures for screening and evaluation as well as training materials for pediatricians and family physicians.

Center for Disease Control (CDC, http://www.cdc.gov/ncbddd/autism/index.html): The autism section on the CDC Web site provides up to date information on the prevalence, early identification, diagnosis, research on causality, and help for families. It is a trustworthy and balanced resource for reports and fact sheets on the most recent findings, including controversial topics such as the role of immunizations in causality, various diets, and alternative interventions.

American Academy of Pediatrics (AAP, http://aappolicy.aappublications.org/cgi/content/full/pediatrics;107/5/1221): Learn the Signs: Act Early Campaign materials are available here. AAP has a focused initiative to continue to inform physicians of the red flags for ASD to increase early identification. They also inform physicians of the importance of early interventions and make recommendations for referral.

Autism Society of America (ASA, http://www.autism-society.org): One of the many national and international professional organizations devoted to supporting individuals with autism and their families through information, resources, referrals, and advocacy. Membership is a minimal annual cost and provides benefits in professional conferences, publications, and contributions to research.

First Words (http://firstwords.fsu.edu): Connects to Autism Speaks for the Video Glossary and provides additional resources and research for early communication and language development integral to the identification and intervention for young children at risk for or with ASD. Free download for the Infant Toddler Checklist, a standardized screening tool, and cutoff scores are maintained here. Additional tools for early identification are posted as available.

References

American Academy of Pediatrics, Council on Children with Disabilities (AAP-CCD). (2006). Identifying infants and young children with developmental disorders in the medical home: An algorithm for developmental surveillance and screening. *Pediatrics, 118*(1), 405–420. Published correction (2006) appears in *Pediatrics, 118*(4), 1808–1809.

American Psychiatric Association. (2000). *Diagnostic and statistical manual of mental disorders* (4th ed., text revision). Washington, DC: American Psychiatric Association.

Bayley, N. (2005). *Bayley Scales of Infant-Toddler Development* (3rd ed.). San Antonio, TX: Pearson.

Bishop, S., Gahagan, S., & Lord, C. (2007). Re-examining the core features of autism: A comparison of autism spectrum disorder and fetal alcohol spectrum disorder. *Journal of Child Psychology and Psychiatry, 48*, 1111–1121.

Bishop, D. V., Maybery, M., Wong, D., Maley, A., & Hallmayer, J. (2006), Characteristics of the broader phenotype in autism: A study of siblings using the children's communication checklist-2. *American Journal of Medical Genetics Part B: Neuropsychiatric Genetics, 141B*, 117–122.

Bishop, S. L., Richler, J., & Lord, C. (2006). Association between restricted and repetitive behaviors and nonverbal IQ in children with autism spectrum disorders. *Child Neuropsychology, 12*(4), 247–267.

Bono, M., Daley, T., & Sigman, M. (2004). Relations among joint attention, amount of intervention and language gain in autism. *Journal of Autism and Developmental Disorders, 34*, 495–505.

Boulware, G., Schwartz, I., Sandall, S., & McBride, B. (2006). Project DATA for toddlers: An inclusive approach to very young chidlren with autism spectrum disorders. *Topics in Early Childhood Special Education, 26*, 94–105.

Carnahan, C., Musti-Rao, S., & Bailey, J. (2009). Promoting active engagement in small group learning experiences for students with autism and significant learning needs. *Education and Treatment of Children, 32*(1), 37–61.

Centers for Disease Control and Prevention. (2009). Prevalence of Autism Spectrum Disorders. *Morbidity and Mortality Weekly Report, 58*(SS10), 1–20.

Centers for Disease Control and Prevention Department of Health and Human Services (CDC-HHS). (2007). Prevalence of autism spectrum disorders: Autism and developmental disabilities monitoring network, 14 sites, United States, 2002. *Morbidity and Mortality Weekly Report Surveillance Summaries, 56*(1), 12–28.

Charman, T., Baron-Cohen, S., Swettenham, J., Baird, G., Drew, A., & Cox, A. (2003). Predicting language outcome in infants with autism and pervasive developmental disorder. *International Journal of Language and Communication Disorders, 38*, 265–285.

Dawson, G., Rogers. S. Munson, J., Smith, M., Winter, J., Greenson, J., et al. (2010). Randomized, controlled trial of an intervention for toddlers with autism: The Early Start Denver Model. *Pediatrics, 125*(1), 17–23.

Dawson, G., Toth, K., Abbott, R., Osterling, J., Munson, J., Estes, A., & Liaw, J. (2004). Early social attention impairments in autism: Social orienting, joint attention, and attention to distress. *Developmental Psychology, 40*, 271–283.

Filipek, P., Accardo, P., Baranak, G., Cook, E., Dawson, G., Gordon, B., et al. (2000). The screening and diagnosis of autistic spectrum disorders. *Journal of Autism and Developmental Disorders, 29*(6), 439–484.

Fox, L., Dunlap, G., & Cushing, L. (2002). Early intervention, positive behavior support, and transition to school. *Journal of Emotional and Behavioral Disorders, 10*(3), 149–157.

Garfinkle, A. N. & Schwartz, I. S. (2002). Peer imitation: Increasing social interactions in children with autism and other developmental disabilities in inclusive preschool classrooms. *Topics in Early Childhood Special Education, 22*(1), 26–38.

Greenspan, S., & Weider, S. (2006). *Engaging autism: Using the floortime approach to help children relate, communicate, and think.* Cambridge, MA: DiCopa Press.

Howlin, P., Goode, S., Hutton, J., & Rutter, M. (2004). Adult outcome for children with autism. *Journal of Child Psychology and Psychiatry, 45*, 212–229.

Hume, K., Bellini, S., & Pratt, C. (2005). The usage and perceived outcomes of early intervention and early childhood programs for young children with autism spectrum disorder. *Topics in Early Childhood Special Education, 25*, 195–207.

Johnson, C. P., & Myers, S. M. (2007). American Academy of Pediatrics, Council on Children with Disabilities: Identification and evaluation of children with autism spectrum disorders. *Pediatrics, 120*(5), 1183–1215.

Kasari, C., Freeman, S., & Paparella, T. (2006). Joint attention and symbolic play in young children with autism: a randomized controlled intervention study. *Journal of Child Psychology and Psychiatry, 47*, 611–620.

Kasari, C., Paparella, T., Freeman, S., & Jahromi, L. B. (2008). Language outcome in autism: Randomized comparison of joint attention and play interventions. *Journal of Consulting and Clinical Psychology, 76*, 125–137.

Kashinath, S., Woods, J., & Goldstein, H. (2006). Enhancing generalized teaching strategy use in daily routines by caregivers of children with autism. *Journal of Speech, Language, and Hearing Research, 49*, 466–485.

Klin, A., & Volkmar, F. (2003). Asperger syndrome: Diagnosis and external validity. *Child and Adolescent Psychiatric Clinics of North America, 12,* 1–13.

Landa, R., & Garrett-Mayer, E. (2006). Development in infants with autism spectrum disorders: A prospective study. *Journal of Child Psychology and Psychiatry, 47,* 629–638.

Laurent, A., & Rubin, E. (2004). Challenges in emotional regulation in Asperger syndrome and high-functioning autism. *Topics in Language Disorders, 24*(4), 286–297.

LeCouteur, A., Lord, C., & Rutter, M. (2003). *Autism Diagnostic Instrument—Revised.* Los Angeles: Western Psychological Services.

Lord, C., & Paul, R. (1997). Language and communication in autism. In D. J. Cohen & F. R. Volkmar (Eds.), *Handbook of autism and pervasive developmental disorders* (2nd ed., pp. 195–225). New York: Wiley.

Lord, C., Risi, S., DiLavore, P. S., Shulman, C., Thurm, A., & Pickles, A. (2006). Autism from 2 to 9 years of age. *Archives of General Psychiatry, 63*(6), 694–701.

Lord, C., Rutter, M., DiLavore, P. C., & Risi, S. (1999). *Autism diagnostic observation schedule.* Los Angeles: Western Psychological Services.

Mandell, D. S., Listerud, J., Levy, S. E., & Pinto-Martin, J. A. (2002). Race differences in the age at diagnosis among Medicaid-eligible children with autism. *Journal of the American Academy of Child and Adolescent Psychiatry, 41*(12), 1447–1453.

Massey, N. G., & Wheeler, J. J. (2000). Acquisition and generalization of activity schedules and their effects on task engagement in a young child with autism in an inclusive preschool classroom. *Education and Training in Mental Retardation and Developmental Disabilities, 35*(3), 326–335.

McGee, G., Morrier, M., & Daly, T. (1999). An incidental teaching approach to early intervention for toddlers with autism. *Journal of the Association for Persons with Severe Handicaps, 24,* 133–146.

Meadan, H., Ostrosky, M., Zaghlawan, H., & Yu, S. (2009). Promoting the social and communicative behavior of young children with autism spectrum disorders: A review of parent-implemented intervention studies. *Topics in Early Childhood Special Education, 29*(2), 90–104.

Miller, L. J., Robinson, J., & Moulton, D. (2004). Sensory modulation dysfunction: Identification in early childhood. In R. DelCarmen-Wiggins & A. Carter (Eds.), *Handbook of infant, toddler, and preschool mental health assessment* (pp. 247–270). London: Oxford University Press.

Mitchell, S., Brian, J., Zwaigenbaum, L., Roberts, W., Szatmari, P., Smith, I., & Bryson, S. (2006). Early language and communication development of infants later diagnosed with autism spectrum disorders. *Developmental and Behavioral Pediatrics, 27,* S69–S78.

Mullen, E. M. (1995). *Mullen scales of early learning.* San Antonio, TX: Pearson.

Mundy, P., & Burnette, C. (2005). Joint attention and neurodevelopmental models of autism. In F. Volkmar, R. Paul, A. Klin, & D. Cohen (Eds.), *Handbook of autism and pervasive developmental disorders* (3rd ed., pp. 650–681). New York: Wiley.

Mundy, P., Delgado, J., & Block M. (2003). *Early social communication scales.* University of Miami.

Mundy, P., Sigman, M., & Kasari, C. (1990). A longitudinal study of joint attention and language development in autistic children. *Journal of Autism and Developmental Disorders, 20,* 115–128.

National Research Council (NRC). (2001). *Educating children with autism*. Washington, DC: National Academy Press.

Osterling, J., & Dawson, G. (1994). Early recognition of children with autism: A study of first birthday home videotapes. *Journal of Autism and Developmental Disorders, 24*, 247–257.

Osterling, J., Dawson, G., & Munson, J. (2002). Early recognition of one year old infants with autism spectrum disorder versus mental retardation: A study of first birthday party home videotapes. *Development and Psychopathology, 14*, 239–252.

Paul, R., Chawarska, K., Cicchetti, D., & Volkmar, F. (2008). Language outcomes of toddlers with autism spectrum disorders: A two year follow-up. *Autism Research, 1*, 97–107.

Powell, D., Dunlap G., & Fox, L. (2006). Prevention and intervention for the challenging behaviors of toddlers and preschoolers. *Infants and Young Children, 19*(1), 25–35.

Prizant, B., Wetherby, A., Rubin, E., & Laurent, A. (2007). *The SCERTS Model manual: Enhancing communication and socioemotional abilities of young children with ASD*. Baltimore: Paul H. Brookes.

Prizant, B., Wetherby, A., Rubin, E., Laurent, A., & Rydell, P. (2007). *The SCERTS Model: A comprehensive educational approach for children with Autism Spectrum Disorders, Volume II—Intervention*. Baltimore: Paul H. Brookes.

Robins, D. L., Fein, D., Barton, M., & Green, J. A. (2001). The *Modified Checklist for Autism in Toddlers*: An initial study investigating the early detection of autism and pervasive developmental disorders. *Journal of Autism and Developmental Disorders, 31*, 131–144.

Rogers, S., Hayden, D., Hepburn, S., Charlifue-Smith, R., Hall, T., & Hayes, A. (2006). Teaching young nonverbal children with autism useful speech: A pilot study of the Denver Model and PROMPT interventions. *Journal of Autism and Developmental Disorders, 36*(8), 1007–1024.

Rogers, S. J., & Vismara, L. A. (2008). Evidence-based comprehensive treatments for early autism. *Journal of Clinical Child and Adolescent Psychology, 37*, 8–38.

Rutter, M., Bailey, A., & Lord, C. (2003). *Social Communication Questionnaire*. Los Angeles: Western Psychological Services.

Schertz, H., and Odom, S. L. (2007) Promoting joint attention in toddlers with autism: A parent-mediated approach. *Journal of Autism and Developmental Disorders, 37*, 1562–1575.

Sigman, M., & Ruskin, E. (1999). Continuity and change in the social competence of children with autism, Down syndrome, and developmental delays. *Monographs of the Society for Research in Child Development, 64*.

Sparrow, S. S., Cicchetti, D. V., & Balla, D. A. (1984). *The Vineland Adaptive Behavior Scales*. Bloomington, MN: Pearson Assessments.

Sperry, L. A., Whaley, K. T., Shaw, E., & Brame, K. (1999). Services for young children with autism spectrum disorder: Voices of parents and providers. *Infants and Young Children, 11*, 17–33.

Stone, W. L., Coonrod, E. E., & Ousket, O. Y. (2000). Brief report, *Screening Tool for Autism in Two-Year-Olds* (STAT): Development and preliminary data. *Journal of Autism and Developmental Disorders, 30*(6), 607–612.

Stone, W. L., Coonrod, E. E., Turner, L. M., & Pozdol, S. L. (2004). Psychometric properties of the STAT for Early Autism Screening. *Journal of Autism and Developmental Disorders, 34*(6), 691–701.

Stone, W. L., McMahon, C. R., & Henderson, L. M. (2008). Use of the *Screening Tool for Autism in Two-Year-Olds* (STAT) for children under 24 months: An exploratory study. *Autism, 12,* 557–573.

Strain, P., McGee, G., & Kohler, F. (2001). Inclusion of children with autism in early intervention environments. In M. J. Guralnick (Ed.). *Early childhood inclusion: Focus on change* (pp. 337–363). Baltimore: Paul H. Brookes.

Westby, C. (2009). Considerations in working successfully with culturally/linguistically diverse families in assessment and intervention of communication disorders. *Seminars in Speech and Language, 30,* 279–289.

Wetherby. A., & Prizant, B. M. (2002). *Communication and symbolic behavior scales developmental profile.* Baltimore: Paul H. Brookes.

Wetherby, A., Watt, N., Morgan, L., & Shumway, S. (2007). Social communication profiles of children with autism spectrum disorders in the second year of life. *Journal of Autism and Developmental Disorders, 37*(5), 960–975.

Wetherby, A., & Woods, J. (2006). Effectiveness of early intervention for children with autism spectrum disorders beginning in the second year of life. *Topics in Early Childhood Special Education, 26,* 67–82.

Wetherby, A., & Woods, J. (2008). In K. Chawarska, A. Klin, & F. Volkmar (Eds.), *Autism spectrum disorders in infants and toddlers: Diagnosis, assessment, and treatment* (pp. 170–206). New York: Guilford Press.

Wetherby, A., Woods, J., Allen, L., Cleary, J., Dickinson, H., & Lord, C. (2004). Early indicators of autism spectrum disorders in the second year of life. *Journal of Autism and Developmental Disorders, 34,* 473–493.

Whalen, C., & Schreibman, L. (2003). Joint attention training for children with autism using behavior modification procedures. *Journal of Child Psychology and Psychiatry, 44,* 456–468.

Wimpory, D. C., Hobson, R. P., Williams, J. M. G., & Nash, S. (2000). Are infants with autism socially engaged? A study of recent retrospective parental reports. *Journal of Autism and Developmental Disorders, 30,* 525–536.

Wolery, M., & Garfinkle, A. (2002). Measures in intervention research with young children who have autism. *Journal of Autism and Developmental Disorders, 32,* 463–478.

Woods, J., Kashinath, S., & Goldstein, H. (2004). Effects of embedding caregiver-implemented teaching strategies in daily routines on children's communication outcomes. *Journal of Early Intervention, 26,* 175–193.

Woods, J., & Wetherby, A. (2003). Early identification and intervention for infants and toddlers at-risk for autism spectrum disorders. *Language, Speech, and Hearing Services in Schools, 34,* 180–193.

Yeargin-Allsopp, M., Rice, C., Karapurkar, T, Doernberg, N., Boyle, C., & Murphy, C. (2003). Prevalence of autism in a US metropolitan area. *Journal of the American Medical Association, 289*(1), 49–55.

Yoder, P., & Stone, W. (2006). Randomized comparison of two communication interventions for preschoolers with autism spectrum disorders. *Journal of Consulting and Clinical Psychology, 74,* 426–435.

Zimmerman, I. L., Steiner, V. G., & Pond, R. E. (2002). *Preschool language scale, Fourth Edition (PLS-4).* Harcourt Assessment.

Chapter 10

Supporting Children with Visual Impairment, Hearing Loss, and Severe Disabilities

Rashida Banerjee, Sandy K. Bowen, and Kay Alicyn Ferrell

The Individuals with Disabilities Education Act (IDEA, 2004) defines low-incidence disabilities as:

A visual or hearing impairment, or simultaneous visual and hearing impairments; a significant cognitive impairment; or any impairment for which a small number of personnel with highly specialized skills and knowledge are needed in order for children with that impairment to receive early intervention services or a free appropriate public education. (IDEA, 2004, § 1462[c][3])

Low-incidence disabilities include blindness, low vision, deafness, hard-of-hearing, deaf-blindness, significant developmental delay, complex health issues, orthopedic impairments, multiple disability, autism, and acquired brain injury, which together comprise less than 1 percent of the estimated resident school-age population of the United States (U.S. Department of Education, 2009). Because infants and toddlers are not reported by disability category, the prevalence of low-incidence disabilities in early childhood is unknown, but is likely similar to the school-age rate.

This chapter focuses on three low-incidence disabilities that have significant implications for services during early childhood: (1) visual impairment, (2) deaf and hard of hearing, and (3) severe disabilities. Although there are some similarities in the services provided, the unique characteristics, attributes, and needs of young children from each of these categories merit individual attention. With the intent to provide a basic understanding of early intervention and preschool issues for infants and young children with these three low-incidence disabilities, each disability category is explored through the lens of families that have been part of the early intervention process. Following a similar outline, each section briefly defines the disability, reviews the service delivery process, provides a brief synthesis of research-based or promising practices, suggests strategies for professionals and families, and identifies some contemporary controversial issues in working with young children with these significant disabilities and their families.

VISUAL IMPAIRMENT

Ryan. Sue-Ellen's pregnancy and birth of 6 lb.–9 oz. Ryan were uneventful. She and daddy Rick were delighted with their little boy, who was absolutely perfect in their opinion! He was an engaging baby who responded with huge smiles to his parents' voices and seemed particularly interested in the sounds around him. Sometimes Ryan seemed startled when one of them picked him up without saying something to him first, but it wasn't until he started reaching for his bottle that they noticed that he sometimes missed. As Ryan grew, his parents began to notice different behaviors, such as frequent blinking in sunlight, and they realized that unlike most babies, he never turned toward a bright light. He passed his well-baby checkups with flying colors, however, so they told themselves that they were simply first-time parents who worried too much.

As Ryan approached 10 months of age, Sue-Ellen's anxiety increased. Ryan did not seem interested in playing with toys, and he still startled when she approached him silently from the side. When she explained these concerns to Ryan's pediatrician, he told her that Ryan was fine, but if it would ease her fears, he would refer them to a pediatric ophthalmologist. Ryan saw the pediatric ophthalmologist about two months later, and was diagnosed with bilateral optic nerve hypoplasia (ONH), an underdeveloped optic nerve. ONH is characterized by reduced visual acuity and, in Ryan's case, a reduced visual field.

Definition of Visual Impairment

Visual impairment incorporates a range of visual abilities, from total blindness to near-normal visual functioning. The legal definition of blindness, used to qualify for government entitlement programs, uses a clinical measurement of visual acuity. To be diagnosed as legally blind, an individual must be measured with a distance visual acuity of 20/200 or less in the best eye with correction, or a field loss of

20 degrees or less. (A measure of 20/200 means that the person who is legally blind sees at 20 feet what an individual with typical vision sees at 200 feet; a field loss of 20 degrees is about one-third of the normal horizontal field of vision.) Although this represents a significant visual loss, individuals who are legally blind may have enough remaining vision to be able to read print. Obtaining a distance visual acuity measurement in infants and young children, of course, is difficult. Thankfully, IDEA (2004) supports a more liberal interpretation of vision loss and defines visual impairment as "an impairment in vision that, even with correction, adversely affects a child's educational performance" (Individuals with Disabilities Education Act [IDEA] Regulations, 2006, § 300.8[c][13]). This educational definition places the emphasis on performance and how effectively vision is used, rather than on a clinical diagnosis that may have no relationship to how a child functions in the home, school, or community.

There are a range of terms used to describe visual impairment. The most commonly used in educational contexts are *blindness*, which usually refers to total loss of vision, with or without light perception (the ability to perceive light); *low vision*, referring to a range of visual abilities from typical vision to severe vision loss, including visual learners, tactual learners, and those who learn using both modalities; and *visual function*, referring to how an individual uses the visual sensory system. In this chapter, because Ryan is diagnosed with optic nerve hypoplasia (ONH), the terms *visual impairment* and *low vision* are used to describe his type of visual impairment. Children with ONH demonstrate a wide range of visual function, ranging from normal visual acuity to no light perception and from generalized loss of detail to subtle peripheral field loss (Blind Babies Foundation, 1998). ONH is sometimes accompanied by endocrine and neurological complications as well.

The pediatric ophthalmologist referred Ryan for further medical testing to rule out any complications. There were no signs of any midline brain anomalies on a CT scan, and the pediatric endocrinologist determined that Ryan did not have any growth hormone deficiencies, although she suggested periodic consultations over the next few years.

Although the incidence of visual impairment in infants is unknown, estimates of the number of children ages 3–21 with visual impairments range from 0.04 percent, based on the number of children reported as served under IDEA (U.S. Department of Education, 2009), to 0.1 percent, based on the National Health Interview Survey (Benson & Marano, 1994). These small proportions support Congress's designation of visual impairment as a low-incidence disability and emphasize the necessity of ensuring that appropriate personnel with expertise in visual impairment are involved in the delivery of services.

Service Delivery

Services for infants with visual impairments began in the 1930s with home counseling and training services for families (Ferrell, 2000; Koestler, 2004). During the 1950s, with the growth in the number of children with congenital blindness due to prematurity, many parents created their own services in cities across the country (Turnbull, Turnbull, Erwin, & Soodak, 2006). Several of these parent-created services have evolved into private agencies, providing a variety of services to children and adults with visual impairment. Visual impairment is considered an established risk condition under Part C of IDEA (2004), and children qualify for early intervention services based on a diagnosis of visual impairment.

In Ryan's case, the pediatric ophthalmologist referred his family to the lead agency in the state for early intervention services under Part C. Because a specialized agency for children with visual impairments was located in Ryan's community, Ryan's parents called and asked for more information about visual impairment. At the parents' request, a developmental specialist from the agency worked with the early intervention program to assess Ryan's development and to develop an Individualized Family Service Plan (IFSP) for Ryan and his family.

The mean age at which young children are diagnosed with a visual impairment is approximately 5 months, although referral for services generally does not occur until six months later (Ferrell, 1998; Hatton, 2001). Some eye conditions, such as retinopathy of prematurity, are diagnosed before discharge from the hospital after birth, while others may not be discovered until the child misses a developmental milestone. Parents often notice more subtle vision abnormalities sooner than the medical community, primarily because they spend so much more time with their children. Many parents report that their concerns are often dismissed by their pediatricians until the visual impairment interferes more with the child's daily routines (Tompkins, 1998). Still other eye conditions seem to be secondary to other, more severe neurological insults. The proportion of children with visual impairment who also have another disability is estimated to be approximately 60 percent (Ferrell, 1998; Hatton, 2001; Pogrund, 2002). More precise estimates of young children with disabilities in addition to visual impairment are difficult to determine, since they are reported to the U.S. Department of Education by their primary disability only. There is general agreement in the fields of early intervention and early childhood special education that services must be provided to an infant, toddler, or preschooler with visual impairment by a teacher certified or licensed to teach children with visual impairment in the state, and by an orientation and mobility (O&M) specialist whose primary function is related to movement within and orientation to the child's environment. The O&M specialist may or may not be state certified; some states adopt the professional organization's certification process as their own, while other states treat O&M as a related service and do not require a separate teaching license. However, states also have different standards for licensing teachers of students with visual impairment. Colorado, for example, licenses visual impairment specialists for children birth to 21 years, while other states only license for K–12. Personnel preparation programs are significantly different as a result, and while K–12 certified teachers may have expertise in visual impairment, they may not have training with infants and preschoolers. A transdisciplinary approach to service delivery is thus critical for optimum family support.

Synthesis of Research and Promising Practices

Research in early education of children with visual impairment has generally fallen victim to the urgency of providing services. Developmental studies found no significant differences in development of milestones among children with and without visual impairment in the 1940s and 1950s (Maxfield & Buchholz, 1957; Norris, Spaulding, & Brodie, 1957). Fraiberg's work in the 1960s demonstrated delays in several developmental domains, which she theorized were largely due specifically to vision loss (Fraiberg, 1977). With this work as a basis, the prevailing philosophy postulated that children with visual impairment and children with vision were "more alike than different," and that children with visual impairment simply needed more time to learn the skills that their vision loss did not allow them to learn incidentally (Ferrell, 2000, p. 121). Ferrell (2000) has challenged this approach, suggesting that the "premise of comparability was faulty" (p. 121), and has proposed an individual-differences approach to examining the development of children with visual impairment. As Ferrell (1997) stated:

Children with blindness and visual impairment learn differently, for no other reason than the fact that in most cases they cannot rely on their vision to provide information. The information they obtain through their other senses is *inconsistent* (things do not always make noise or produce an odor), *fragmented* (comes in bits and pieces), and *passive* (not under the child's control). It takes practice, training, and time to sort all this out. (p. v)

Following an exploratory study (Ferrell et al., 1990) that seemed to suggest a difference in the sequence of milestone acquisition among some children with visual impairment, a federally funded prospective study known as Project PRISM was initiated in 1991. Findings from this study (Ferrell, 2010), the largest developmental study since 1957, suggest that:

There is great variability in how young children with visual impairments develop. There was a large difference in time between the earliest age when a child acquired a skill and the latest age when a different child acquired the same skill. These differences became greater as children grew older.

Children with visual impairment appear to follow a different developmental sequence. It has been assumed that the order in which children with visual impairments learn developmental skills is the same as the order in which children without disabilities learn the same skills. PRISM demonstrated that some milestones (such as language and communication) were acquired earlier than children with typical development, while others were acquired later.

Better vision does not necessarily mean better performance. Conventional wisdom believed that the more severe the visual impairment, the greater the impact on early child development. Yet, PRISM found that children with the "best" vision were not always doing as well as the children with poorer vision. This finding is also supported by Hatton's research (Hatton, Bailey, Burchinal & Ferrell, 1997; Hatton, Erickson, & Lee, 2009).

Some children develop at the same rate as children without disabilities. Children with visual impairment who did not have additional disabilities and who were born at term acquired skills within the same age range as children without disabilities.

Additional disabilities have more impact on a child's development than does visual impairment itself. Particularly in infancy, additional disabilities posed more difficulties for children than did visual impairment alone, particularly when families received early intervention services that addressed their vision loss.

As children with visual impairment grow older, additional disability may have less of an impact. The effects of mild additional impairment seem to dissipate with age, while more severe disabilities may continue to pose difficulties for children.

The visual function of children with visual impairment may or may not improve over time. PRISM (Ferrell, 1998) demonstrated that visual function improved simply with the passage of time, regardless of any visual stimulation program that was implemented. As children grew older, they were better able to understand what they were seeing, and thus performed better. If children were medically diagnosed as totally blind, visual function did not improve over the course of the study.

Delineating "best practice" in the face of so little evidence-based research seems somewhat precarious. As in other areas of visual impairment, too few people are doing too little research in early intervention, and the studies that have been conducted have not replicated past studies to the point where one can confidently state that a practice is "best." The Division on Visual Impairments (DVI) of the Council for Exceptional Children (CEC) has adopted a position paper that recommends several components of an early intervention program, many of which are similar to CEC's Division for Early Childhood (DEC) Recommended Practices (Sandall, Hemmeter, Smith, & McLean, 2005). Key elements *not* included in DEC's recommended practices are:

- Assessment of the unique sensory capabilities and preferences of the child to identify appropriate environmental adaptations and intervention strategies, including the use of low-vision devices that promote accessibility and effective use of all senses.
- Facilitation of emergent literacy skills (Braille and print) based on the child's sensory preferences and individual learning style.
- Provision of services by specialists who are appropriately trained to enhance the development and early learning of infants and young children with visual impairments, including assessment, intervention and education planning, and the development or modification of developmentally and functionally appropriate support and services (DVI, 2003).

Strategies for Professionals and Families

The following strategies are helpful to both families and early interventionists when working with young children with visual impairment, regardless of age (Ferrell, 2010):

Create opportunities for learning. Most learning occurs naturally during typical daily routines and activities, without having to be specifically taught. When children are visually impaired, however, there is no assurance that learning occurred or that the child was even aware that there was something to learn. Incidental learning primarily occurs through observation and experience, but vision loss limits the opportunity to observe, imitate, and practice. Adults can help structure experiences to make sure the child with visual impairment does not miss out on what is going on around him.

Provide repeated exposures and experiences. Children with visual impairment do not have the luxury of seeing objects and events repeatedly. Repetition is a key element of brain-based learning and should be created when it does not happen naturally.

Use concrete objects. Expose children frequently to real objects rather than representations or models. Once a child knows what a dog *really* is, then the stuffed animal can *represent* the real dog. Until then, from the child's perspective, they are two different things and two different concepts.

Build experiences from parts to wholes. Help children use what is known (the parts) to put together a concept of the whole. Although vision works the opposite way (you see the whole object before you break it down into smaller details), children with visual impairment have to put the whole together from the parts. Sometimes they are limited by what they can actually touch at one time—such as the family pet, where they can only feel the ears, the tail, the paws, and the nose individually. Repeated exposure to these parts helps the child to understand that it all belongs to one dog. Make comparisons and point out relationships between what is known and what needs to be learned.

Provide structure when it does not exist. Vision itself provides structure to the environment because the relationships of the parts are clear.

Look at the situation from the child's point of view and figure out how you would do a particular task before you ask a child to do it.

Use consistent language. It can be difficult for a child with visual impairment to understand that different words actually refer to the same object (for example, pants, jeans, trousers, slacks, cutoffs, and overalls). Applying the strategies of repetition and making no assumptions can assist adults in structuring language experiences that eliminate confusion and build understanding.

Do not assume that better vision leads to better performance. Children with better vision are often assumed to need minimal specialized instruction and/or accommodations, but research has demonstrated that children with low vision may be at greater risk than children who are totally blind.

Use daily routines to reinforce concepts. Predictability is difficult when the result of your actions cannot always be seen. Use the predictability of everyday occurrences to teach children about positional, tactile, and auditory concepts. These natural interaction times build structure, predictability, and anticipation while creating opportunities to practice skills.

Introduce families to adults with visual impairment so they know the possibilities for the future and what lies ahead.

Make "do'ers" instead of "done-to'ers." Sometimes it is easier and faster simply to do things for a child instead of giving him the time and opportunity to do it on his own. Young children with visual impairment need to know that there are expectations—not excuses—for his performance. This helps to build self-esteem and a sense of accomplishment.

Ryan's mom worried that the aspirin she took during her first trimester of pregnancy was the cause of Ryan's ONH. She read online that it was often associated with substance abuse, and while aspirin wasn't anything like substance abuse, well, still, maybe it was her fault.

It is also important to recognize that visual impairment is embedded in the Judeo-Christian tradition, where blindness was administered as a punishment for past sins, or where people who are blind were viewed benevolently as individuals requiring care and protection. It is difficult to escape this history. Families hold different religious beliefs; some may think their child's visual impairment is their fault, either consciously or unconsciously, even if the condition is not inherited. Other spiritual beliefs may interfere with the recommended medical treatment, such as prescription lenses. While these beliefs can be present for any disability, visual impairment seems to be particularly vulnerable to misperceptions about abilities and potential. A benevolent approach can be detrimental to a child, however, because it transmits the subtle message that the individual needs constant care and that independence is not expected.

Sue-Ellen's mother was particularly upset by the diagnosis of Ryan's visual impairment. Her experience with visual impairment was not particularly positive—there was one classmate with a visual impairment in her high school, but he was socially isolated because he didn't play sports or drive a car. He attended the high school reunion, and she discovered that he now had a family of his own, but had never held a job and received Supplemental Security Income (SSI) just because he had a disability! She feared that Ryan, if he went to school at all, would end up without friends, begging on the street.

Controversial Issues

Persistent issues seem to dominate the national discourse about young children with visual impairment. These issues generally involve service delivery, but they are rooted in the concept of specialized services for unique educational needs.

Natural Environments

IDEA (2004) states that early intervention services should be provided in home or community settings where children without disabilities participate, to the maximum extent appropriate. However, the concept of natural environments is much broader than simply a place. Unfortunately, natural environments have been interpreted as meaning that programs developed specifically for children with vision loss are not natural and therefore not appropriate. Ferrell (2010) suggests that the discussion around natural environments should focus more on the educational context of the child. For an infant with visual impairment, for example, the natural environment is certainly the home environment; but as the child grows, the educational context will change. Valid questions then center on (1) the frequency and type of interactions available with peers, (2) the opportunities for learning through other sensory modalities (e.g., balls that beep), (3) safety, (4) literacy opportunities (books in Braille or large print), (5) accommodations that provide access to the preschool curriculum, and (6) access to other families of children with visual impairments. If the environment does not make accommodations for visual impairment—that is, if the environment is organized from a visual perspective—the natural environment may be anything but natural for a child with visual impairment.

Assessment and Expectations

IDEA (2004) requires children to be assessed periodically using valid instruments designed to measure developmental skills. There are no valid developmental instruments for children with visual impairment. Clinicians struggle with what to do: administer an instrument that was developed or standardized on children with normal vision (thus, invalid), or base recommendations entirely on clinical judgment. This is one reason why it is critical to involve professionals with expertise in visual impairment as part of the educational team. If a standardized instrument is administered, the visual impairment specialist can help to interpret the results; if clinical judgment must be relied upon, the visual impairment specialist is likely to have more experience with children who are visually impaired than other members of the team.

Tied into the issue of assessment are expectations. The visual impairment specialist usually brings a lifespan perspective to the discussion, familiar with many successful adults who are visually impaired, employed, and active members of the community. The visual impairment specialist, through training and experience, sees the possibilities of visual impairment rather than the limitations. When interpreting developmental tests that presume visual competency, some professionals might find the apparent gaps overwhelming and, as a result, fail to expect children with visual impairment to accomplish typical preschool skills. Worse yet, without expertise in visual impairment, some early childhood educators have attributed what is really visual test bias to the child's developmental delay or mental retardation, even in the absence of medical confirmation. This can establish a downward spiral for young children with visual impairment, where the adults in their lives judge them to be incapable of learning a particular skill, so the skill is not taught. Yet, without deliberate exposure, the child never learns what is expected because the visual impairment does not permit acquisition of the skill by observation and imitation. It is a conundrum. Young children with visual impairment are often handicapped more by society's attitude toward them than they are by the visual impairment itself.

Today, Ryan attends school with his same-age peers. He attended a Montessori-based child care program from 3 to 5 years, where teachers from the specialized agency and an O&M specialist from the school district visited frequently to help the staff make accommodations for Ryan's visual impairment. While the school district initially believed that Ryan was doing well, statewide testing in Grade 3 demonstrated that he was falling behind in reading and math. Ryan was referred for a low-vision evaluation with an optometrist who prescribed a stand magnifier for working at his desk and a telescope for outdoor activities. Software was purchased that enlarged the screen on the classroom computers, and Ryan's parents bought the same software for their home computer. Sue-Ellen and Rick are confident about Ryan's future, and Ryan seems healthy and happy, enjoying his friends, hating his homework, and thinking about trying out for track next year.

DEAF AND HARD OF HEARING

Norma's eyes glisten with tears as she recalls the day she discovered that her daughter Lissette was deaf. Norma's pregnancy and delivery of her second child was normal. As part of the hospital new-baby routine, Lissette was screened for a variety of developmental, genetic, and metabolic disorders, including hearing loss. The day Norma was to take Lissette home, the nurse stood by her bed and, through a Spanish interpreter, informed Norma that while most of Lissette's screenings were normal, she had failed her newborn hearing screening. The nurse encouraged Norma to follow up with the pediatrician at her next appointment.

The next few weeks brought more testing and finally a confirmation that Lissette had a bilateral sensorineural profound hearing loss. Norma wondered how this could have happened and often blamed herself. No other family members, immediate or extended, had any kind of hearing loss. Then, suddenly, before Norma made any other decision for Lissette, life changes forced the family to move to a new state. The responsibilities of the move and setting up a new household, coupled with the growing realization that her perfect Lissette could not hear, caused Norma to postpone immediate follow-up with an audiologist in her new home while she was lost to the system in her previous state.

Like Lissette, 24,000 (6 per 1,000) newborns are diagnosed with a hearing loss each year (Beginnings for Parents of Children Who Are Deaf or Hard of Hearing, 2008). The type and degree of hearing loss varies, from mild to profound; high or low frequency; conductive (external, canal, or middle ear) or sensorineural (inner ear or nerve); and in one or both ears. If not detected early, hearing loss can have a profound lasting effect on a child's overall development, resulting in "life-long deficits in speech and language acquisition, poor academic performance, personal-social maladjustments, and emotional difficulties" (Harlor & Bower, 2009, p. 1253).

Definition of Deaf and Hard of Hearing

The Individuals with Disabilities Act (IDEA, 2004) includes two separate, distinct categories for children with hearing loss who may be eligible for special education and related services: deafness and hearing impairment. Deafness is defined as "a hearing impairment that is so severe that the child is impaired in processing linguistic information through hearing, with or without amplification that adversely affects a child's educational performance" (IDEA, 2006, § 300.8[c][5]). As a more global term, hearing impairment is defined as "an impairment in hearing, whether permanent or fluctuating, that adversely affects a child's educational performance but that is not included under the definition of deafness" (IDEA, 2006,§ 300.8[c][3]).

Although defined specifically by IDEA for educational purposes, the terms hearing impairment, deafness, and hearing loss have particular political and cultural implications. Hearing impairment is often used as a global term to discuss all types and ranges of hearing loss; however, it connotes a medical view of impairment or may be perceived as a deficit. In contrast, individuals who are deaf may choose to belong to a cultural group that distinguishes itself socially from individuals who are hearing. A Deaf person has a sense of pride regarding his or her identity. Deaf culture, denoted with a capital D, refers to a group of individuals who share a common language (American Sign Language) and fundamental beliefs and practices in social codes of behavior, art, history recreation, entertainment, and worship (Moore & Levitan, 1993).

Individuals who possess usable residual hearing and appropriate amplification prefer the term hard of hearing. Individuals who are hard of hearing generally use audition and spoken language as their primary mode of communication (Hearing Loss Association of America, 1997).

Service Delivery

These opposing views (medical versus cultural) have influenced early intervention and educational opportunities for infants and preschoolers who are deaf or hard of hearing. Depending on the philosophy that one espouses, the choices for communication, amplification, and even education will be influenced. Due to the potentially debilitating delays found in children who were identified with hearing loss as a toddler or young child, the National Institutes of Health (NIH, 1993) concluded that all infants should be screened for hearing loss as part of neonatal screenings at birth. Today, this mandate has expanded to include processes for screening, referral, diagnosis, and intervention. Individual states have comprehensive state plans for screening infants prior to hospital discharge. Although each state program is unique and individual to the respective state, they all share a similar goal: to ensure that infants who fail the newborn hearing screening are evaluated by a diagnosing audiologist and receive follow-up services from an early interventionist with expertise in hearing loss and deafness to promote development in areas of language, social-emotional development, and cognition. The American Academy of Pediatrics (2007) in its most recent update on hearing loss reiterated the importance of receiving appropriate intervention by 6 months of age from professionals with expertise and training in hearing loss specific to infants and young children. Once identified with a hearing loss, infants qualify for early intervention services because hearing loss is considered an established risk condition under Part C.

At age 7 months, during a well-baby checkup with the pediatrician, Norma mentioned that Lissette had failed the newborn screening. The pediatrician immediately referred Lissette to an audiologist who confirmed the hearing loss and recommended that Lissette be fitted with binaural hearing aids. The audiologist also contacted the local early childhood (Part C) director to arrange early intervention services for Lissette and her family. Following state guidelines, the director contacted Norma and assigned an early intervention specialist trained to work with infants who are deaf to meet with the family to assess the family's needs and determine what services would be provided to ensure that Lissette had every opportunity to optimize her overall development.

Synthesis of Research and Promising Practices

Early identification coupled with appropriate amplification for infants with hearing loss has demonstrated the ability to improve many of the academic and language delays seen prior to universal newborn hearing screening (American Speech-Language-Hearing Association [ASHA], 2008; Miyamoto, Hay-McCutcheon, Kirk, Houston, & Bergeson-Dana, 2008; Moeller, 2000; Yoshinaga-Itano, Sedey, Coulter, & Mehl, 1998). "Families with infants whose hearing loss is identified through a newborn hearing screening program are able to make the most of their babies' first months of life by providing an optimal foundation for language, cognition, and social-emotional development" (Sass-Lehrer, 2002, p. 1). Early intervention guidelines specifically related to children who are deaf or hard of hearing have been identified by several professionals and professional organizations (see, for example, Alexander Graham Bell Association, 2002; Colorado Home Intervention Program, 2003; Colorado Home Intervention Program & New Mexico School for the Deaf, 2004; National Agenda, 2005; Sass-Lehrer, 2002).

In 2005, a group of experts in early intervention for infants with hearing loss convened to make recommendations for appropriate interventions for children who are deaf or hard of hearing (Marge & Marge, 2005). The final recommendations for exemplary practices include five areas that have also been promoted by the other professional organizations: (1) effective child find efforts, (2) key decision making by the family about choice of services, (3) choices of services that are specific to the needs and capabilities of the child and family, (4) ongoing monitoring of outcomes as a basis for educational planning, and (5) certified and qualified service providers with expertise in working with infants and young children who are deaf or hard of hearing.

To ensure that the child and family receive the maximum benefit from early childhood special education services, one of the most important considerations when providing early intervention services for children who are deaf or hard of hearing is hiring qualified personnel with specialized preparation. It has been recommended that "qualified professionals have knowledge and expertise in general education, education of individuals with a hearing loss, early childhood education, families, and the impact of deafness on development" (Sass-Lehrer, 2002, p. 17). In addition to content knowledge, professionals should demonstrate competencies in the language(s) that the child and family are using. In this way, the interventionist is able to provide an appropriate language model for the family (Sass-Lehrer, 2002). These professionals may include teachers of the deaf, speech-language pathologists, and audiologists. Building on the strengths and knowledge of the family, the interventionist provides materials and resources to assist the family in making the decisions that will best meet the child's needs.

Sass-Lehrer (2002) has identified three areas of inquiry for families seeking effective early intervention services and for early intervention programs who are seeking to develop a quality model for service delivery: (1) family-centered services, (2) communication and language acquisition, and (3) collaboration in program development and evaluation. Family-centered services build on the family's unique strengths and provide support and resources that will enhance the child's development and the family's competence. Communication and language acquisition not only ensure that families receive information regarding all communication choices, but also that the interventionist is fluent in language and communication modes used by the child and family. In this way, the interventionist provides an appropriate language model for the parents and the child. The third area, collaboration, suggests an interdisciplinary approach to intervention to provide quality services and to ensure that families are an integral part of the intervention and ongoing evaluation process.

Strategies for Professionals and Families

After completing an Individual Family Service Plan (IFSP) with Lissette and her family, an early interventionist was assigned to begin working with the family in their home. The interventionist spoke Spanish and was knowledgeable about children with hearing loss, how to develop language and speech, and how to enhance audition within the daily routines of the child and her family. The interventionist met with the family on a weekly basis to teach American Sign Language (ASL) and to promote the development of Lissette's auditory skills.

Calderon and Greenberg (1997) reviewed the literature to examine the effectiveness of early intervention and concluded that little evidence existed to support specific conditions or interventions for successful outcomes for families and children who are deaf or hard of hearing. These results are not unexpected considering the complexity of variables that combine when working with families: degree of hearing loss, age of identification and amplification, type of amplification, communication and language choice, and cultural characteristics of the home. Notwithstanding the lack of evidence to establish specific outcomes-based interventions for children, several areas have been identified that do make a difference (Colorado Home Intervention Program, 2003; Colorado Home Intervention Program & New Mexico School for the Deaf, 2004; Sass-Lehrer, 2003).

Family-Centered Approach

Family involvement is critical for the child's overall development. The purpose of family-centered intervention is to empower the family in making choices for the child. In a family-centered approach, the interventionist joins the family and works in the context of the family unit, using the family's preferred communication mode. In this way, the parents begin to feel competent in their abilities and confident in their decisions.

Identifying Daily Routines

Model programs focus on family-centered intervention through daily routines. Family-centered programs must "focus on natural daily routines as the medium for communication interaction and language growth" (Marge & Marge, 2005, p. 18). The goal of the interventionist is to provide parents with the opportunities to integrate strategies for communication and play skills into the daily routines and unique setting of the family. In this way, the family's cultural values and beliefs will be supported. Sass-Lehrer has stated, "through routine and caring interactions young children acquire both the language and social mores that link them to their family, culture, and community" (2002, p. 8).

Natural Environments

The concept of natural environments for children who are deaf or hard of hearing may have additional meanings than those generally defined under IDEA for children with disabilities. A joint committee of the American Speech-Language-Hearing Association (ASHA) and the Council on Education of the Deaf (CED) developed guidelines for selecting and advocating for appropriate natural environments for infants and toddlers who are deaf or hard of hearing (ASHA-CED, 2006). The reason for these recommendations is that the environment should provide the fewest language and communication barriers possible. The joint committee determined that "natural environments include the home, child care center, school, or other setting where the child's language(s) and communication modality (or modalities) are used by fluent adult users and where peers are using and/or acquiring the same languages through similar modalities" (ASHA-CED, 2006, p. 1). Providing social and academic opportunities for direct communication, in the child's preferred communication mode with family members, peers, and professionals, allows the child full and equal access for natural development.

Utilizing Family Needs, Concerns, Priorities, Strengths, Resources, and Interests in Planning Intervention

Because parental involvement is a key contributor to outcomes for children, it is vital that parents have input at the beginning and in the development and implementation of their child's program of intervention and have the opportunity to eventually lead the process. (Marge & Marge, 2005, p. 17)

Whereas parents should be recognized as the primary decision makers, professionals have a responsibility to strengthen "the parent's competence and confidence to positively effect [sic] their child's development" (p. 17). Interventionists working with parents should identify the positive things the parents are doing to reinforce and generalize skills and to help the parents assess if what they are doing is successful. The interventionist serves as a coach, observing and monitoring what parents are doing, and encouraging, reinforcing, and educating parents to support the development of their child.

Professionals must honor and support the decisions parents make for their child. Interventionists should value family cultures, decisions, and choices and set aside personal opinions and judgments. Parents should be provided with opportunities and resources to make informed decisions; facilitators should support the parents and child in bringing those choices to a successful completion.

Transitioning to Preschool

At age 3, Lissette was eligible to attend preschool. Norma visited the preschool programs in the area and in collaboration with the transition team from the sending and receiving programs determined that the preschool for students who were deaf or hard of hearing best met Lissette's linguistic, social, and academic needs. Although Lissette had a cochlear implant, she still used sign language for a majority of her receptive and expressive language. The preschool program had six other 3- to 5-year-olds who were deaf and used sign language as a preferred mode of communication. Additionally, two students with normal hearing ability, who had parents who were deaf, were in the class. Both the teacher of the deaf and the instructional aide used a combination of signed language and spoken English to communicate with the children. The setting provided Lissette with full access to the teachers and her peers in a language and a communication mode that she used.

Moving from the early intervention system to the education system can be a difficult transition for families and children. For children who are deaf or hard of hearing, one of the most important considerations is access to an environment that allows them to communicate with adults and peers in their preferred language(s) or modality (modalities) of communication. The National Agenda (2005) is a grassroots movement designed to provide guidance to professionals working with families and children who are deaf or hard of hearing to significantly improve the quality of services to the children and families. The National Agenda has as its third goal the establishment of a collaborative system to fully inform families regarding all service and program options for their children, and to ensure that parents are equal partners in making decisions for their child. The National Agenda also strongly proposes the following:

Deaf and Hard of Hearing children will have as an integral, required part of their educational program, access to a critical mass of age, cognitive, and communication/language peers and teachers and educational staff who are proficient in the individual child's language and communication mode. (p. 21)

Controversial Issues

When Lissette was 21 months old, she received a cochlear implant. This decision was one of the most difficult that Norma had ever made. It was clear that Lissette was not making progress in speech, language, or audition. These significant communication delays impacted every aspect of Lissette's life. Although Lissette could not access the sounds of spoken language, Norma had been using a combination of spoken Spanish and signed language with Lissette. After receiving her implant, Norma continued signing with Lissette as a way to bridge development in spoken language to known concepts in signed language.

Cochlear implantation is one of the most controversial issues for professionals, Deaf adults, and families. As of April 2009, approximately 25,500 children in the United States had received a cochlear implant (U.S. Department of Health & Human Services, 2009). The U.S. Food and Drug Administration has approved cochlear implantation for children ages 12 months to 17 years of age if the child has a profound, bilateral sensorineural hearing loss and receives little to no benefit from hearing aids. At the center of the debate is whether an implant for a child is ethically justifiable. The National Association of the Deaf (NAD, 2000) has issued a Position Statement on Cochlear Implants based on "a wellness model" to show that many adults who are deaf have achieved high levels of wellness in all areas of their life with and without cochlear implants. NAD encourages parents to gather information with respect to many options for their child who is to experience a full life and "recognizes the rights of parents to make informed choices for their deaf and hard of hearing children, respects their choice to use cochlear implants and all other assistive devices, and strongly supports the development of the whole child" (p. 10).

Language and communication choice is a second issue that can be controversial for parents and professionals. Parents have choices regarding the way(s) they will communicate with their child. Choices may include spoken language, American Sign Language, Signed English, cued speech, or a combination of options. Although parents should make a communication choice early on to optimize language development for the child, this decision may evolve based on child preference, family involvement, and amplification options. There is no research that definitively supports any one of these options over others for *all* children who are deaf or hard of hearing.

A final area of controversy that may exist for some families centers on educational options. IDEA (2004) requires that each public agency must ensure that:

> 1) To the maximum extent appropriate, children with disabilities . . . are educated with children who are non-disabled; and 2) special classes, separate schooling or other removal of children with disabilities from the regular educational environment occurs only if the nature or severity of the disability is such that education in regular classes with the use of supplementary aids and services cannot be achieved satisfactorily. (IDEA Regulations, 2006, § 300.114[a][2])

However, for individuals who are deaf and hard of hearing, it is critical that professionals understand that "the continuum of placement options must be made available to all students who are deaf and hard of hearing, with the recognition that natural and least restrictive environments are intricately tied to communication and language" (National Agenda, 2005, p. 11). When determining what is the least restrictive environment for a child who is deaf or hard of hearing, professionals must take into account the child's communication, language, and educational needs. In other words, those working with students who are deaf or hard of hearing should refer to the LRE not as the *least restrictive environment*, but rather as a *language-rich environment*.

SEVERE DISABILITIES

At 36 years of age, Benny's mom, Carla, was pregnant for the second time, 10 years after Billy was born. Just as in the previous pregnancy, she had taken all the necessary steps to remain healthy—no smoking, no drinking, and no coffee. However, at 26 weeks, complications occurred, and Carla had to be flown via helicopter from her small mountain town to the city nearby where she could receive adequate care. Benny was born through C-section at 26 weeks' gestation, weighed 1 lb., 3 oz., and was 11 inches long. In less than 24 hours after his birth, doctors had informed his parents that Benny was "too tiny and was fighting for his life" in the neonatal intensive care unit (NICU). They were advised to make plans for the funeral. Even if Benny lived, doctors said, he was likely to have brain damage, the extent of which could not be known at the time. However, Benny survived his first 24 hours and many more days and weeks. Ten surgeries and seven months later, Benny went home on oxygen support, with a tracheostomy (trach) tube, and a list of nurses who would stay with him 24/7 to support his intensive medical needs. Today, while Benny continues to use a trach tube and requires intense medical care including support from nursing staff, he is a feisty young boy, who according to his mom, behaves as all typical 3-1/2-year-olds do, "attends" preschool at home, enjoys playing with and teasing his brother, is a fussy eater, and loves to "sing" his favorite song, "The Wheels on the Bus." Benny's team of professionals have helped Benny and his family overcome personal and agency barriers and provided continued support to enhance their outcomes.

Although most preterm infants overcome acute problems with few lasting effects, a minority, like Benny, do sustain long-term medical and neurodevelopmental complications (Rais-Bahrami & Short, 2007). This section focuses on these significant long-term impacts of prematurity and other conditions that result in severe disabilities in children.

Definition of Severe Disabilities

The term "severe disabilities" has been defined by professionals, family members, and self advocates to include a number of characteristics (Sontag & Haring, 1996). Early childhood services usually link severe disabilities and multiple disabilities into a single program to serve children with extensive mental retardation and related disabilities (Turnbull, Turnbull, & Wehmeyer, 2007). IDEA defines *multiple* disabilities as:

> concomitant impairments (such as mental retardation–blindness or mental retardation–orthopedic impairment), the combination of which causes such severe educational needs that they cannot be accommodated in special education programs solely for one of the impairments. Multiple disabilities does not include deaf-blindness. (IDEA Regulations, 2006, § 300.8[b][6])

According to Kennedy (2004), the descriptive label of "severe disabilities" includes (1) moderate, profound, or severe intellectual disability as measured by the interaction of intelligence and adaptive behavior; (2) disability that is present throughout a person's life; and (3) disability that requires support from other people to enhance an individual's capability. People with severe or multiple disabilities may exhibit a wide range of characteristics depending on the combination and severity of disabilities and the person's age. There are, however, some traits they may all share, including limited speech or communication, difficulty in basic physical mobility, significant impairments in intellectual functioning, and/or a need for support in major life activities such as domestic, recreational, and vocational (Turnbull et al., 2007). The American Association on Intellectual and Developmental Disabilities (AIDD) stresses that when working with individuals with significant needs:

> [P]rofessionals must take additional factors into account, such as the community environment typical of the individual's peers and culture. Professionals should also consider linguistic diversity and cultural differences in the way people communicate, move, and behave. Finally, assessments must also assume that limitations in individuals often coexist with strengths, and that a person's level of life functioning will improve if appropriate personalized supports are provided over a sustained period. (AAIDD, 2009)

Some of the known genetic and environmental causes that may lead to severe disabilities include Fragile X syndrome, autism, Down syndrome, fetal alcohol syndrome, deaf-blindness, traumatic brain injury, and other nonspecific intellectual disabilities (Kennedy, 2004; Westling & Fox, 2009). However, these conditions do not always result in severe disabilities. The delays in children due to severe disabilities have a pervasive impact on child and family beyond the early childhood years because of the intensity of the disabling conditions (Chen, 1997).

Service Delivery

Overall, the context, curriculum, and philosophy of educational service delivery for individuals with severe disabilities have evolved over the years (Jackson, Ryndak, & Wehmeyer, 2010; Westling & Fox, 2009). Before the 1950s, children with significant disabilities were housed in institutions soon after birth. The few services that were available were provided privately by parent organizations and religious groups (Westling & Fox, 2009). Further, while federal legislation in 1975 (P.L. 94-142, the precursor to IDEA) brought compulsory education to school-aged children with significant needs within the public school system, it was not until 1986 that amendments were made to the legislation to create a voluntary program for states to provide services to infants and toddlers with special needs and their families to maximize the children's development. Currently, the federal grant program, Part C of the Individuals with Disabilities Education Act (IDEA, 2004), assists states in providing statewide early intervention services for infants and toddlers with disabilities, ages birth through 2 years, and their families. Similar programs for preschool-aged children are offered through Section 619, Part B of IDEA.

Typically, if the well-baby checkups reveal potential complications, the medical and special education professionals conduct a more thorough evaluation of the medical, physical, sensory, cognitive, and adaptive needs to identify the extent of disabling conditions and supports that are necessary to provide effective interventions for children with severe disabilities and their families (Horn, Chambers, & Saito, 2009).

Since Benny had an established risk condition, he was directly eligible to receive Part C services under IDEA. Once he was somewhat medically stable, the pediatrician referred Benny to the local early intervention (EI) contact person. His EI team met with Carla at the hospital and conducted an authentic assessment of his abilities, using observation, interview, and some direct tests in Benny's natural environment, the hospital at that time. His mom gave input to identify Benny's strengths and developmental needs as well as the family's resources, strengths, concerns, and needs. The assessments conducted by his early intervention team over time have allowed Benny to demonstrate his strengths and have accommodated for his disabilities. For example, since Benny cannot speak due to the trach tube, the early intervention team modified the test to allow him to use gestures or guttural sounds. The team, which includes his mom, used this information to plan Benny's next goals and intervention on his IFS. Once out of the hospital, Benny's EI team provided home-based services to Benny and his family. Later, when Benny was close to 3 years of age, his team helped plan the transition process so he could begin attending a Head Start program, which also provided early childhood special education services. When Benny turned 3, the early childhood team decided to continue to provide twice-a-week home-based services to Benny because he has a highly suppressed immune system and needs to be in a highly sanitized environment with easy access to oxygen and urgent medical care in case of emergency.

Synthesis of Research and Promising Practices

Historical and contemporary issues in research on intervention and practices for individuals with severe disabilities have focused on three broad categories: access, equity, and quality (Jackson et al., 2010). The following synthesis of literature on working with young children with severe disabilities is provided within this broad framework.

Approaches to Assessment

Increasingly, in early childhood, there is a call for service delivery to follow a linked system, whereby the assessment guides the goal development, intervention, progress monitoring, and further evaluation (Bagnato, Neisworth, & Munso, 1997; Pretti-Frontczak, 2002). A well-developed and implemented assessment must enhance children's learning and developmental outcomes within the context of their family's culture and natural routines. However, the assessment procedures for students with severe disabilities are often not equitable and target child deficits and accentuate what the child cannot do, rather than emphasizing the strengths of the child, thus resulting in low expectations for success (Downing & Demchak, 2002). Further, assessments that are normed on children who are typically developing often provide a negative picture of a child with severe disabilities, because the assessment may not utilize skills in the natural environment or may not emphasize the skills that are valued by the individual, family, or the community. Therefore, authentic assessment that documents the learning and development of children during real life activities and routines has been emphasized and is especially true for children with severe disabilities (Neisworth & Bagnato, 2004). Assessments must (1) measure the child's learning with respect to the IFSP outcomes or Individual Education Program goals (IEP), and (2) be more broadly based on the child's development and learning gains, in order to make inclusion in the community and access to general curriculum the focus for designing services provided to young children (Horn et al., 2009).

Assistive Technology

To provide equity and access for children with severe disabilities to least restrictive environments, IDEA (2004) requires that assistive technology (AT) be considered and provided for a child with disabilities if it is determined that the child needs such technology to access and participate in everyday learning activities (Judge & Parette, 1998). AT services include any service that directly assists a child with a severe disability in the selection, acquisition, and use of an AT device. Services may also include training and coordinating with other service providers and family members. However, early childhood professionals must consider child and family preference as a prerequisite for any assistive technology solutions (Plunkett, Banerjee, & Horn, 2010).

The extended stay at the hospital was stressful for Benny's mom. The early intervention (EI) provider met with Carla to provide support and suggest resources available to the family. The AT she suggested helped Carla to provide support to Benny and allow him to experience positive interactions with family members. Through trial and error, Carla discovered that placing Benny in the swing and turning on the vibrator element calmed him. He was able to tolerate his family members holding his hand, talking to him, and stroking his face. Between the ages of 1 and 2, the occupational therapist (OT) and EI provider suggested low-tech AT that allowed Benny to gain strength and mobility and to roam safely in his home. The OT also suggested special positioning and a seating system for Benny to better support his body during play and daily living skills, such as bathing, dressing, feeding, and toileting.

When Benny was older, the speech therapist introduced him and his mom to medium-tech assistive devices, such as switch-activated sound and vibrating toys to encourage Benny to communicate his daily needs, preferences, and choices, and to interact with his peers and adults, who could not understand his vocalizations, gestures, and signs. Benny currently uses a 16-switch voice output device to communicate his needs, initiate conversations, and interact with adults and peers.

Family-Centered Practices

Recently, to enhance the quality of services provided, the delivery of early childhood intervention services has shifted from professional, clinical models to a family-centered model in all areas of service delivery (Keilty & Galvin, 2006). Due to the intensity of the services and support required for children with significant needs, early childhood professionals must also support family-centered services such as family training, social work, and respite care, as well as the child-focused services of occupational therapy, speech therapy, and physical therapy. Increasing diversity in the United States has further underscored the need for family-centered services with families from diverse cultural and linguistic backgrounds.

Collaboration

Multiple professionals and agencies are involved in providing educational, physical, medical, and social-emotional services to children with severe disabilities and their families in various learning environments—home, school, and community. Collaboration between parents, related service providers such as speech language pathologists, occupational and physical therapists, early interventionists, and educators is critical to effectively support children with severe disabilities (Horn, Thompson, & Nelson, 2004).

Over the years, Carla has interacted with numerous professionals to ensure the best services possible for Benny. Carla is thankful that most professionals, representing different areas of expertise including a social worker, visual impairment specialist, nurse, early interventionist, occupational therapist, and speech therapist, worked as a team with Carla to identify her and her family's needs and researched and implemented strategies to solve them. For example, when Benny was in the hospital, the EI team was able to raise money for her and provide her with information on Medicaid and other similar options to aid in paying the hospital bills.

Strategies for Professionals and Families

Some strategies that have been listed in the literature as promising for young children with severe disabilities are:

Supporting access to and progress in the general curriculum. The primary function of early intervention and early childhood special education services is to promote children's learning and development (Wolery, 2005). Further, though health and genetic inheritance are important, children's social and physical environments are crucial to children's learning and development. Accordingly, children's access to and progress in a high-quality classroom within the general curriculum is critical for serving children with severe and multiple disabilities (Horn et al., 2009). To provide high-quality learning environments to young children that enhance their learning, Wolery suggests adults must (1) "design environments to promote children's safety, active engagement, learning, participation, and membership; (2) individualize and adapt practices for each child based on ongoing data to meet children's needs; and (3) use systemic procedures within and across environments, activities, and routines to promote children's leaning and participation" (p. 31).

Naturalistic approaches. Early childhood professionals have increasingly embraced the use of naturalistic approaches, also called activity-based instruction or incidental teaching, to support meaningful outcomes for the child with disabilities and their families (Horn & Banerjee, 2009). Naturalistic instructional approaches are particularly relevant for children with severe disabilities as they are age-appropriate and can be implemented in a variety of child learning environments and service delivery models, including home visiting, child care, community preschools, and public schools; as well as across professionals, including teachers, therapists, school counselors, and social workers. Furthermore, naturalistic instructional procedures can be applied to address a variety of skills and promote development in children across a variety of developmentally important domains. *For example, the early interventionist taught Benny the names of colors during meal times and suggested to Carla how she might reinforce and generalize these concepts during naturally occurring communication at home.*

Utilizing family needs, concerns, priorities, strengths, resources, and interests in planning intervention. Parents' opinions and suggestions are critical in understanding the needs and preferences of young children with multiple and severe disabilities. As the main decision makers for their children, parents must have opportunities to participate in the eligibility determination, goals to be addressed, and the specific services to be provided to their children. Further, families of children with a severe disability need large amounts of formal and informal supports that can help attenuate the stress and loneliness these families may already feel. Formal supports may include support from professionals, parent groups, and agencies. Informal supports may include extended family, friends, or neighborhood communities, participation in church or other institutions of social, spiritual, or religious nature. The importance of considering cultural values and family expectations to optimize the young child's ability to engage in developmentally appropriate activities and experiences is underscored. Research has shown that families that utilize coping strategies, such as developing professional and social networks and finding meaning through reframing, have shown greater family resilience, strengths, and positive outcomes (Childre, 2004).

Carla has been actively involved in the community to ensure that parents of children receiving new services adequately understand and utilize the services afforded to them under the law. She volunteers with the hospital and local and state agencies to present parent perspectives in training professionals who work with families of young children with severe needs.

Controversial Issues

Current debate among professionals and policy makers who work with students with severe disabilities has been around the provision of least restrictive environment and inclusion for children with severe disabilities in educational programs and community settings. The question is not "whether teachers used specific forms of instruction and not others, but whether students even had access to the educational opportunities afforded to all other students" (Jackson et al., 2010). Using theory, historical records, and empirical research, Jackson and colleagues (2010) argue that "inclusive education, in which students experience significant proportions of their day in the age-appropriate contexts and curriculum of general education, is a research-based practice with students who have extensive support needs" (p. 175).

Researchers argue that least restrictive environment for children with severe disability, afforded under IDEA to all individuals with disabilities, is the environment that is designed or experienced by children without disabilities. These early childhood settings may include special education and related services provided in regular kindergarten classes, public or private preschools, Head Start centers, child care facilities, preschool classes offered to an eligible prekindergarten population by the public school system, home/early childhood combinations, home/Head Start combinations, and other combinations of early childhood settings. However, placement in high-quality inclusive early childhood settings alone does not guarantee a level of instruction needed to address the needs of children with severe disabilities. To optimize outcomes for young children with severe disabilities, the early childhood professionals must ensure equity, access, and quality by (1) setting meaningful goals for children that are functional in a variety of contexts; (2) planning appropriate adaptations and modifications to enable children to participate fully in the curriculum; and (3) adopting and implementing a well-defined, research-based curriculum that allows children to make progress across all developmental domains. It is insufficient to simply place a child in a general education classroom without facilitating meaningful opportunities for learning and interaction within the daily routine (Horn & Banerjee, 2009; Horn et al., 2009).

CONCLUSION

Although low-incidence disabilities affect only a small proportion of children, the impact of the disability on the child can be overwhelming for the family. This chapter has provided an overview of three different disabilities under the category of low incidence. Each of these is unique in the way the disability is identified and early intervention and preschool services are offered, yet they are similar in that children and families with low-incidence disabilities face similar hurdles—communication, supportive and enriching environments, and the understanding of the professionals and communities in which they live.

Although it may be a legal assurance that students who have visual impairment, deafness or hearing loss, or severe disabilities are entitled to early intervention services, it should not be taken for granted that these services are necessarily provided by highly qualified individuals who understand and adhere to best practices. The goal of early intervention and early childhood special education is to alleviate the delays often attributed to a disability and to provide services and resources to the family to establish a strong environment of learning and growth that will support children throughout their lives. A quality program that provides individualized, family-centered, instructional services in "natural" environments, supports collaboration, and focuses on a child's strengths rather than weaknesses is critical to ensuring that children with low-incidence disabilities are active participants in all aspects of life and are making meaningful progress towards valued life outcomes.

REFERENCES

Alexander Graham Bell Association for the Deaf and Hard of Hearing. (2002). *Best practice model*. Retrieved from http://nc.agbell.org/NetCommunity/Page.aspx?pid=737

American Academy of Pediatrics Joint Committee on Infant Hearing. (2007). Position statement: Principles and guidelines for early hearing detection and intervention programs. doi:10.1542/peds.2007-2333

American Association on Intellectual and Developmental Disabilities. (AAIDD) (2009). Retrieved from http://www.aamr.org/content_100.cfm

American Speech-Language-Hearing Association (ASHA) (2008). *Roles and responsibilities of speech-language pathologists in early intervention: Technical report*. Retrieved from http://www.asha.org/docs/html/TR2008-00290.html

ASHA-CED. (2006). *Natural environments for infants and toddlers who are deaf or hard of hearing and their families*. Retrieved from American Speech-Language-Hearing Association, http://www.asha.org/advocacy/federal/idea/nat-env-child-facts.htm

Bagnato, S. J., Neisworth, J. T., & Munso, S. M. (1997). LINKing assessment and early intervention. Baltimore: Paul H. Brookes.

Beginnings for Parents of Children Who Are Deaf or Hard of Hearing. (2008). *The importance of early diagnosis/intervention*. Retrieved from http://www.ncbegin.org/early_intervention/early_intervention.shtml

Benson, V., & Marano, M. A. (1994). Current estimates from the National Health Interview Survey, 1992. *Vital Health Statistics, 10*(189), 1–269.

Blind Babies Foundation. (1998). *Pediatric visual diagnosis factsheet: Optic nerve hypoplasia*. Retrieved from http://www.tsbvi.edu/seehear/spring99/opticnerve.htm

Calderon, R., & Greenberg, M. (1997). The effectiveness of early intervention for deaf children and children with hearing loss. In M. J. Guralnick (Ed.), *The effectiveness of early intervention* (pp. 445–482). Baltimore: Paul H. Brookes.

Chen, D. (1997). *Effective practices in early intervention: Infants whose multiple disabilities include both vision and hearing loss* [report for OSEP Grant NO. H025D30002]. Northridge: California State University. (Eric document Reproduction Service No. ED406795)

Childre, A. (2004). Families. In C. H. Kennedy, & E. M. Horn (Eds.), *Including students with severe disabilities* (pp. 78–99). New York: Pearson.

Colorado Home Intervention Program. (Producer) (2003). *Early intervention illustrated: The home team* [DVD]. Boys Town Press.

Colorado Home Intervention Program and the New Mexico School for the Deaf (Producer). (2004). *Early intervention illustrated: The art and science of home visits* [DVD]. Boys Town Press.

Division on Visual Impairments (DVI), Council for Exceptional Children. (2003). *Position statement: Family-centered practices for infants and young children with visual impairments*. Retrieved from http://www.cecdvi.org/Postion%20Papers/family_centered.htm

Downing, J. E., & Demchak, M. (2002). In J. E. Downing (Ed.), *Including students with severe and multiple disabilities in typical classrooms: Practical strategies for teachers* (2nd ed., pp. 37–70). Baltimore: Paul H. Brookes.

Ferrell, K. A. (1997). Preface. In P. Crane, D. Cuthbertson, K. A. Ferrell, & H. Scherb (Eds.), *Equals in partnership: Basic rights for families of children with blindness or visual impairment* (pp. i–v). Watertown, MA: The Hilton/Perkins Program and the National Association for Parents of the Visually Impaired.

Ferrell, K. A. (1998). *Project PRISM: A longitudinal study of developmental patterns of children who are visually impaired* [final report]. Greeley, CO: University of Northern Colorado, National Center on Severe & Sensory Disabilities. Retrieved from http://www.unco.edu/ncssd/research/PRISM/default.html

Ferrell, K. A. (2000). Growth and development of young children. In M. C. Holbrook & A. J. Koenig (Eds.), *Foundations of education*. Vol. 1: *History and theory of teaching children and youths with visual impairments* (2nd ed., pp. 111–133). New York: AFB Press.

Ferrell, K. A. (2010). *Reach out and teach* (2nd ed. rev.). New York: AFB Press.

Ferrell, K. A., Trief, E., Deitz, S., Bonner, M. A., Cruz, D., Ford, E., & Stratton, J. (1990). The visually impaired infants research consortium (VIIRC): First year results. *Journal of Visual Impairment and Blindness, 84*, 404–410.

Fraiberg, S. (1977). *Insights from the blind*. New York: Basic Books.

Harlor, A. D. B., Jr., & Bower, C. (2009) Hearing assessment in infants and children: Recommendations beyond neonatal screening. *Pediatrics, 124*, 1252–1263. doi:10.1542/peds.2009-1997

Hatton, D. D. (2001). Model registry of early childhood visual impairment. *Journal of Visual Impairment & Blindness, 95*, 418–433. Retrieved from http://www.afb.org/jvib/jvib_main.asp

Hatton, D., Bailey, D. B., Burchinal, M., & Ferrell, K. A. (1997). Developmental growth curves of preschool children with vision impairments. *Child Development, 64,* 788–806.

Hatton, D., Erickson, K., & Lee, D. B. (2009, November). *Phonological awareness and concepts about print in young children with visual impairments.* Paper presented at 9th Biennial Getting in Touch with Literacy Conference, Costa Mesa, CA.

Hearing Loss Association of America. (1997, November–December). Policy statement on educating hard of hearing children in regular schools. *Hearing Loss Magazine.* Retrieved from http://www.hearingloss.org/advocacy/hardofhearingchildren.asp

Horn, E., & Banerjee, R. (2009). Understanding curriculum modifications and embedded learning opportunities in the context of supporting all children's success. *Language, Speech, and Hearing Services in Schools, 40,* 406–415.

Horn, E., Chambers, C., & Saito, Y. (2009). Techniques for teaching young children with moderate/severe or multiple disabilities. In S. A. Raver (Ed.), *Early childhood special education—0–8 years: Strategies for positive outcomes* (pp. 255–278). New Jersey: Merrill.

Horn, E., Thompson, B., & Nelson, C. (2004). Collaborative teams. In C. H. Kennedy & E. M. Horn (Eds.), *Including students with severe disabilities* (pp. 17–32). New York: Pearson.

Individuals with Disabilities Education Act [IDEA], 20 U.S.C. 1400 (2004).

Individuals with Disabilities Education Act [IDEA] Regulations, 34 C.F.R. Parts 300–304 (2006).

Jackson, L., Ryndak, D., & Wehmeyer, M. (2010). The dynamic relationship between context, curriculum, and student learning: A case for inclusive education as a research-based practice. *Research and Practice for Persons with Severe Disabilities, 33*(4), 175–195.

Judge, S. L., & Parette, H. L. (1998). Family centered assistive technology decision making. *Infant-Toddler Intervention, 8,* 185–206.

Keilty, B., & Galvin, K. M. (2006). Physical and social adaptations of families to promote learning in everyday experiences. *Topics in Early Childhood Special Education, 26,* 219–233.

Kennedy, C. H. (2004). Students with severe disabilities. In C. H. Kennedy & E. M. Horn (Eds.), *Including students with severe disabilities* (pp. 3–16). New York: Pearson.

Koestler, F. A. (2004). *The unseen minority: A social history of blindness in the United States* (reissued). New York: AFB Press.

Marge, D. K., & Marge, M. (2005). *Beyond newborn hearing screening: Meeting the educational and health care needs of infants and young children with hearing loss in America.* Report of the National Consensus Conference on Effective Educational and Health Care Interventions for Infants and Young Children with Hearing Loss, September 10–12, 2004. Syracuse, New York: Department of Physical Medicine and Rehabilitation, SUNY Upstate Medical University. Retrieved from http://www.upstate.edu/pmr/beyond_newborn.pdf

Maxfield, K. E., & Buchholz, S. (1957). *A social maturity scale for blind preschool children: A guide to its use.* New York: American Foundation for the Blind.

Miyamoto, R. T., Hay-McCutcheon, M. J., Kirk, K. I., Houston, D. M., & Bergeson-Dana, T. (2008). Language skills of profoundly deaf children who received cochlear implants under 12 months of age: A preliminary study. *Acta Oto-Laryngologica, 128,* 373–377.

Moeller, M. P. (2000). Early intervention and language development in children who are deaf and hard of hearing. *Pediatrics, 106*(3), e43.

Moore, M. S., & Levitan, L. (2001). *For hearing people only* (3rd ed.). MSM Productions.

National Agenda: Moving forward on achieving educational equality for deaf and hard of hearing students. (2005). Retrieved from National Agenda: Deaf and Hard of Hearing, http://www.ndepnow.org/pdfs/national_agenda.pdf

National Association of the Deaf (NAD), Cochlear Implant Committee. (2000). NAD position statement on cochlear implants. Retrieved from the National Association of the Deaf, http://www.nad.org/issues/technology/assistive-listening/cochlear-implants

National Institutes of Health. (1993). *Early identification of hearing impairment in infants and young children.* Consensus development conference statement. Retrieved from http://consensus.nih.gov/1993/1993HearingInfantsChildren092html.htm

Neisworth, J. T., & Bagnato, S. J. (2004). The mismeasure of young children: The authentic assessment alternative. *Infants and Young Children, 17,* 198–212.

Norris, M., Spaulding, P. J., & Brodie, F. H. (1957). *Blindness in children.* Chicago: University of Chicago Press.

Plunkett, D., Banerjee, R., & Horn, E. (2010). Supporting early childhood outcomes through assistive technology. In Seok, S. (Ed.), *Handbook of research on human cognition and assistive technology: Design, accessibility and transdisciplinary perspectives* (pp. 339–358). Hershey, PA: IGI Global.

Pogrund, R. L. (2002). Refocus. In R. L. Pogrund & D. L. Fazzi (Eds.), *Early focus: Working with young children who are blind or visually impaired and their families* (2nd ed., pp. 1–15). New York: AFB Press.

Pretti-Frontczak, K. L. (2002). Using curriculum-based measures to promote a linked system approach. *Assessment for Effective Intervention, 27*(4), 15–27.

Rais-Bahrami, K., & Short, B. L. (2007). Premature and small-for-dates infants. In M. K. Batshaw, L. Pellegrino, & N. J. Roizen (Eds.), *Children with disabilities* (6th ed., pp. 107–122). Baltimore: Paul H. Brookes.

Sandall, S., Hemmeter, M. L., Smith, B. J., & McLean, M. E. (Eds.). (2005). *DEC recommended practices: A comprehensive guide.* Longmont, CO: Sopris West.

Sass-Lehrer, M. (2002). *Early beginnings for families with deaf and hard of hearing children: Myths and facts of early intervention and guidelines for effective services.* Retrieved from Laurent Clerc National Deaf Education Center, Gallaudet University, http://clerccenter.gallaudet.edu/Clerc_Center/Information_and_Resources/Info_to_Go/Help_for_Babies_(0_to_3)/Early_Intervention/Early_Beginnings_Contents.html

Sass-Lehrer, M. (2003). Programs and services for deaf and hard of hearing children and their families. In B. Bodner-Johnson & M. Sass-Lehrer (Eds.), *The young deaf or hard of hearing child: A family-centered approach to early education* (pp. 153–180). Baltimore: Paul H. Brookes.

Sontag, E., & Haring, N. G. (1996). The professionalization of teaching and learning of children with severe disabilities: The creation of TASH. *Journal of the Association for Persons with Severe Handicaps, 21,* 39–45.

Tompkins, C. (1998). Goal 1: Students and their families will be referred to an appropriate education program within thirty days of identification of a suspected visual impairment. In A. L. Corn & K. M. Huebner (Eds.), *A report to the nation: The national agenda for the education of children and youths with visual impairment, including those with multiple disabilities* (pp. 7–12). New York: AFB Press.

Turnbull, A., Turnbull, R., Erwin, E. J., & Soodak, L. C. (2006). *Families, professionals, and exceptionality: Positive outcomes through partnerships and trust* (5th ed.). Princeton, NJ: Merrill.

Turnbull, A., Turnbull, R., & Wehmeyer, M. (2007). *Exceptional lives: Special education in today's schools* (5th ed.). Princeton, NJ: Merrill.

U.S. Department of Education, Office of Special Education and Rehabilitative Services, Office of Special Education Programs. (2009). *Twenty-eighth annual report to Congress on the implementation of the Individuals with Disabilities Education Act, 2006.* Washington, DC: Author.

U.S. Department of Health and Human Services, National Institutes of Health, National Institute on Deafness and Other Communication Disorders. (2009, August). *NIDCD fact sheet Cochlear implants* [Publication No. 09-4798]. Retrieved from http://www.nidcd.nih.gov/staticresources/health/hearing/FactSheetCochlearImplant.pdf

Westling, D. L., & Fox, L. (2009). *Teaching students with severe disabilities.* New Jersey: Merrill.

Wolery, M. (2005). DEC recommended practices: Child-focused practices. In S. Sandall, M. L. Hemmeter, B. J. Smith, & M. E. McLean (Eds.), *DEC recommended practices: A comprehensive guide for practical application in early intervention/early childhood special education* (pp. 71–106). Longmont, CO: Sopris West.

Yoshinaga-Itano, C., Sedey, A. L., Coulter, D. K., & Mehl, A. L. (1998). Language of early- and later-identified children with hearing loss. *Pediatrics, 102,* 1161–1171.

Chapter 11

What It Means to Be Literate from the Perspective of Young Children: Exploring the Domains of Literacy and Mathematics in Early Childhood

Efleda Tolentino

Early childhood is a time when the foundations of literacy and mathematics are built. Educational systems in countries such as the United States, Canada, France, Germany, Italy, Japan, the Russian Federation, and the United Kingdom recognize the importance of providing programs of education for children at least 3 years of age that involve structured, center-based, and instructional activities (National Center for Education Statistics, March 2009). Research indicates that children who participate in early care and education tend to score higher in mathematics and reading assessments as compared to their peers who had no preprimary care and education prior to kindergarten entry (National Center for Education Statistics, October 2009). Although preprimary education is not compulsory in the United States (with the exception of a few states), children who do attend nursery school, prekindergarten, and kindergarten are immersed in activities that foster emergent literacy and numeracy skills (National Center for Education Statistics, March 2009).

Increasing attention is drawn towards providing literacy and mathematics education in the preschool (Neuman & Roskos, 2005; U.S. Department of Education, 2003). In New York state, standards for mathematics and literacy are in place as early as prekindergarten (University of the State of New York & the State Education Department, 2002). Head Start has also modified its standards to address areas such as mathematics and literacy in accordance with the Child Outcomes

Framework (Head Start Bureau, 2001). In a recent report by the National Center for Education Statistics and the U.S. Department of Education, the findings revealed that the children who entered kindergarten in the fall of 2006 and the fall of 2007 appeared to be equipped with literacy and mathematical knowledge (Flanagan, McPhee, & Mulligan, 2009). The aforementioned cohort of children was diverse in race, ethnicity, socioeconomic status, primary language, family type, as well as range and quality of early care and education experiences (Flanagan et al., 2009).

In a society where literacy and mathematics are considered important, it is essential to draw children as co-participants in the process of cultural transmission, immersing them in mastery and application of concepts and skills early in life as a way to support them in organizing knowledge and experience. Eisenhauer and Feikes (2009) signify the importance of math in young children's lives as they naturally compare, count, quantify, collect data, and "monitor their position in space" (p. 22). In the same vein, literacy is embedded in young children's daily encounters, enabling them to internalize "attitudes, knowledge, and skills about reading, writing, listening, and speaking" (Millard & Waese, 2007, p. 3). Mathematics and literacy simply intersect in children's experiences as they engage in acts of meaning, such as gesturing, drawing, storytelling, conversation, and play. Because children participate in sociocultural practices valued by members of their families and the wider community, they develop concepts of literacy and mathematics long before they enter school (Sarama & Clements, 2009). As they become part of the web of interactions within their immediate environment, they become reflective and deliberate in their use of print, symbols, and marks to represent meaning. Interactions within the environment enable children to acquire and apply knowledge about print, symbols, and stories.

This period is also known as emerging literacy. This term captures the "little-by-little" accumulation of early knowledge upon which the child will build when he enters formal instruction (Clay, 1991). From an emergent literacy perspective, children construct their own literacy. From an emergent numeracy perspective, children are emerging with a working understanding of mathematics as applied in their lives. In other words, because children are constructors, problem solvers, and theorists, they realize the potential of literacy and mathematics as a means to communicate, invent, create, construct, and extend their working schema of the world.

This chapter is an invitation to broaden our understanding of literacy and mathematics in early childhood. The field of early childhood education summons its teachers to strengthen and support preschool literacy (International Reading Association and National Association for the Education of Young Children, 1998) and mathematics (Clements, 2004; National Association for the Education of Young Children and National Council of Teachers of Mathematics, 2002). Embedded within this chapter are children's acts of meaning in the form of conversations, drawings, and written artifacts. In this investigation, it is essential to view literacy and mathematics from a child-centric perspective, which encompasses fully listening to the words and paying attention to the symbols, marks, patterns, and gestures that children incorporate into their acts of meaning. Children's acts of meaning are made with intentionality; that is, children deliberately represent their ideas in graphic, oral, and written narrative forms.

A child-centric perspective necessitates a shift in the ways that we, as adults and child advocates, view mathematics and literacy: What do mathematics and literacy mean to young children? Hence, rather than viewing mathematics and literacy learning as end goals in the lives of young children, literacy and mathematics serve as a means to a greater end. Children perhaps use literacy and mathematics as tools to generate meaning that will enable them to successfully thrive within their social worlds. This requires the ability to construct, deconstruct, and reconstruct knowledge structures on a personal level and apply knowledge constructs on a social level.

The chapter begins with a personal story and is then followed by documentation generated from an observational field study that was conducted in a classroom of emergent readers and mathematicians. The common thread that binds the stories is the children's voice, and how children demonstrate their knowledge of math and literacy through their acts of meaning.

OVERCOMING A SPEECH BARRIER: MAKING MEANING VISIBLE

Our child was diagnosed with speech delay at 31 months of age. While it appeared that our child was bright, sociable, and receptive towards interactions initiated by members of our family and our circle of friends, his speech articulation was not clear, making it difficult for him to be understood. Because my husband and I were also our child's primary caregivers, we were the only ones who could decipher his speech. He would say "oo" for "juice" and "uh" for truck. He would call the ice cream van "ay—eem—en" and would express phrases such as "Things that go" as "ee-ah-ow." After much thought and reflection, my husband and I shared our concerns with the early intervention service coordinator. A team of professionals evaluated our child and recommended speech therapy and group intervention through a play-based early childhood center.

For a year, our child received one-on-one support and instruction from a speech therapist twice during every week and was also a participant in a play group facilitated by an early childhood teacher. As his parents, we were given some guidance in supporting our child's speech development; but because we wanted to understand the essence of our child's speech, we also encouraged him to explore other modes of communication. One of the things we encouraged our child to do was to write and draw. We restructured his play space to include a table that contained writing implements. As soon as we had set up a writing space, we noticed that the space itself and the writing implements within served as tools as well as provocations for our child to pursue varied ways of representing his thinking. The first time he encountered markers was when he was 28 months of age. He produced the following representation (see Figure 11.1).

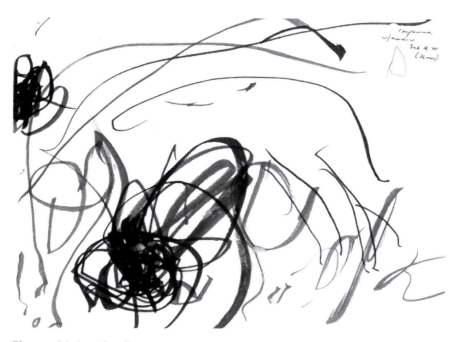

Figure 11.1   The first attempts using a marker.

It is hard to tell whether children are intentional in creating representations when they first use writing implements or simply find pleasure in the movement of the pen or the marks that they produce (Harris, 1963; Kellogg, 1969). With our son, holding the marker seemed to help him gain control over ways that he could express his ideas.

Around the same time, our child was at his table drawing what appeared to be circular figures. Right by his sheet of paper were a number of toy cars and trucks. As he was making circular motions with his marker, he was also engaged in private speech, saying to himself, "weee...." To our son, there was meaning in the marks that he was making; in essence, the speech and the marks on paper served to represent running ideas, or his thinking. As the minutes wore on, the marks progressively appeared to be more and more deliberate. Upon completion of his drawing, he showed me his work, saying "Weee." Because I was not certain what this meant, I asked him, "I see that you made a lot of circles. Can you tell me what they are?" He then leads me to his table and points out the wheels of his cars and trucks. And once more, he said, "Weee." It was then that I realized what it was that he produced. The circular figures were actually wheels (see Figure 11.2). Almost intuitively, he used writing/drawing as a means to be understood. Our child used his writing tools on a regular

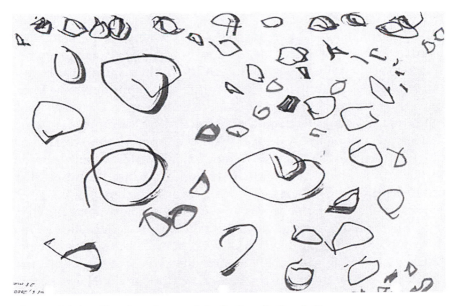

Figure 11.2 Circular shapes labeled as "wheels."

basis, initially satisfying his personal needs and intuitively using his representations as a way to communicate with the rest of our family. Engaged in a process of creation and re-creation, he repeatedly draws wheels on another sheet of paper, perhaps as a way to develop mastery in creating the figure.

Three things struck me about this particular episode. First was my child's desire to convey meaning. His use of various forms of representation was a skillful way to express his thoughts and reveal his intent to be understood. In his desire to be understood, he verbally said the word "wheels," gesturing with his fingers, representing them through his drawings, and *using* concrete examples to convey meaning. Second, I was fascinated with his persistence in drawing the same subject repetitively, as if it were a rehearsal of some sort. Wolf and Perry (1988) would characterize children's repetitive attempts to create figurative representations as a means to develop mastery. Third, I was struck with my child's ability to serve as a scaffold for me, drawing my attention to various representations of a word that apparently had significance for him at that moment. He appeared to have found a medium that enabled him to express ideas that his speech could not fully convey. *My child had figured out an alternative path to communicate his thinking.*

Reflecting upon this experience, I realized that my child was a protagonist in his own learning, and to support my child as a communicator, it was important for me to step back and to listen, to know his area of interest, to know his strengths, and to know his challenges. In other words, it was important for me to know him intimately as a learner. It was also around this age when my child would mark his paper in a flurry of back-and-forth gestures, creating what appeared to be lines, dots, and curves (see Figure 11.3).

Seemingly exercising control over his tool, he attempts to develop mastery in creating lines on paper. He would spend hours working on his sketches that appeared to us as random marks. Just when we began to inquire into whether the marks had meaning for him, he surprised us one day with his first representation of a truck (refer to Figure 11.4). It happened one evening, as he was drawing at his table. Among the writing implements on his table was his truck. Upon completion of his drawings, he approached me and shared his sketch, excitedly saying, "Ah-ow." It was difficult for me to understand his speech, but because his words were accompanied by a visual representation, I was able to understand what he meant to convey. His sketch was a truck that had wheels, a body, an arm, and a claw at the tip. Put together, the lines,

Figure 11.3 A flurry of lines, dots, and curves.

circles, and curves that he repetitively drew in previous drawings appeared to have been combined and configured to take the form of a backhoe, a subject of interest since he was 1 1/2 years old. Golomb (1981) stipulated that children's attempts to create a visual representation are part of the process of searching for meaning and likeness. *The sketch indeed resembled a backhoe.* Then, he pointed to the dark circle underneath the body of the backhoe and said, "weee." It occurred to

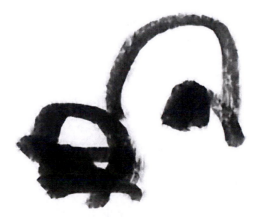

Figure 11.4 First sketch of a backhoe.

us that the repetition of lines, circles, and curves were prerequisites to a big idea, almost as if they were a prelude to a play. This is a simple but clear demonstration of an act of building from within. *Our child used his knowledge of lines, circles, and curves to create a picture that represented an idea, making his thoughts visible.*

Prior to this episode, our child had a fascination for cars and trucks. Like a researcher, he would closely examine his toy, look at its parts, and observe how it moved. To support his investigations, we made trips to construction sites within the neighborhood. He would count and name every truck that he could see while observing how they moved. We also read fiction and nonfiction books that covered trucks and forms of transport. We spent amounts of time during the day in conversation about his favorite topic. In retrospect, the context that includes the activities, the relationships within, and the mode of representations served as a support in his meaning-making process. As his parents and primary caregivers, we provided an environment that acknowledged his questions and interests and created opportunities for furthering his knowledge. Revisiting the same books seemed to have given him opportunities to process what he was learning and to master the concepts that were unfolding on every page.

During our truck investigations, we noticed that we were also incorporating various disciplines such as literacy, mathematics, science, social studies, art, music, and movement. At 29 months, our child had become an expert on the subject of trucks. He was able to name and classify trucks of all kinds, pointing out their uses and their importance in the world that revolved around him. At the same time, he was demonstrating his understanding of mathematical concepts such as symmetry, one-to-one correspondence, patterns, shapes, size, open and closed space, angles, and the relationship between parts to a whole. Excited with this newfound ability to create objects of interest, our child returned to the writing space provided and drew a number of backhoes on the same sheet (see Figure 11.5 for this drawing). It was as if our child was engaged in a recursive cycle of intimate discovery of visual literacy and artistic ability. Research shows that in capturing the visual aspects of an object, children pay attention to the shape, spatial arrangements, the proportions, and the size of their subject (Matthews, 1984).

Hence, our child was honing mathematical skills, drawing figures, composing parts to create the whole picture, counting the number of wheels, and demonstrating one-to-one correspondence between the wheels of his toy trucks and the wheels that were represented on the printed page. Goodnow (1977) would describe this process as a child's

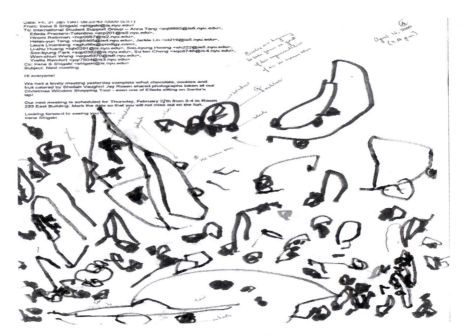

Figure 11.5   First sketch of "many backhoes."

way of searching for equivalents. With every sketch, our child was exploring the concept of quantity, translating concrete concepts into abstract form, and developing the ability to think deductively and inductively with the creation of parts of a whole. Every sketch appeared to have a story embedded. Even as speech articulation was progressing, our child shared stories, sometimes recalling and acting out episodes from books that we had read over and over again, a process known as reenactment of texts. Participating in the act of storytelling, our child would compose personal narratives, sharing text-to-life connections during dialogue. Our child's print awareness was reflected in ways that he incorporated environmental print into his representations.

Children's representations draw our attention to how observant and reflective they are as literate individuals. The sketch that follows show trains of different colors (see Figure 11.6). Every train had a letter or number embedded on it, just like the trains that are found in our local subways. Our child had brought his observations of symbols and environmental print into his drawings, a sophisticated ability for a 2-year-old that reflected (in part) his emerging literacy. Creating marks developed alongside creating print. Children's deliberate acts

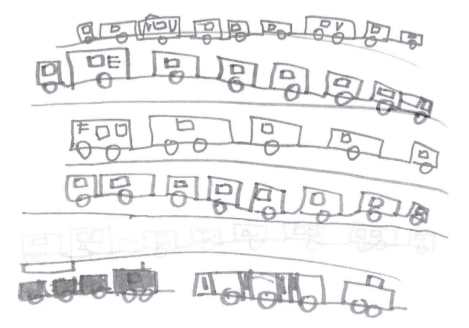

Figure 11.6   Trains in the subway.

of writing or drawing convey their strong desire to tell about something (Schickedanz & Casbergue, 2004). Experimenting with print not
only facilitated writing development, but more importantly, it gave
our child a mode of representation to make his ideas visible.

As our child received speech support services, we also provided him
with opportunities to enrich his learning. In other words, together with
our child's support team, we created supportive contexts within which
he thrived as a learner. Through representations and conversations, it
became apparent that a speech delay was not a barrier to literacy and
mathematical development as well as conceptual development. It was
apparent that a network of social support and consistent, two-way scaffolding were just as important to overcome this challenge.

EMERGENT LITERACY AND MATHEMATICS FROM
A SOCIOCULTURAL PERSPECTIVE

Children's acts are meaning-driven. Their attempts to understand the
world and to use available tools and resources are ways in which they
build upon what they know so that they can fully participate in social

acts that are meaningful in their culture. Literacy and mathematics are a natural part of everyday life. Viewing children from a sociocultural lens enables us to understand how members of a child's culture make an impact on their emerging knowledge of literacy and mathematics.

The Context of Home

As demonstrated in the introductory anecdote, children grow in the context of a social semiotic network of meanings within the culture that enables them to master the systems that are valued by the members of their environment (Halliday, 1978). Initially using cries, gestures, and symbolic representations, young children become literate in the systems of communication that their culture embraces. Even in the crib, infants are already exposed to objects and various forms of representation. Antell and Keating (1983) indicate that in the first weeks of life, infants begin to notice the distinction between small and large quantities. This research is supported by Lipton and Spelke (2003) as they observed 5-month-old infants noticing the difference between small quantities. Young children are at the beginning of their journey of understanding what objects signify, the meaning of the marks that they create, and the print that abounds in their environment. Very young children tend to be more inventive in their attempts to communicate as they are not always "able to clearly express themselves verbally" (Wright, 1997, p. 361). Because of their desire to communicate, they create and invent alternative ways to make their thoughts visible: through words, gestures, and signs (Wright, 1997).

Language is a form of symbolic representation that serves as a tool for learning and communication within social contexts (Britton, 1970). For children, language enables them to jointly construct meaning with others (Vygotsky, 1978). The context in which the communicative act takes place and the shared understanding between participants support the meanings carried by language. As such, the role the immediate environment plays is crucial in promoting language development. Because "language learning is a self-generated, creative process" (Jaggar, 1985, p. 4), children learn language through everyday experiences.

The adults and older siblings who converse with young children often take the responsibility of filling in much of the conversational structure and context by acknowledging and elaborating messages made by young language users to achieve mutual understanding (Lapadat, 1994). As very young children interact with caregivers, they build upon their meaning-making skills (Bruner, 1996; Halliday, 1978). Meaning-making involves bringing together what children know about their world as they encounter new situations and apply them in appropriate cultural contexts (Bruner, 1996).

Guided by at least one adult who serves as the child's primary caregiver or mentor, children participate in acts of meaning that are characterized by "diverse interactional exchanges, mutual reciprocity, differential competence, and strong emotion" (Thompson, 2006, p. 7). Wood, Bruner, and Ross (1976) introduced the term "scaffolding" to refer to adult- or expert-facilitated process that enables a child or novice to solve a problem, carry out a task, or achieve a goal that would be beyond his or her unassisted efforts. The scaffolding provided by an adult to a young child is critical to concept development. In fact, the scaffolding provided by adults serves as a model to children, who in turn develop the capability to play the role of expert in supporting the learning of a novice. "The literacy environment is the social construction of families and the impact of daily experiences on children's lives" (Neuman & Celano, 2001, p. 12). It is in the heart of relational contexts that children learn to make meaning (Halliday, 1978). Meaning-making is the act of giving meaning to events by making connections with them (Wells, 1986).

There is a plethora of literature that attests to the impact of parent-child conversations on young children's concept development. Ruffman, Slade, and Crowe (2002) conducted a longitudinal study that documented mother-child conversations and their impact on children's language development and the emergence of theory of mind. Theory of mind is a cognitive ability that refers to children's awareness of their own thought processes and the thinking of others (Gelman, 2009). The study revealed that children's development of theory of mind were influenced and supported by their mothers' use of mental state languages, or words that describe their feelings or state of being. When children are engaged in conversations with adults, they are exposed to words that serve as semantic referents for emotions, experiences, concepts, and events (Bartsch & Wellman, 1995). Furthermore, when adults provide explanations for events as they transpire in meaningful contexts, they open doors of opportunities for young children to reflect, examine, and organize their understanding of concepts, experiences, and natural phenomena (Thompson, 2006).

Children's comprehension as well as understanding deepens especially when adults direct their attention to specific aspects of a situation (Nelson & Fivush, 2004). "Shared reminiscing contributes to the child's retrieval of significant aspects of past experiences and provides narrative coherence and structure to the child's representation of past events" (Nelson & Fivush, 2004, p. 5). Hence, it can be deduced that prior to school entry, children have had significant experiences with literacy and mathematics (Bodrova, Leong, & Paynter, 1999). The vignette cited earlier in the chapter reveals how emergent knowledge of literacy and mathematics were manifested in the different modes of representation used by a child to communicate his thinking. The role of the adult as listener, observer, and scaffold is key when providing the kind of feedback that will respond to the children's attempts to uncover, discover, and process their emergent knowledge in literacy and mathematics.

The Context of School

Prior to entering preschool, children are equipped with their own concepts of how mathematics and literacy are used in the context of everyday life. These concepts evolve based on their encounters with literacy and mathematics along with the practices that are associated with their use in the home and immediate environment. Children have a literacy set (Holdaway, 1979) which embodies early concepts, attitudes, and skills associated with forms and functions of language and texts necessary for reading and writing (Van Kraayenoord & Paris, 1996). Research indicates that prior to kindergarten entry, children have varying degrees of knowledge in "letter recognition, letter-sound knowledge, recognition of simple words, phonological awareness, receptive and expressive vocabulary and print conventions" (Flanagan et al., 2009, p. 18). Applying the same principle in the context of mathematics, children also develop a mathematical set, which embodies the concepts, attitudes, and skills associated with the use of symbols, concepts, and operations that are necessary for computation, problem solving, and concept development. Kindergarten children have mathematical skills such as "number sense, counting, basic operations, measurement, patterns, and geometry, and spatial sense" (Flanagan et al., 2009, p. 19).

As young children become acculturated to the context of school, they become familiar with school discourse. They learn to act out the social structure within the school, take on roles and responsibilities, follow rules, and participate in practices that are valued within their classroom community. They learn to ask questions and negotiate help as they learn. They participate in literate acts and engage in problem solving that challenge their mathematical and literate abilities. As young children are acclimated to school, they become familiar with school discourse. When school discourse and practices are similar to their primary discourse and literacy practices and mathematical applications in the home, children will build upon their literacy and mathematical sets. In other words, *children will be extending their current understanding of literacy and mathematics easily if there is continuity of experience and learning between home and the child's school.* Kennedy and Surman (2003) reiterated the importance of welcoming children's current understanding and accommodating their meaning-making efforts to facilitate a smooth transition between home and school.

The language children use mirrors the language of their parents and their community (Clay, 1991). Children who have a home language other than English and a cultural background that is different from the dominant culture may experience dissonance and may have difficulty applying their competencies in the context of school. This applies particularly to cultures that have very different traditions regarding the use of written language and mathematical abstractions, and whose living and working circumstances do not promote literacy and mathematics (Leseman, 1999). Research reveals that children whose primary home language was English were able to attain higher scores in reading and mathematics than their peers whose primary home language was not English (Flanagan et al., 2009). The differences in preliteracy and prenumeracy skills place the children of such families at a disadvantage compared to the children of families within the dominant culture. Since reading, writing, and mathematics are cultural constructs, it is important to acknowledge that cultural differences can exist between practices in school and at home (Au, 1980; Purcell-Gates, 1996; Scollon & Scollon, 1981). As early as kindergarten, low achievement in mathematics and literacy appears evident among children from families who are culturally and linguistically diverse (Flanagan et al., 2009).

Another factor that could affect children's success in their transition into a school setting is the absence or lack of resources in their home. The disparities in literacy and numeracy development as reflected between social classes and literate-rich homes become evident in the ways children respond to classroom practices that relate to mathematics and literacy. Neuman and Celano (2001) indicate that children from white, middle-class homes will thrive, while children with low socioeconomic status will start school behind and stay behind. Research has shown that children who come from low-socioeconomic-status homes enter school at a disadvantage as they are ill equipped academically in comparison with their peers who are more privileged (Stipek & Ryan, 1997). Researchers have traced differences in the frequency of book reading for children from middle- and low-income homes (Anderson-Yockel & Haynes, 1994; Pellegrini, Galda, Jones, & Perlmutter, 1995; Sonnenschein, Brody, & Munsterman, 1996). Symons, Szuszkiewicz, and Bonnell (1996) revealed how parental print exposure may predict children's emergent literacy. Since adults with little print exposure may be infrequent readers, their children may receive less exposure to literacy activities. Flanagan et al. (2009) report that children whose household incomes were at or above poverty attained higher scores in reading and mathematics as compared to children who lived in poverty.

Given this reality, there will be children who seem better prepared to learn in school, and there will also be others who may be ill equipped or have skills that are unacknowledged in school settings (Neuman & Celano, 2001), resulting in underachievement (Fryer & Levitt, 2004; Natriello, McDill, & Pallas, 1990). In a study conducted by Lee and Ginsburg (2007), early childhood teachers of children coming from low socioeconomic status recognized that students are disadvantaged and therefore need to prepare their children for kindergarten by providing literacy and mathematics education. In contrast, early childhood teachers of children coming from middle socioeconomic status believe that play and socialization take precedence over academics and emphasized the importance of modifying curriculum to fit the pace and level of the children (Lee & Ginsburg, 2007).

Early childhood teachers need to be cognizant of such differences so that they can create ways to build and strengthen partnerships between the child's home and the school. When teachers and parents work in partnership, children will most likely succeed as efforts are collaboratively directed towards ensuring coherence in learning at home and in school (Benigno & Ellis, 2004). Because school is a sociocultural context, it will benefit children greatly when adults within the environment give children opportunities to share their ways of making meaning and ways in which they incorporate their knowledge of literacy, mathematics, and other content areas in their own lives. Through engaging in an exchange of ideas (whether in the form of dialogue, signs, or gestures) within a co-constructed space, both adults and children within the school context will be creating a space that offers opportunities to internalize concepts and to organize experiences. The extent of understanding and depth of meaning that children take away from interactions will depend on the quality of responses provided by the adult, the level of engagement of the young child participating in the interaction, and the value of the information to the child at that moment.

Children's knowledge of literacy and mathematics often emerges in the context of interactions with others. To view children from a sociocultural lens is to see them as part of a web of interactions and encounters with divergent perspectives among members of their culture as they are immersed in meaning-making of valued beliefs and practices, using tools that enable them to participate in co-constructing understanding. The documentation that follows tells social stories that take place in the context of school. The events reveal children's ways of participating in their social worlds.

DATA COLLECTION AND ANALYSIS

The three episodes featured in the following sections were generated from an observational field study grounded in the qualitative method of inquiry that examined the role of talk in children's learning (Guba & Lincoln, 1989). In this study, I investigated the nature of talk among preschoolers who were engaged in various activities during their work time. Since the focus of this chapter is on children's emerging knowledge in literacy and mathematics as they are engaged in play and self-selected activities, the documentation presented in subsequent sections will reveal the ways that children naturally incorporate literacy and mathematics in the context of the classroom. In other words, of the class members between the ages of 4 and 5 years old, some have had previous experience in an early care and education setting, and a few children were in the process of transitioning between the home environment and the school environment.

The children who participated in this study were based in an independent school located in a multiethnic and multi-economic residential area in an urban setting. Founded in the early twentieth century, the school prides itself in delivering a child-centered education combined with academic rigor. Since observations transpired during children's work time, opportunities to collect data in the form of field notes, video documentation, and transcripts were available during five work time periods every week for an entire school year. Analysis of data began with the first field notes and was carried out recursively in cycles of data collection and analysis. Patterns and themes emerged from field notes, which were then organized into categories.

Using the utterance as the basic unit of analysis for talk episodes, transcripts contained faithful representations of both verbal and non-verbal communication. Transcripts of children's conversations were analyzed using Halliday's (1978) framework, featuring the Social Context of a Situation. This framework acknowledges the influence of three components within a context that determine the texts and narratives that unfold within the situation. Talk transcripts examined what participants talked about, the roles that they played during their interaction, and ways that they used language to communicate intent.

After doing the threefold analysis, I examined my findings in the light of the research questions posed, giving attention to how the topics, roles, and functions of language affect the meanings that emerge for the children. Written artifacts included in this documentation were analyzed by identifying resonating patterns and themes, and interpreted based on the meaning that the child writer wished to convey. To check for trustworthiness of data analyzed, a group of researchers reexamined and counterchecked data and addressed areas that appeared ambiguous.

INTENTIONALITY AND THE YOUNG WRITER

Writing was a popular choice among the children in the prekindergarten classroom that I observed. Supplied with writing implements and materials, children communed at the writing table, engaged in self-initiated projects, and worked independently or in collaboration with peers. There were pencils, crayons, and markers on a supply shelf filled with writing materials. The children shared the common space but maintained respect for personal space. Children went to other areas of the classroom whenever they needed writing implements or supplies that were not available in their area. Children also used classroom resources such as name cards, picture dictionaries, and environmental print as they worked on writing-related activities. Although the practice of writing took place in other areas that had writing implements available, such as the block area or the dramatic play area, most children communed at the writing table. The writing table was a social space that welcomed experimentation, learning, and exchange of ideas among peers. Work time provided abundant opportunities and adequate space for children to engage in various forms of explorations. Within the structure of work time, children at the writing table worked with a personal agenda. For instance, children were found

Table 11.1   Irina and Mindy—Name Writing

Irina:	Which one do you want me to make your name in? [Refers to color of the crayon preferred by Mindy.]
Mindy:	Red . . . in a pattern . . . like red-blue, red-blue.
Irina:	Mindy . . . [Searches for Mindy's name card and finds it among 13 others.]
Mindy:	M . . . I . . . N . . . D . . . Y . . . [Spells her name for Irina.]
Irina:	M . . . I . . . N . . . [Writes letters using the colored pattern described by Mindy.] D . . . [Writes the letter D in reverse.]
Mindy:	Did you know that's backwards? [Refers to the letter D written by Irina.]
Irina:	[Irina is engrossed with picking a specific color of crayon.] I'm gonna make the Y a special color. I'm gonna make it rainbow. [Instead of writing a Y, however, Irina ends up writing the letter A]
Mindy:	A?! [Mindy is unable to conceal her disappointment. Irina attempts to conceal her mistake by coloring the letter A with green crayon.]
Irina:	This is some grass between. [In an attempt to conceal the letter A, she writes the letter Y in black and outlines it.]
Mindy:	[Remains quiet as she works on her book.]

composing stories, generating lists, making signs, inventing secret codes, and writing letters. As children engaged in writing, they talked about what they were writing and *how* they were writing. In the following transcript, Irina and Mindy are working on separate writing projects. As Mindy worked on writing her book, Irina was writing up a birthday list that contained names of their classmates whom she planned to invite to her birthday party. She used name cards as a reference to spell and copy the names of her friends. Since Mindy was her best friend, she wrote her name first (see Table 11.1).

Although Irina meant to write Mindy's name accurately, she ended up writing one of the letters in her friend's name in reverse. Why did it matter to Mindy whether or not her name is spelled correctly and the letters faithfully encoded? Irina discovered that *writing her friend's name beautifully was just as valuable as writing it accurately.* In spite of Irina's attempts to remedy her mistake, Mindy's disappointment, though silent, appeared quite pronounced.

This transcript reveals how emergent writers like Mindy and Irina are aware of conventional ways of writing letters and words, particularly their peer's name. Name writing was a common practice in the prekindergarten classroom observed in this study. Berk (2000) indicated that by the age of 2, children have begun to develop a sense of self, which helps them to classify themselves as the same or different from others. Aside from self-identification, name writing gives us a glimpse into the emergent literacy skills of young children (Haney, 2002). Irina's use of name cards reveals her resourcefulness as a writer as well as her desire to write the names of her peers accurately. Her knowledge of patterns and one-to-one correspondence were apparent as she copied the letters in Mindy's name. Hence, when Irina accidentally reversed and misrepresented the last two letters in Mindy's name, she made an attempt to conceal her error by decorating around the letters.

In this classroom, children made an effort to consult their friends or refer to classroom resources such as name cards to check the spelling of their friends' name (Tolentino, 2004). Spelling their name accurately has begun to matter. Their literate acts reflect how their knowledge of literacy has moved toward more conventional forms. In this particular episode, children consulted their peers about spelling the letters in their names to further enrich their work and fulfill their intent. They also seemed to be aware that print conveyed a message, and that it was important to be accurate.

In this episode, writing was a means to fulfill a bigger agenda— generating a birthday list. Children like Irina were bringing their knowledge of letters, sounds, and patterns into the interpersonal plane (Vygotsky, 1978). Emergent writers are at different points in their literacy development (Clay, 1991). This was true of Mindy and Irina. Mindy knew letter names, sound-letter relationships, the direction of letters, and the order of letters in words. Irina, on the other hand, had developed literate behaviors such as consulting environmental resources that enable them to fulfill intent. Some emergent writers recognize the shapes of letters and their equivalent sound; others may be able to write them in conventional forms; while still others may invent their own representations. Therefore, coming together and exchanging ideas through talk gives emergent writers opportunities to learn and transform each other's schema. Rosenblatt (1969) acknowledged that emergent writers are equipped with "linguistic and life experiences" (p. 42) that prepare them for the act of reading and writing. Conversations reveal how young children construct or transform their knowledge as well as their linguistic and life experiences while interacting with peers.

CHILDREN AND THEIR SOCIAL WORLD: ESTABLISHING CONNECTIONS

The talk episode that follows depicts the same participants, Irina and Mindy, working side by side at the writing table the next day. While Mindy continued to pursue her writing project, Irina continued generating a list of people whom she planned to invite to her birthday party. As Irina worked on her list, she used an organizing system that distinguished friends whom she intended to invite to her birthday party and those whom she did not plan to invite. Irina was sorting name cards among two piles: a "Yes" pile and a "No" pile. She designed a system wherein she matched the number of letters in each child's name to determine whether or not they would match as friends. She paired up the name cards of friends who had the same number of letters in their names. A perfect match between the number of letters among the names of children established their connection as friends, and their name cards would be placed together on what Irina labeled the Yes pile (see Table 11.2).

Table 11.2 Irina and Mindy—Finding Equivalence

Irina:	1 . . . 2 . . . 3 . . . 4 . . . 5 . . . 6 [Counts the letters in Jeremy's name.]
	1 . . . 2 . . . 3 . . . 4 . . . 5 . . . 6 [Counts the letters in Jilian's name and realizes that it has the same number as Jeremy's. She then puts Jeremy's and Jilian's namecards together, the first pair in a pile]
	1 . . . 2 . . . 3 . . . 4 . . . [Counts the letters in Mindy's name but remains uncertain when she gets to the last letter. Previously, when Irina wrote Mindy's name, she had made a mistake as she wrote the last letter and proceeded to conceal the error with some grass and rewriting the last letter in Mindy's name.]
	1 . . . 2 . . . 3 . . . 4 . . . [Counts the letters of Mindy's name once more and appears to remain uncertain as she missed counting the last letter.] Mindy: Five. [Points to the last letter in her name.]
Irina:	Five? [Repeats to herself, and realizes that she missed counting the last letter in Mindy's name.]
	Goody. [Satisfied.]
	That's four. [Referring to the equivalence in number of paired names: Jilian and Jeremy; Mindy and Irina.]
	1 . . . 2 . . . 3 . . . 4 . . . 5 . . . [Counts the letters in her own name.]
	Five? [To herself.]

(Continued)

Table 11.2   (Continued)

	Five. [Confirms that her name has the same number as Mindy's; then draws a line that connects the letters of her name with Mindy's.]
	So we connect if there's five.
	We connect if there's 1 . . . 2 . . . 3 . . . 4 . . . [Counts the letters in Joan's name; Joan is Mindy and Irina's best friend.]
	We connect if there's 1 . . . 2 . . . 3 . . . 4 . . . [Counts the letters in Joan's name once more.]
	Nope. [Shakes her head with a look of disappointment.]
	We do *not* connect to Joan.
Irina:	Yes, Chen, thank you. [Puts Chen's name on the Yes pile.]
	C . . . H . . . E . . . N . . . [Copies Chen's name onto her list]
	And Evan . . . [Copies Evan's name onto her list]
	Evan! [Puts Chen's and Evan's name cards on top of the Yes pile.]

According to Eisenhauer and Feikes (2009), counting is part of children's natural world. Irina was counting almost throughout this episode, but she was also engaged in a self-initiated process of problem solving. As Irina refined her organizing system, she had created categories in the form of piles: on the Yes pile contained the name cards of children whom she planned to invite to her birthday party, and on the other pile were name cards of children whose names did not match. At the same time, she organized the piles in such a way that the name cards were organized in pairs; each pair would constitute the names of children who had the same number of letters in their names. For example, because Jilian and Jeremy both had six letters in their names, their name cards would be paired together and placed on the Yes pile; and Chen and Evan's names, each containing four letters, would be paired together and placed on the same pile. Worth noting in this vignette was the initial peer support provided by Mindy when Irina was experiencing disequilibrium. Looking back at the vignette, Irina was counting the letters in Mindy's name and stopped shortly when she thought that there were only four letters in Mindy's name. Mindy had to point out the fifth letter in her name that Irina missed. Initially stuck, Irina was able to move forward because of the peer support provided by her friend, Mindy. It appeared as though Irina was relieved that the number of letters in Mindy's name matched her own. The match seemed to signify something important to Irina, which was friendship. If one were to examine Irina's organizing system, it would appear that she had a sophisticated understanding of categories within subcategories: One category would contain pairs of cards, and a pair would constitute a match in the number of letters of a name unit. While demonstrating one-to-one correspondence between the letters in each name, she was also accurately counting letters and coordinating number words with letter names in a collection.

Through this episode, Irina demonstrates emergent numeracy skills: she was counting, sorting, categorizing, and establishing one-to-one correspondence. Aside from building numerical competence, she was demonstrating emergent literacy skills. She was referring to each child's name card and reading the name on each card; copying the letters in each name accurately onto her list; and demonstrating directionality by writing each name from left to right, and top to bottom. Her list served her personal needs, as it contained the names of children whom she classified under the Yes pile, the pile that had the names of children whom she had planned to invite to her party whose names matched by virtue of the number of letters. It appeared that names, connections, and friendships were important to Irina as she established her organizing system and as she prepared her invitation list. While emergent literacy skills enabled Irina to develop lists of her friends' names, emergent numeracy skills empowered her to determine correspondences between names. At the same time, she was fulfilling multiple tasks: generating a list, thinking through her decisions, justifying her reasons for classifying elements within categories and subcategories, and engaging in higher-order thinking of mathematical and literacy concepts. The vignette reveals how children like Irina incorporate both mathematical and literacy skills in the context of everyday tasks. She was gathering data, comparing quantities, configuring patterns, and making symbols. Preschool children like Irina are capable of spontaneously and creatively engaging in advanced mathematical activities (Ginsburg, Inoue, & Seo, 1999). As Ginsburg, Inoue, and Seo (1999) pointed out, preschool children, even in the context of free play, "create and extend complex patterns, building intricately balanced and symmetrical structures, and solve multistep problems" (p. 92). Irina demonstrated her ability to engage in mathematical discourse (Harper, Boggan, & Tucker, 2008). At the same time, she was engaged in reading and writing, both of which are literacy skills. Even as a 4-year-old, children like Irina have already come to value and apply mathematical and literacy concepts in the context of daily life and to fulfill personal needs.

WHERE MATH AND LITERACY INTERSECT: CHILDREN'S STORY WRITING

The children in the classroom I observed also engaged in book making and story dictation. It was common to see children at the writing table, writing their story or illustrating their texts. Book writers had the opportunity to share their book with their classmates during story time at the end of the day. They were given time to work on their books during work time. Thus, work time was a venue for book writers to continue working on their material. If children needed assistance, they were encouraged to consult their peer or seek help from a teacher. What follows is a story entitled "My Basketball Book," composed and illustrated by Jilian and shown in Figures 11.7 through 11.13. Jilian had watched a live basketball game with his father and wanted to share his story with the rest of the class. Guided by his teacher, he worked on "My Basketball Book" for a week. He first illustrated the events that he recalled from the basketball game and then dictated the words of his story to his teacher, who in turn, transcribed the text for Jilian.

Jilian's familiarity with basketball as a sport seems clear. He appeared to know the objective of the game—to shoot as many baskets as possible; he noted the scores on the scoreboard; and he appeared to be aware that the scores reflected the performance of the team members. Jilian also

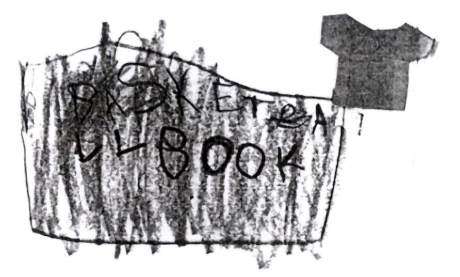

Figure 11.7   Title: My Basketball Book.

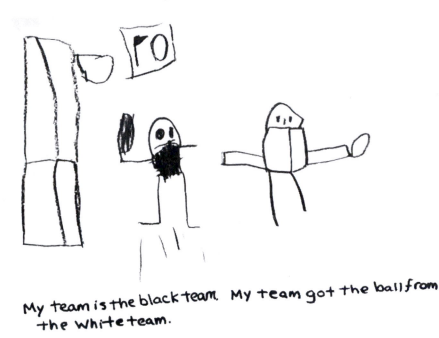

My team is the black team. My team got the ball from the white team.

Figure 11.8　Page 1: My team is the Black Team. My team got the ball from the White Team.

used language that was common to sports spectators: "The game is tied up—2 to 2!" Jilian's ability to recount events and retell them in the form of a text narrative is impressive. This requires reminiscing and rehearsal of events on his part, thoughtful attention to detail, and awareness of audience. As he recounted the events, he also had to retell them in a way that was clear and comprehensible to his listeners and readers. His dictated text entitled "My Basketball Book" had a beginning, middle, and end. It had the elements of a story—namely, setting, characters, plot, rising action, conflict, and resolution. Jilian's text also revealed his understanding of grammatical structures of language and conventions of text. He had a cover page, which contained the title, and an end page for his text. He demonstrated print awareness and appeared to know that the print on the page conveyed the meaning of his illustrations. His pages were arranged in sequence, making the story both logical and cohesive to his readers.

At the same time, Jilian seemed to make a conscious effort in making his story as authentic as possible to his readers. His illustrations appear

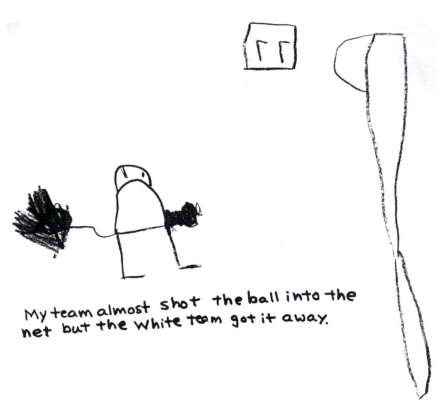

My team almost shot the ball into the net but the White team got it away.

Figure 11.9   Page 2: My team almost shot the ball into the net but the White Team got it away.

to faithfully represent parts of the game that he was able to recount. Authenticity appears to be a characteristic valued by novice writers as they seek to create a trustworthy representation of their story (Tolentino, 2004). Jilian's book reveals that he is a writer who is aware of story genre and is able to use his knowledge of literacy as a means to tell his story. Looking at the same book from a mathematical lens, it appears that Jilian is confident in his ability to apply math in his own life. He used numbers in a highly specific situation: to keep score. He demonstrated his awareness of the importance of the increase in the scores and in the consequence of every change of numbers. On his own, Jilian was intuitively applying mathematical principles (Krogh & Slentz, 2001). The story composed by Jilian reveals that he is becoming mathematically literate and developing the voice of a writer.

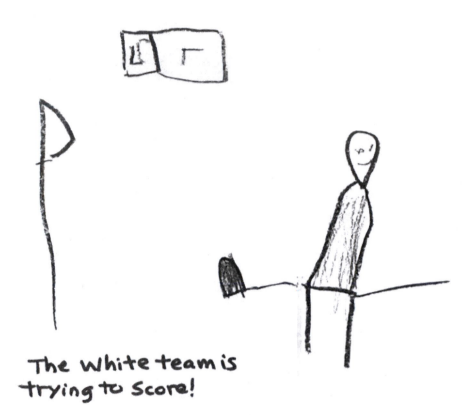

The white team is trying to score!

Figure 11.10   Page 3: The White Team is trying to score!

THE ENVIRONMENT AS "THE THIRD TEACHER": CONTEXTS THAT NURTURE YOUNG CHILDREN'S PURSUIT OF LITERACY AND MATHEMATICS

The seeds of mathematics and literacy are planted long before children enter the realm of school (Bodrova, Leong, & Paynter, 1999). As demonstrated in the four episodes within this chapter, the artifacts and dialogue produced by the children reveal their "growing understanding of written language and the conventions of print" (Millard & Waese, 2007, p. 9). They also demonstrate young children's natural ability to incorporate mathematical concepts in everyday context. The episodes unfolded naturally and spontaneously; but worth considering is how each context was structured to provoke the kind of dialogue, artifacts,

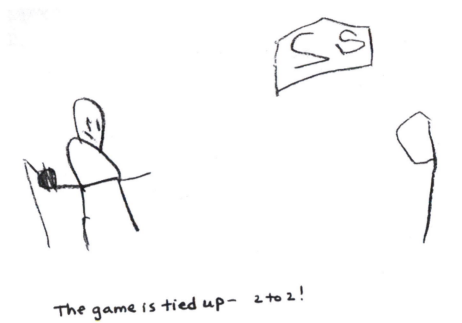

The game is tied up— 2 to 2!

Figure 11.11   Page 4: The game is tied up—2 to 2!

and interactions among the participants. In what ways did the environment teach?

The concept of environment as the third teacher is rooted in the Reggio Emilia approach to early care and education. The Reggio Emilia approach originated in Italy and was inspired by constructivist perspectives of Jean Piaget; social constructivist ideas of Lev Vygotsky, Jerome Bruner, and John Dewey; and the revolutionary ideas of Paolo Freire (Malaguzzi, 1996). The Reggio Emilia approach is rooted in the belief that children are protagonists in their learning and that teachers and parents work in partnership to support the development and well-being of young children (Malaguzzi, 1998). It is an approach that makes children's ideas visible and their questions central to the development of curriculum. The Reggio Emilia approach capitalizes on the value of space and materials within the learning environment and their instructional potential. The learning environment can be structured in ways that provoke inquiry, encourage investigation, and invite dialogue.

This chapter provided documentation that was generated from two different environments: home and school. In both contexts, children

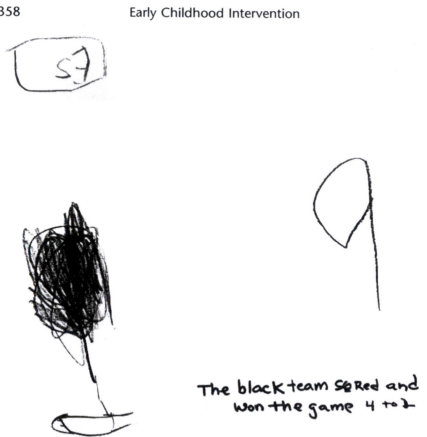

The black team scored and
won the game 4 to 2

Figure 11.12   Page 5: The Black Team scored and won the game 4 to 2.

gravitated toward the writing space and used the materials within the space to carry out their personal agenda. In the home context, materials served as tools to enable a young child to represent ideas that his speech could not clearly articulate. In the context of the classroom, the children used the time and space provided to pursue writing projects such as creating a list and writing a story. In both contexts, children were constructing and sharing ideas and interpreting meaning both socially and cognitively. Halliday (1978) described this exchange of meanings as a creative process of using language as a "symbolic resource" (p. 3) within a social structure. As children interact with their environment, they become part of a semiotic system, where meanings are constructed and exchanged. The semiotic structure can be interpreted on three dimensions: field or ongoing activity, tenor or the roles and relationships involved, and mode or field of action in which meanings are

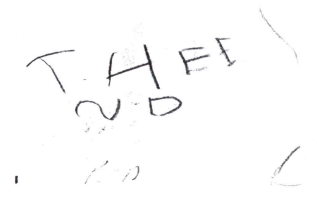

Figure 11.13   Page 6: The End.

expressed. These three components determine the nature of texts (verbal and nonverbal) that emerge from the participants. In the contexts of dialogue at home, young children learn to participate in communicative acts that are valued by the members of the child's culture. In the context of school, young children learn to participate in activities that are valued within the classroom. Children come to realize that they play a part in the meaning-making that transpires in the home and in school.

The Learning Environment: Field

Field refers to the learning environment: the activity, setting, and materials. In both the home context and the school context, the writing table served as a space for children to fulfill their personal agenda. Providing children with resources, tools, and concrete objects empower them as learners (Bennett, Elliot, & Peters, 2005). Because children were equipped with materials and tools, they were able to draw representations of their ideas, generate a birthday list, and write a story.

Beyond the physical space, the tone of the environment conveys the beliefs and attitudes toward mathematics and literacy learning. In both contexts, children were deeply engaged in their work because they were fulfilling a personal need and realized that their work had value. Across all the contexts, the children had an innate desire to make sense of the world, to figure things out, and to make connections. As noted earlier, the children made an effort to be authentic in their representations, whether they were drawing a backhoe, spelling their friend's name, matching the letters to establish a connection between pairs, or recounting the sequence of events in a basketball game. From the way they responded to the resources provided, it was apparent that they have seen how materials such as writing implements, birthday invitations, and stories are created and used by the members of their culture (Varol & Farran, 2006). It is then safe to say that providing children with opportunities to develop mathematical and literacy concepts within an environment that actively encourages them to engage in literacy acts and problem solving can transform a space in ways that will advance both mathematical and literacy learning (Aram & Biron, 2004; Bodrova, Leong, & Paynter, 1999; Nel, 2000). The activities in which the children engaged were open-ended, choice-driven, and self-initiated. The children's mathematical and literacy understandings emerged through their interactions and playful activities in their natural world, whether in a nurturing home environment or in the context of a classroom (Eisenhauer & Feikes, 2009; Sarama & Clements, 2009). In the same vein, early childhood teachers believe in the importance of fostering literacy and mathematics skills by providing materials and resources that provoke literacy and mathematics learning (Lee & Ginsburg, 2007).

Tenor: Relationships and Roles

Tenor is the relationship between the participants (Halliday, 1978). In every relationship, participants take on a role. The nature of the social interaction and the meanings produced are influenced by the roles that participants play within the context. At the heart of the learning environments presented in this chapter are relationships: parent-child, peer-to-peer, expert-novice, and teacher-child. Within the context of parent-child relationships, children are provided the scaffolding needed to enable them to go a step further in their learning. Children are highly motivated to convey their ideas clearly to another. In the case of my child, he proactively created strategies to represent his ideas. He had opportunities to feel like an expert, one who feels competent in his skills. He had opportunities to develop ownership for his learning.

Because learning is a social process, it is natural for children to gravitate toward a fellow participant within the context. In the classroom episodes, Irina was in close proximity to Mindy as she wrote her birthday list. They engaged in dialogue even as they were doing different writing projects. At times, Mindy provided Irina with the support that she needed to enable her to continue her work. Jilian, on the other hand, worked in collaboration with his teacher. While it appeared that he knew how powerful his illustrations were in telling a story, he intuitively knew that words were just as important in writing a book. Jilian took the initiative to ask for assistance from his teacher to complete his project. As illustrated in the examples, learning is a social process. Children learn from their parents, teachers, and peers, but because they are also participants in various activities of their culture, they can be each other's teachers and provide just as much support as adults can. Children can be conversational partners, literacy scaffolds, and problem solvers.

Mode: Children's Talk, Play and Stories

A child-centered environment is a nurturing, playful environment that encourages children to use various modes of representation. This environment acknowledges children's natural interests, unique learning styles, and academic capacities (Project Zero & Reggio Children, 2001). An environment that encourages play, dialogue, drawing, gesturing, and signing conveys to the children that their ideas can be expressed in a hundred languages (Malaguzzi, 1996). The children featured in the various contexts were clearly equipped with an understanding of their world and their own ideas of space, relationships, and quantity (Baroody & Wilkins, 1999; Copley, 2000). Through their drawings, conversations, lists, and books, they were constructing mathematical and literacy concepts on their own, incorporating them into their natural world.

IN PURSUIT OF A CHILD-CENTRIC APPROACH TO LITERACY AND MATH INSTRUCTION

The children presented in this chapter were emergent readers, writers, and mathematical thinkers. Up to the point the study was undertaken, they had no previous exposure to formal literacy or mathematics instruction. Nevertheless, the children were already expressing their knowledge of literacy and mathematics in a way that came naturally. This is most likely because young children are curious and creative. In the context of their daily lives, they apply insight and inquiry as they solve problems and various situations that involve quantities, relationships, symbols, and story. The true question is: how much have we capitalized on the knowledge that children have? Are our educational and care contexts open and accepting of children's ideas and dispositions about learning? When children enter school, are knowledge and concepts accessible to them? Are they presented within their zone (Vygotsky, 1978)? When teaching methods, content, and approaches do not align with the children's knowledge, strategies, and learning approaches, they are unable to find meaning and use in what they are taught. They experience dissonance as they seek to connect what is taught with what is known.

With the advent of No Child Left Behind, there has been a movement toward teacher accountability and for student academic achievement. Unfortunately, the standards-based accountability movement has created unnecessary pressure on academic achievement among children. As a result, instruction is driven by curriculum models that address outcomes and standards rather than an approach to curriculum that is child-initiated and child-generated. This gives children little time to think, process, and reflect upon what they are learning. Teachers and children also find themselves caught in a tug-of-war between a skills-emphasis view and a meaning-emphasis view of reading and writing.

As far as reading and writing instruction are concerned, there does not need to be one method of teaching that separates skill instruction from meaning-centered instruction. Instead, teachers need to be equipped with as many methods as is possible to support children as literacy learners. Perhaps instead of imposing what children need to learn about reading and writing and expecting them to regurgitate the information, teachers can build upon what children already know about reading, writing, and ways of making meaning. If this is made possible by every teacher in every classroom of emergent readers and writers, then perhaps the process of becoming literate will be a more meaningful experience.

Early childhood teachers can create a balance between adult-directed and child-initiated activities (Bodrova & Leong, 1995). Teachers can create spaces within their classroom that strengthen children's competence while also nurturing their imagination, energy, and curiosities (Andrews & Trafton, 2002). Early childhood teachers can build upon the foundations of knowledge that young children have started to build on their own. As teachers, we are in a position to start from where the children are, allowing them to continue investigating questions that are important to them, building from what they know and furthering their knowledge (Eisenhauer & Feikes, 2009). Most of all, we need to foster secure relationships that will see children through the challenges of the real world.

REFERENCES

Anderson-Yockel, J., & Haynes, W. O. (1994). *Joint book-reading strategies in working class African-American and white mother-toddler dyads*. Norwood, NJ: Ablex.

Andrews, A., & Trafton, P. R. (2002). *Little kids—powerful problem solvers: Math stories from a kindergarten classroom*. Portsmouth, NH: Heinemann.

Antell, S., & Keating, D. (1983). Perception of numerical invariance in neonates. *Child Development, 54,* 695–701.

Aram, D., & Biron, S. (2004). Joint storybook reading and joint writing interventions among low SES preschoolers: Differential contributions to early literacy. *Early Childhood Research Quarterly, 19,* 588–610.

Au, K. (1980, Summer). Participation structures in a reading lesson with Hawaiian children: Analysis of a culturally appropriate institutional event. *Anthropology and Education Quarterly, 11*(2), 91–115.

Baroody, A. J., & Wilkins, J. L. M. (1999). The development of informal counting, numbers, and arithmetic skills and concepts. In J. V. Copley (Ed.), *Mathematics in the early years* (pp. 48–65). Reston, VA: National Council of Teachers of Mathematics.

Bartsch, K., & Wellman, H. M. (1995). *Children talk about the mind*. New York: Oxford University Press.

Benigno, J., & Ellis, S. (2004). Two is greater than three: Effects of older siblings on parental support of preschoolers' counting in middle-income families. *Early Childhood Research Quarterly, 19,* 4–20.

Bennett, P., Elliot, M., & Peters, D. (2005). Classroom and family effects on children's social and behavioral problems. *Elementary School Journal, 105*(5), 461–499.

Berk, L. E. (2000). *Child Development* (5th ed.). Needham Heights, MA: Allyn & Bacon.

Bodrova, E., & Leong, D. J. (1995). *Tools of the mind: A Vygotsian approach to early childhood education*. New York: Prentice Hall.

Bodrova, E., Leong, D. J., & Paynter, D. E. (1999). Literacy standards for preschool learners. *Educational Leadership, 57*(2), 42–46.

Britton, J. (1970). *Language and learning*. London: Penguin Press.

Bruner, J. S. (1996). *The culture of education*. Cambridge, MA: Harvard University Press.

Clay, M. M. (1991). *Becoming literate: The construction of inner control*. Auckland, New Zealand: Heinemann.

Clements, D. H. (2004). Perspective on "The Child's Thought and Geometry." In T. P. Carpenter, J. A. Dossey, & J. L. Koehler (Eds.)., *Classics in mathematics education research* (p. 60). Reston, VA: National Council of Teachers of Mathematics.

Copley, J. V. (2000). *The young child and mathematics*. Washington, DC: National Association for the Education of Young Children.

Eisenhauer, M., & Feikes, D. (2009). Dolls, blocks, and puzzles: Playing with mathematical understandings, *Young Children, 64*(3), 18–24.

Flanagan, K. D., McPhee, C., & Mulligan, G. (2009). The children born in 2001 at kindergarten entry: First findings from the kindergarten data collections of the Early Childhood Longitudinal Study, Birth Cohort (ECLS-B) NCES 2010-005. National Center for Education Statistics, Institute of Education Sciences, U.S. Department of Education.

Fryer, R. G., & Levitt, S. D. (2004, May). Understanding the Black-White test score gap in the first two years of school. *Review of Economics and Statistics, 86*(2), 447–464.

Gelman, S. A. (2009). Learning from others: Children's construction of concepts. *Annual Review of Psychology* (Vol. 60). Palo Alto, CA: Annual Reviews.

Ginsburg, H. P., Inoue, N., & Seo, K. (1999). Young children doing mathematics: Observations of everyday activities. In J. V. Copley (Ed.), *Mathematics in the early years* (pp. 88–99). Reston, VA: National Council of Teachers of Mathematics.

Golomb, C. (1981). Representation and reality: The origins and determinants of young children's drawings. *Review of Research in Visual Art Education, 14*, 36–48.

Goodnow, J. J. (1977). *Children drawing.* Cambridge, MA: Harvard University Press.

Guba, E. G., & Lincoln, Y. (1989). *Fourth generation evaluation.* Newbury Park, CA: Sage Publications.

Halliday, M. A. K. (1978). *Language as a social semiotic: The social interpretation of language and meaning.* Maryland: University Park Press.

Haney, M. R. (2002). Name writing: A window into the emergent literacy skills of young children. *Early Childhood Education Journal, 30*(20), 101–105.

Harper, S., Boggan, M. K., & Tucker, C. (2008, Fall). Using children's literature to teach math. *Southeastern Teacher Education Journal, 1*(1), 77–83.

Harris, D. B. (1963). Children's drawings as measures of intellectual maturity. San Diego, CA: Harcourt, Brace, & World.

Head Start Bureau. (2001). Head Start Child Outcomes Framework. *Head Start Bulletin, 70*, 44–50.

Holdaway, D. (1979). *The foundations of literacy.* South Portsmouth, NH: Heinemann Educational Books.

International Reading Association & National Association for the Education of Young Children. (1998). *Overview of learning to read and write: Developmentally appropriate practices for young children.* A joint position of the International Reading Association (IRA) and the National Association for the Education of Young Children (NAEYC). Washington, DC: NAEYC

Jaggar, A. M. (1985). On observing the language learner: Introduction and overview. In A. M. Jaggar & M. T. Smith-Burke (Eds.), *Observing the language learner* (pp. 1–7). Newark, DE: International Reading Association.

Kellogg, R. (1969). *Analyzing children's art.* Palo Alto, CA: National Press Books.

Kennedy, A., & Surman, L. (2003). Literacy transitions. In L. Makin & C. J. Diaz (Eds.), *Literacies in early childhood: Changing views, challenging practice* (pp. 104–117). Sydney, NSW, Australia: MacLennan and Petty.

Krogh, S., & Slentz, K. (2001). *The Early Childhood Curriculum.* Mahwah, NJ: Lawrence Erlbaum Associates.

Lapadat, J. (1994). *Learning language and learning literacy construction of meaning through discourse.* University of Northern British Columbia.

Lee, J. S., & Ginsburg, H. P. (2007). Preschool teachers' beliefs about appropriate early literacy and mathematics education for low- and middle-socioeconomic status children. *Early Education and Development, 18*(1), 111–143.

Leseman, P. P. M. (1999). Home and school literacy in a multicultural society. In L. Eldering & P. P. M. Leseman (Eds.), *Effective early education: Cross-cultural perspectives*. New York: Falmer Press.

Lipton, J. S., & Spelke, E. S. (2003). Origins of number sense: Large number discrimination in human infants. *Psychological Science, 14*, 396–401.

Malaguzzi, L. (1996). *The hundred languages of children: Narrative of the possible*. Reggio Emilia, Italy: Reggio Children.

Malaguzzi, L. (1998). History, ideas, and basic philosophy: An interview with Leila Gandini. In C. Edwards, L. Gandini, & G. Forman (Eds.), *The hundred languages of children: The Reggio Emilia approach—advanced reflections* (2nd ed.). Greenwich, CT: Ablex.

Matthews, J. (1984). Children drawing: Are young children really scribbling? *Early Child Development and Care, 18*(1–2), 1–39.

Millard, R., & Waese, M. (2007). *Language and Literacy, from birth . . . for life* [Research summary]. Ontario: Canadian Language and Literacy Research Network.

National Association for the Education of Young Children (NAYEC) and the National Council of Teachers of Mathematics. (2002). *Early childhood mathematics: Promoting good beginnings*. Retrieved from http://www.naeyc.org/files/naeyc/file/positions/psmath.pdf

National Center for Education Statistics. (2009, March). *Comparative indicators of education in the United States and Other G-8 Countries: 2009*. Institute of Education Sciences, U.S. Department of Education.

National Center for Education Statistics. (2009, October). The children born in 2001 at kindergarten entry: First findings from the kindergarten data collections of the early childhood longitudinal study, birth cohort (ECLS-B). Institute of Education Sciences, U.S. Department of Education.

Natriello, G., McDill, E., & Pallas, A. (1990). *Schooling disadvantaged students: Racing against catastrophe*. New York: Teachers College Press.

Nel, E. (2000). Academics, literacy and young children: A plea for a middle ground. *Childhood Education, 76*(3), 136–141.

Nelson, K., & Fivush, R. (2004, April). The emergence of autobiographical memory: A social cultural developmental. *Psychological Review, 111*(2), 486–511.

Neuman, S. B., & Celano, D. (2001). Access to print in low-income and middle-income communities: An ecological study of four neighborhoods. *Reading Research Quarterly, 32*, 10–32.

Neuman, S. B., & Roskos, K. (2005). The state of state prekindergarten standards. *Early Childhood Research Quarterly, 20*(2), 125–145.

Pellegrini, A. D., Galda, L., Jones, I., & Perlmutter, J. (1995). *Joint reading between mothers and their Head Start children. Discourse Processes, 19*(3), 441–463.

Project Zero & Reggio Children. (2001). *Making learning visible: Children as individual and group learners*. Reggio Emilia, Italy: Reggio Children.

Purcell-Gates, V. (1996). Stories, coupons, and the TV Guide: Relationships between home literacy experience and emergent literacy knowledge, *Reading Research Quarterly, 31*(4), 406–428.

Rosenblatt, L. M. (1969, Winter). Towards a transactional theory of reading. *Journal of Reading Behavior, 1*, 31–49.

Ruffman, T., Slade, L., & Crowe, E. (2002, May–June). The relation between children's and mothers' mental state language and theory-of-mind understanding. *Child Development, 73*(3), 734–751.

Sarama, J., & Clements, D. H. (2009). Building blocks and cognitive building blocks: Playing to know the world mathematically. *American Journal of Play, 1* (3), 313–337.

Schickedanz, J., & Casbergue, R. M. (2004). *Writing in preschool: Learning to orchestrate meaning and marks.* Newark, DE: International Reading Association.

Scollon, R., & Scollon, S. B. K. (1981). *Narrative, literacy, and face in interethnic communication.* Norwood, NJ: Ablex.

Sonnenschein, S., Brody, G., & Munsterman, K. (1996). The influence of family beliefs and practices on children's early reading development. In L. Cohen, P. Afflerbach, & D. Reinking (Eds.). *Developing engaged readers in school and home communities* (pp. 3–20). Mahwah, NJ: Lawrence Erlbaum Associates.

Stipek, D. J., & Ryan, R. H. (1997). Economically disadvantaged preschoolers: Ready to learn but further to go. *Developmental Psychology, 33,* 711–723.

Symons, S., Souskiewicz, T., & Bonnell, C. (1996). Parental print exposure and young children's language and literacy skills. *Alberta Journal of Educational Research, 42,* 49–58.

Thompson, R. A. (2006, January). Conversation and developing understanding: Introduction to the special issue. *Merrill-Palmer Quarterly, 52*(1), 1–16.

Tolentino, E. P. (2004). "I don't know if I can read this, but I can read the pictures": The role of talk in emergent literacy. Unpublished doctoral dissertation, New York University.

University of the State of New York and the State Education Department. (2002). *Mathematics core curriculum.* New York: Author.

U.S. Department of Education. (2003). Good start, grow smart. Retrieved from http://www.acf.hhs.gov/programs/ccb/initiatives/gsgs/gsgs_guide/guide .htm

Van Kraayenoord, C. E., & Paris, S. G. (1996, March). Story construction from a picture book: An assessment activity for young learners. *Early Childhood Research Quarterly, 11*(1), 41–61.

Varol, F., & Farran, D. C. (2006, June). Early mathematical growth: How to support young Children's mathematical development. *Early Childhood Education Journal, 33*(6), 381–387.

Vygotsky, L. S. (1978). *Mind in society: The development of higher psychological processes* (M. Cole, V. John-Steiner, S. Scribner, & E. Souberman, Eds. & Trans.). Cambridge, MA: Harvard University Press. [Original work published 1934].

Wells, G. (1986). *The meaning makers.* Portsmouth, NH: Heinemann.

Wolf, D., & Perry, M. D. (1988). From endpoints to repertoires: Some new conclusions about drawing development. *Journal of Aesthetic Education, Special Issue: Art and Mind Education, 22*(1), 17–34.

Wood, D., Bruner, J. S., & Ross, G. (1976, April). The role of tutoring in problem-solving. *Journal of Early Child Psychology, 17*(2), 89–100.

Wright, S. (1997). Learning how to learn: The arts as core in an emergent curriculum. *Childhood Education, 73,* 361–365.

About the Editor and Contributors

EDITOR

Susan P. Maude, PhD, is an Associate Professor in the Department of Human Development and Family Studies, College of Human Sciences at Iowa State University. Her research interests include inclusive personnel preparation, program evaluation in early intervention and early childhood special education, and innovative ways to evaluate diversity within programs. She has worked as a practitioner, researcher, faculty member, and/or program evaluator across multiple states (Connecticut, Illinois, Indiana, Iowa, Oregon, Pennsylvania, and Vermont) and has evaluated statewide as well as national professional development initiatives. Dr. Maude is a past-president of the International Division for Early Childhood (DEC) at the Council for Exceptional Children (CEC). DEC is a national organization dedicated to promoting policies and practices that aid the development of young children with special needs and their families.

CONTRIBUTORS

Rashida Banerjee, PhD, is an Assistant Professor and Early Childhood Special Education Program coordinator in the School of Special Education at the University of Northern Colorado. Her main emphasis has been acting as a catalyst to promote quality services for children with disabilities and their families in early intervention/early childhood programs. Her research areas and interests include: effective inclusive intervention for young children with multiple and severe disabilities; teacher preparation and effective community, family, and professional partnerships. She is an alumnus of the Ford Foundation International Fellowships program and is a recipient of the J. David Sexton Doctoral

Student Scholarship Award from the Division for Early Childhood of the Council for Exceptional Children and the Division for Research Award (Quantitative methods) of the Council for Exceptional Children.

Sandy K. Bowen, PhD, is a Professor in the School of Special Education at the University of Northern Colorado. Her area of emphasis is in the education of students who are deaf or hard of hearing. She has worked with infants, children, and youth who are deaf/hard of hearing in Utah, Texas, Arizona, and Colorado for 20 years. Her research interests include: teacher preparation, literacy development, early intervention, and Hispanic deaf/hard of hearing students and families, and multicultural issues in deafness. She is fluent in American Sign Language and Spanish. In addition to her university assignments, she is an early interventionist in the Colorado Early Intervention Program working with infants and toddlers who are deaf or hard of hearing and their families. She publishes in the field of deafness and is a contributing author to the *SKI-HI* Curriculum Manual for interventionists working with infants and toddlers who are deaf.

Cornelia Bruckner, PhD, is an Adjunct Faculty at San Francisco State University. Dr. Bruckner's research focus is in autism (e.g., early symptoms of autism in the younger sibling of children with autism and prelinguistic communication in young children with autism). She is currently a research associate with the Desired Results Access Project to measure young children's with disabilities development across the country. Her research in collaboration with Paul Yoder has been published in the *American Journal of Mental Retardation* and in international journals including *Autism*.

Susan B. Campbell, PhD, is Professor of Psychology and Psychiatry and Chair of the Developmental Program in the Department of Psychology at the University of Pittsburgh. Her research interests include social and emotional development in children with an emphasis on the early detection of behavior and developmental problems; her work also examines parent-child relationships and family risk, most notably maternal depression. Dr. Campbell's current research focuses on the early social development of infants and toddlers at familial/genetic risk to develop autism. She is a former Editor of the *Journal of Abnormal Child Psychology* and a former Chair of the Publication Committee of the *Society for Research in Child Development*.

Lynette K. Chandler, PhD, is Associate Chair and Professor in the Department of Teaching and Learning at Northern Illinois University where she teaches courses in early childhood special education and applied behavior analysis. Her research interests and publications have focused on early language and literacy, Response to Intervention, functional assessment, inclusion, social skills, and transition. She is a past-president of the International Division for Early Childhood of the Council for Exceptional Children. She currently collaborates with several preschools programs on Response to Intervention models to promote early language and literacy skills.

Nasiah Cirincione Ulezi, EdD, is an Assistant Professor at Chicago State University. Dr. Cirincione-Ulezi has worked extensively in the field of early childhood special education since 1995 as both a classroom teacher and a developmental therapist. She specializes in children with Autism Spectrum Disorders, and believes in working from a strength-based, family-centered philosophy. Dr. Cirincione-Ulezi serves as a Trustee on the Executive Board for the Illinois Developmental Therapy Association, a nonprofit professional organization that supports the interests of developmental therapists. Additionally, she is President of the Illinois Division for Early Childhood, a subdivision of the national DEC/CEC.

Patricia Morris Clark is an Instructor of Mental Health and Human Services at the University of Maine at Augusta, where for 10 years, she has led the Early Childhood Studies program teaching courses in early childhood and exceptionality mostly through interactive television and distance education. In 2007, Professor Clark earned a prestigious yearlong national fellowship to work at the Office of Head Start in Washington, D.C., in the Division of Training and Technical Assistance. She has more than 20 years of experience teaching in preschool, kindergarten, middle school, and adult education. Her research focuses on literacy in Head Start and preschool, and she recently completed research in London on Sure Start, the English equivalent of Head Start.

Rob Corso, PhD, is Project Coordinator for the Center on the Social and Emotional Foundations for Early Learning (CSEFEL) and an Assistant Research Professor at Vanderbilt University. Dr. Corso has also coordinated the evaluation of SpecialQuest Birth–Five project. He has conducted many large-scale evaluations of programs serving children and families and has developed outcomes frameworks for measuring the impact of in-service training for national efforts aimed at improving the capacity of Early Head Start, Migrant and Seasonal Head Start, and child care.

Sharon Doubet, PhD, is an Assistant Professor in Special Education at Illinois State University. Her research focuses on children's social/emotional skill development. She is also interested in early childhood assessment, curriculum, and teachers' support of young learners. Dr. Doubet has served as an educational consultant for the implementation of program-wide positive behavior support (early childhood) at several levels: child care centers, schools, communities, and state-level systems.

Winnie Dunn, PhD, OTR, FAOTA, is a Professor and Chair of Occupational Therapy Education, School of Allied Health, University of Kansas. Dr. Dunn is a member of the Academy of Research, and received the Ayres Research Award. She has developed the *Sensory Profiles*, measures for infants/toddlers, adolescents, and adults; these tests are used internationally. Dr. Dunn was honored as the Eleanor Clark Slagle Lecturer, the highest academic honor for Occupational Therapists in the United States in 2001. Most recently, she wrote: *Living Sensationally*, which translates her research for the public; it has been highlighted in Time magazine, on Canadian Public Radio, and in the London Times newspaper among others.

Kay Alicyn Ferrell, PhD, is Professor of Special Education and Executive Director of the National Center on Severe and Sensory Disabilities at the University of Northern Colorado. She has coordinated teacher preparation programs in both early childhood special education and visual impairment at University of Northern Colorado and at Teachers College, Columbia University. She has conducted federally-funded research in the early development of young children with visual impairment and published extensively on education of infants, children, and youth who are blind and visually impaired, including the landmark book for families, *Reach Out and Teach*.

Mary McLean, PhD, is a Kellner Professor of Early Childhood Education and Professor in the Department of Exceptional Education at the University of Wisconsin-Milwaukee, where she heads the Early

Childhood Special Education Program and is Director of the Early Childhood Research Center. She is a past-president of the International Division for Early Childhood (DEC) of the Council for Exceptional Children (CEC) and was awarded the Merle B. Karnes for Service to the Division from DEC. Dr. McLean is coauthor of two books on the DEC Recommended Practices (Sandall, McLean, & Smith, 2000; Sandall, Hemmeter, Smith, & McLean, 2005) and also two books on assessment of young children with special needs (McLean, Bailey, & Wolery, 1996; McLean, Wolery, & Bailey, 2004).

Susan M. Moore, JD, MA-SLP, CCC, is the Director of Clinical Education and Services for the Department of Speech, Language and Hearing Science at the University of Colorado, Boulder. Her publications include articles and chapters focused on working with culturally and linguistically diverse children and families, early language, and literacy learning. She has collaborated with the Denver Public Schools in the Early Reading First project to help culturally diverse children. Dr. Moore is an ASHA (American Speech Language Hearing Association) Fellow and holds Specialty Recognition in Child Language.

Clara Pérez-Méndez, Founder and Director of Puentes Culturales, was born in Mexico and has lived in the United States since 1975. Clara is an educator, nationally recognized speaker, and consultant focused on building understanding and competence for those in education who work with linguistically diverse children and families. She is a regular lecturer in both preservice and in-service programs preparing personnel to work with culturally diverse populations. Her involvement and expertise in early education include coordination of a bilingual early Child Find assessment team; consultation and workshop development with the Colorado Department of Education for training cultural mediators, interpreters, and translators; and collaboration with the University of Colorado at Boulder developing El Grupo de Familias (http://www.puentesculturales.com). Ms. Pérez-Méndez has a wealth of experience working with families from traditionally underrepresented backgrounds, especially Spanish-speaking families.

Lynda Cook Pletcher, MEd, is a Technical Assistant Specialist with the National Early Childhood Technical Assistant Center (NECTAC) at the Frank Porter Graham Child Development Institute, University of North Carolina. Her research and training interests are family-centered practices, natural environments, home-based services, service coordination, and systems change. Ms. Pletcher has worked in the field of early childhood/early intervention for over 25 years. She has provided home-based services to children and families, managed numerous outreach and training projects funded by the U.S. Office of Special Education Programs, and has been a regional and state administrator of IDEA Part C programs.

Amanda C. Quesenberry, PhD, is an Assistant Professor at Illinois State University in the Department of Curriculum and Instruction. She has worked in early childhood programs across the country as well as in local Head Start programs as a trainer and technical assistance provider. In 2007, Dr. Quesenberry completed a National Fellowship at the Office of Head Start in Washington, D.C. Her research interests include young children's social and emotional development, educators' professional development, and early childhood policy.

Patricia Snyder, PhD, is the David Lawrence Jr. Endowed Chair in Early Childhood Studies and a Professor in the School of Special Education, School Psychology, and Early Childhood Studies and the Department of Pediatrics at the University of Florida. She was founder and Director of the interdisciplinary Early Intervention Institute at the Louisiana State University Health Sciences Center and has held faculty appointments at LSU Health Sciences Center, Vanderbilt University Medical Center, and Peabody College at Vanderbilt University. She has been a recipient of the Alan A. Copping Excellence in Teaching Award from the Louisiana State University system, the Merle B. Karnes Award for Service to the International Division for Early Childhood (Council for Exceptional Children), the Article of the Year Award from the American Psychological Association (APA) Division 16, and a Service to the Profession Award from the American Occupational Therapy Association. Dr. Snyder served from 2002 to 2007 as the editor of the *Journal of Early Intervention*. She currently serves as Associate Editor, Consulting Editor and board member for several journals, including *Topics in Early Childhood Special Education, Journal of Early Intervention, American Journal on Mental Retardation, Infants and Young Children*, and *Young Exceptional Children*.

Efleda Tolentino is an Assistant Professor in the Department of Curriculum and Instruction and is also the Director of the Early Childhood Education program in the School of Education at Long Island University (C. W. Post). Being a social constructivist, she examines the teaching/

learning context: the participants, the environment, the verbal and non-verbal narratives that unfold within; and the ways that teachers and early care and education providers respond to children. By examining children's narratives, she brings to the fore identities that remain invisible and voices that are drowned by dominant discourse. She believes in the role of teacher educators as agents of change, posing dilemmas that challenge students to think in more critical ways. Inspired by Paolo Freire's work, she asserts that teacher education is challenged to be not only a source of information but a vehicle for transformation. In this scenario, education becomes a space that provides prospective teachers countless opportunities to reinvent themselves, shape their beliefs, as well as define and refine their practice. She also believes that the university classroom has the potential to become a learning laboratory that promotes critical discourse, dialogic inquiry and collaborative work between students and members of the community.

Rachel Whittington Saffo is a PhD candidate at the School of Communication Science and Disorders, College of Communication and Information at Florida State University. Her current research and teaching interests are in neurolinguistics, autism, and bilingual language development.

Juliann Woods, PhD, is a Professor in the School of Communication Science and Disorders at Florida State University. Dr. Woods's research and teaching interests include early identification and intervention for autism, communication delays and disorders, family guided routines-based intervention, and professional development. Her research is conducted in applied settings with children and families and the providers that support them.

Robin Miller Young, EdD, NCSP, is the Student Services Coordinator at Prairie Children Preschool (Indian Prairie SD # 204, Aurora, IL), an inclusive, tuition-based EC/"at-risk"/ECSE school. She serves on the administrative leadership team, overseeing daily operations and guiding development, implementation, and evaluation of school improvement initiatives such a Response to Intervention (RtI) and a birth-to-grade-3 "seamless continuum." Her research interests include explicit early academic and social interventions, professional development frameworks such as coaching and mentoring models, and leadership strategies that move organizations into effective and efficient structures and program practices.

Naomi Younggren, PhD, is the personnel development coordinator for the U.S. Army Educational and Developmental Intervention Services (EDIS) supporting early intervention programs in Europe, Korea, and the United States. She is also an adjunct faculty member with Central Texas College–Europe Campus. Dr. Younggren's early childhood special education experiences include being an early intervention provider and preschool teacher, providing technical assistance, and serving in a program development and leadership capacity. She has presented at national conferences including the OSEP (Office of Special Education Programs) National Early Childhood Conference addressing service delivery models and outcomes measurement in early intervention. Dr. Younggren has authored early intervention handbooks and coauthored the OSEP mission, principles, and practice statements for early intervention services in natural environments (2008).

Advisory Board

Heidi M. Feldman, MD, PhD, is the Ballinger-Swindles Endowed Professor of Developmental and Behavioral Pediatrics at Stanford University School of Medicine. She also serves as the Medical Director of the Developmental and Behavior Pediatric Programs at Lucile Packard Children's Hospital. Dr. Feldman received her BA in Psychology (1970), summa cum laude, and her PhD in Developmental Psychology (1975) from the University of Pennsylvania. She received her MD from the University of California, San Diego (1979). Dr. Feldman has memberships in several professional societies such as the Society for Research in Child Development, the Society for Pediatric Research, and the American Academy of Pediatrics. She has served as President at the Society for the Developmental Behavioral Pediatrics. Her research focuses on developmental-behavioral pediatrics, language development in young children, and language and cognition after prematurity. She has published more than 50 peer-reviewed articles in journals like the *New England Journal of Medicine, Science, Brain and Language, Child Development, Journal of Behavioral Developmental Pediatrics, Developmental Neuropsychology,* and *Pediatrics*. She is one of the editors of the current edition of the premier textbook in her field, *Developmental-Behavioral Pediatrics* (4th ed.), published in 2009. She has served as grant reviewer for the National Institutes of Health (1992–1997 and 2008–2012) and an abstract reviewer for the Pediatric Academic Societies. Dr. Feldman has held several academic appointments: Professor at the Medical Center Line, Stanford University (2006 to present), Professor in Pediatrics, University of Pittsburgh (2000–2006), and Faculty Member at the Center for the Neural Bases of Cognition at the University of Pittsburgh/Carnegie Mellon University (2003–2006). Dr. Feldman has received several awards such as Best Doctors in America (2007–2008 and 2009–2010), Academy of Master Educators, University of Pittsburgh School of Medicine (2006),

Outstanding Alumna, University of California San Diego (2003), Ronald L. and Patricia M. Violi Professor of Pediatrics and Child Development, University of Pittsburgh (2001–2006), Excellence in Education Award, University of Pittsburgh School of Medicine (2000), and the Chancellor's Distinguished Teaching Award (1999).

Marilou Hyson, PhD, is a consultant in early child development and education and an Affiliate Faculty member in Applied Developmental Psychology at George Mason University. Formerly Associate Executive Director and Senior Consultant with the National Association for the Education of Young Children (NAEYC), Marilou contributed to the development of many position statements on issues including early learning standards, professional preparation standards, early childhood mathematics, and curriculum/assessment/program evaluation. She is the author of the recent book *Enthusiastic and Engaged Learners: Approaches to Learning in the Early Childhood Classroom*, published by NAEYC and Teachers College Press. Two book chapters on early childhood professional development and higher education systems were published in 2010. Internationally, Marilou consults in Indonesia, Bangladesh, Bhutan, and Vietnam through the World Bank and Save the Children. In the United States, Marilou consults with organizations including the Families and Work Institute, the Finance Project, the National Center for Children in Poverty, and the Society for Research in Child Development. Prior to joining NAEYC, Marilou was an SRCD Fellow in the U.S. Department of Education and Professor and Chair of the University of Delaware's Department of Individual and Family Studies. The former editor-in-chief of *Early Childhood Research Quarterly*, Marilou's research and publications have emphasized young children's emotional development, parents' and teachers' beliefs and educational practices, issues in linking research with policy and practice, and early childhood teacher preparation.

Robert Silverstein, JD, is a principal in the law firm of Powers Pyles Sutter & Verville, P.C., and he also serves as the director of the Center for the Study and Advancement of Disability Policy. Mr. Silverstein received his BS in economics, cum laude, from the Wharton School, University of Pennsylvania in 1971. He received his JD in 1974 from Georgetown University Law Center. His main areas of interest are public policy issues and the policymaking process focusing in the areas of disability, health care, rehabilitation, employment, education, social security, and civil rights. In his capacity as staff director and chief counsel to the U.S. Senate Subcommittee on Disability Policy and other positions (1986–1997), Mr. Silverstein was the behind-the-scenes architect of more than 20 bills enacted into law, including the Americans with Disabilities Act (ADA), Rehabilitation Act (1992 Amendments), the Early Intervention Program for Infants and Toddlers with Disabilities (1986), and the Individuals with Disabilities Education Act Amendments (1991, 1997 Amendments). He has presented keynotes speeches before national and state organizations and trained leaders and others in more than 40 states regarding various public policy issues and the police making process. He has more than 75 papers, articles and policy briefs on public policy issues from a disability perspective published in journals such as *Behavioral Sciences and the Law, and Iowa Law Review*. Mr. Silverstein has assisted federal, state, and local policymakers and key stakeholder groups to translate research into consensus public policy solutions addressing identified needs.

Sue Swenson is an experienced nonprofit and government leader in the field of advocacy and support for people with developmental disabilities and their families. She is interested in the application of modern management and marketing techniques to help public systems better know and serve the people they are intended to help, with a special interest in interdisciplinary applications and international collaborative efforts. Mrs. Swenson is a frequent public speaker and enthusiastic participant in forums designed to improve the lives of citizens with disabilities. She worked for The Arc of the United States as CEO. She also served as Executive Director of Joseph P. Kennedy, Jr., Foundation. She was appointed by the Clinton White House to serve as Commissioner of the Administration on Developmental Disabilities, U.S. DHHS, and served as a Kennedy Public Policy Fellow at the U.S. Senate Subcommittee on Disability Policy. Mrs. Swenson received her AB in humanities in 1975, and an AM in humanities (1977) from the University of Chicago and an MBA from the Carlson School of Management at the University of Minnesota (1986). She has three adult sons, one of whom has developmental disabilities.

Jane E. West, PhD, currently serves as Senior Vice President for Policy, Programs, and Professional Issues at the American Association of Colleges for Teacher Education (AACTE). West has written broadly on special education, disability policy and teacher preparation. She served as the staff director for the U.S. Senate Subcommittee on Disability Policy in the early 1980s under the chairmanship of Sen. Lowell P. Weicker. She currently leads AACTE's engagement in the education policy discussion related to teacher preparation, the Elementary and Secondary Education Act and the Higher Education Act.

Index

Universal (prevention) level of
multitiered model, 185, 186, 243,
244–46
Universal Preschool, 45
University Centers for Excellence in
Developmental Disabilities
(UCEDD), 5

Valeska Hinton Early Childhood
Education Center (VHECEC):
PBS project, 249–50
Vanderbilt Home Visiting Script
(VHVS), 24
Vineland Adaptive Behavior Scale,
143, 275
Visual function, 299. *See also* Visual
impairment
Visual impairment, 297; controversial
issues, 306–7; defined, 298–300;
developments in, 302–3;
example, 298–307; in infants,

299–300; practices in treating,
301–3; research in, 301–3; service
delivery, 300–301; strategies
for professionals and families,
303–5

War on Poverty, 5, 80, 81–83
Westinghouse Report, Head Start
evaluation, 95
Women, Infants, and Children
(WIC), 6
Workforce, personnel development,
236–37
*Workgroup on Principles and Practices for
Natural Environments*, 149
Writing, 362; and children, 347–49;
intersection of math and literacy,
353–57; name, 349

Zone of Proximal Development
(ZPD), 41

CPSIA information can be obtained at www.ICGtesting.com
Printed in the USA
BVOW011638070213

312625BV00003B/57/P